P9-DBO-072

Mammography
and Early Breast
Cancer Detection

12/29/14

## MCFARLAND HEALTH TOPICS SERIES

*Living with Multiple Chemical Sensitivity: Narratives of Coping.* Gail McCormick. 2001

*Graves' Disease: A Practical Guide.* Elaine A. Moore with Lisa Moore. 2001

*Autoimmune Diseases and Their Environmental Triggers.* Elaine A. Moore. 2002

*Hepatitis: Causes, Treatments and Resources.* Elaine A. Moore. 2006

*Arthritis: A Patient's Guide.* Sharon E. Hohler. 2008

*The Promise of Low Dose Naltrexone Therapy: Potential Benefits in Cancer, Autoimmune, Neurological and Infectious Disorders.* Elaine A. Moore and Samantha Wilkinson. 2009

*Living with HIV: A Patient's Guide.* Mark Cichocki, RN. 2009

*Understanding Multiple Chemical Sensitivity: Causes, Effects, Personal Experiences and Resources.* Els Valkenburg. 2010

*Type 2 Diabetes: Social and Scientific Origins, Medical Complications and Implications for Patients and Others.* Andrew Kagan, M.D. 2010

*The Amphetamine Debate: The Use of Adderall, Ritalin and Related Drugs for Behavior Modification, Neuroenhancement and Anti-Aging Purposes.* Elaine A. Moore. 2011

*CCSVI as the Cause of Multiple Sclerosis: The Science Behind the Controversial Theory.* Marie A. Rhodes. 2011

*Coping with Post-Traumatic Stress Disorder: A Guide for Families,* 2d ed. Cheryl A. Roberts. 2011

*Living with Insomnia: A Guide to Causes, Effects and Management, with Personal Accounts.* Phyllis L. Brodsky and Allen Brodsky. 2011

*Caregiver's Guide: Care for Yourself While You Care for Your Loved Ones.* Sharon E. Hohler. 2012

*You and Your Doctor: A Guide to a Healing Relationship, with Physicians' Insights.* Tania Heller, M.D. 2012

*Autogenic Training: A Mind-Body Approach to the Treatment of Chronic Pain Syndrome and Stress-Related Disorders,* 2d ed. Micah R. Sadigh. 2012

*Advances in Graves' Disease and Other Hyperthyroid Disorders.* Elaine A. Moore with Lisa Marie Moore. 2013

*Cancer, Autism and Their Epigenetic Roots.* K. John Morrow, Jr. 2014

*Living with Bipolar Disorder: A Handbook for Patients and Their Families.* Karen R. Brock, M.D. 2014

*Cannabis Extracts in Medicine: The Promise of Benefits in Seizure Disorders, Cancer and Other Conditions.* Jeffrey Dach, M.D., Elaine A. Moore and Justin Kander. 2015

*Managing Hypertension: Tools to Improve Health and Prevent Complications.* Sandra A. Moulton. Series Editor Elaine A. Moore. 2016

*Mammography and Early Breast Cancer Detection: How Screening Saves Lives.* Alan B. Hollingsworth, M.D. 2016

# Mammography and Early Breast Cancer Detection

## How Screening Saves Lives

ALAN B. HOLLINGSWORTH, M.D.

**MCFARLAND HEALTH TOPICS**

McFarland & Company, Inc., Publishers
*Jefferson, North Carolina*

LIBRARY OF CONGRESS CATALOGUING-IN-PUBLICATION DATA

Names: Hollingsworth, Alan B., author.
Title: Mammography and early breast cancer detection :
how screening saves lives / Alan B. Hollingsworth, M.D.
Description: Jefferson, North Carolina : McFarland & Company,
Inc., Publishers, 2016. | Series: Mcfarland health topics |
Includes bibliographical references and index.
Identifiers: LCCN 2016027129 | ISBN 9781476666105
(softcover : acid free paper) ∞
Subjects: LCSH: Breast—Radiography. | Breast—
Cancer—Diagnosis. | Breast—Imaging.
Classification: LCC RG493.5.R33 H65 2016 | DDC 618.1/907572—dc23
LC record available at https://lccn.loc.gov/2016027129

BRITISH LIBRARY CATALOGUING DATA ARE AVAILABLE

ISBN (print) 978-1-4766-6610-5
ISBN (ebook) 978-1-4766-2588-1

Front cover photograph of mammography machine
© 2016 Mark Kostich / iStock

Printed in the United States of America

*McFarland & Company, Inc., Publishers
Box 611, Jefferson, North Carolina 28640
www.mcfarlandpub.com*

# Table of Contents

# Acknowledgments

I suppose that I've set a Guinness world record for the length of time a surgeon has "officed" with breast radiologists—23 years straight, and counting. I owe a great deal to a long list of these physicians who have shared their experience and knowledge with me, allowing my claim as a quasi-radiologist—not so much with interpretations, but in my study of "Breast Imaging, Theory of."

Most recently, this would be Drs. Rebecca G. Stough, Melanie Pearce, Carol O'Dell, Charles Brekke, James Hendrix, John Bowers, and Angela McCoy, all of them supported, in turn, by our breast center staff, led by manager Nancy Miller, RT.

A high-risk screening program incorporates both *prediction* and *detection*, and our program at Mercy Breast Center has been the springboard for this book. Prediction requires risk analysis that often includes genetic testing in order to determine the probability of breast cancer. To that end, I owe a great deal to my now-retired clinical nurse specialist, Sharon Nall, APRN-CNS, MS, OCN, CBCN (and a few more letters I can't recall), who took her extensive oncology background from years prior, and from 1999 on, focused entirely on breast cancer—first as my clinical nurse, then as our breast cancer nurse navigator (before the term was widely known), then devoting the final phase of her career to risk assessment and genetic testing. Today, that program continues in top-notch form with board-certified genetic counselor Julie Beasley, MS, LCGC, and Marsha Pratt, M.D., board-certified medical geneticist, both of whom bring a unique level of expertise to a community-based breast cancer program.

Keeping us all in line and on time is the administrative director of the high-risk program, Michelle Hauge, who has been with me since my arrival at Mercy in 1999. Imaging research is commandeered by Kathy Tucker, RT, while blood test research coordinator is Debbie Hudson with Michelle doubling as part-time phlebotomist. Research nurses Paige Chiles and Christina Caldwell, along with Ana Carr and the IRB team, were of critical help in the Provista multi-site trial for the blood test. We are also indebted to Ellen Wardlaw, RN, our nurse navigator, who offers universal assistance to our program. Valued administrative assistance is provided by Andrea Bunnitt, Lara Gaston, RN, and Tracy Higgs, RN. And for her graphic design of the illustrations in this book, as well as the same in years past, I am indebted to Nita West.

General thanks go out to all members of the breast cancer team at Mercy Hospital, Oklahoma City, including the physicians from multiple specialties as well as other providers and support staff who work to make the weekly breast conference successful, while delivering high quality patient care. Too, thanks to the administration, notably CEO Jim Gebhart, COO Aaron Steffens and (now retired) Dr. Mark Johnson, M.D., who allowed me to have an academic afterlife, preserving my research goals in the community hospital setting.

Of course, all the work in predicting the probability of breast cancer through risk analysis and genetics would be pointless without effective interventions, and the key here is early detection through multi-modality imaging for the high risk patient. One might think it would be relatively easy to buy a breast MRI, plug it in, and start counting cancers. It is not. Let me rephrase that—it's not easy to do it well. To that end, Dr. Rebecca G. Stough picked up the ball and ran with it, treating the breast MRI program as her baby, with extraordinary efforts at quality assurance, given the wide variation in outcomes being reported across the country. Her efforts in providing a center of excellence for Oklahoma ended up generating a national presence. Once believing that her future was sitting in a dark room interpreting mammograms, Dr. Stough found herself under the lights at the expert's podium, speaking about breast MRI and helping to train other radiologists across the country. Recently, Dr. Stough was joined in leading our breast imaging program by Dr. Melanie Pearce, a fellowship-trained breast radiologist deeply devoted to high quality patient care.

Breast MRI technologists Kim Raymond and Lorri Foster have invested a great deal of time in tracking the MRI data that allowed our program to be one of the earliest accredited breast MRI programs in the country, as well as generating the information we needed for our scientific presentations and publications. Emily Buckelew has been with us from the beginning of the breast MRI program as well, helping to publicize and educate physicians about the benefits of high Sensitivity imaging, always cheerful no matter what the chore.

I would not have written this book if it weren't for the strong staff support noted above that keeps the wheels turning at Mercy Breast Center. Too, I am very grateful to all my patients who have taught me what the screening experience is like, and to the 2,000 women of Oklahoma who have donated blood samples to our ongoing research. Gratitude in advance goes to the thousands of women who will be involved in our clinical trials to improve screening over the next decade as well. And special thanks are due for activist Jill Greene who led the fund-raising campaign for our breast center and cancer center in the new Coletta building.

Heretofore, writing in my spare time has been devoted to novels and non-medical non-fiction, a form of escapism, I suppose. However, the anti-screening social tsunami described in this book prompted me to escape the escapism and do something that might make a difference. This, of course, turned the writing process into something that bore a strong resemblance to work rather than pleasure. I mention this so as to acknowledge my family, starting with wife Barbara, who had to listen to my persistent and annoying answer whenever fun-filled options were proposed: "Sorry, I have to work on the book." Still, I worked to put family first, writing in spurts, before and after the basketball games of Shawn and Clara (children of Susannah and Ryan Bebee), or working around Thomas the Tank Engine's schedule with Luke, Patrick, or Charlotte (children of Emily and Jeff Belisle).

In my previous works, I've always managed to slip in the name of my barber, either as a character or even the name of a fictional dormitory complex (Crim Center in *University Boulevard*), given the important role he plays as a sounding board. But for this book, it just didn't work out. Sorry, Doyle.

# Preface

Medical science is not immune to fads and fashions. We might call them "trends" to maintain a veneer of self-respect, but they are what they are. And, if the trend lingers long enough, it becomes a standard of care. Indeed, the data doesn't necessarily have to change; merely the mind's eye.

A pervasive trend today is the "less is more" philosophy, admittedly overdue when it comes to the treatment of cancers so early that perhaps they shouldn't be called cancer at all. However, when the "less is more" philosophy invades the world of breast cancer screening, we get something else entirely—*less* screening equals *more* breast cancer deaths.

The certainty that mammographic screening saves lives, however, is not universal. Some very bright physicians and researchers contend that the lives saved in clinical trials are largely, if not entirely, artificial by-products of epidemiologic trickery. But if it proves true that screening does, in fact, save lives, then we are left with some uncomfortable realities, the first being that the "less is more" screening tsunami is going to drown a fixed number of women. And it's not too difficult to derive a good approximation of that number.

In spite of this unsettling reality, nearly everywhere one turns today, the "less is more" trend is bleeding its way into screening guidelines. Women and their physicians are being told to learn about the harms of mammography as compared to the small probability of benefit. Okay so far, but what if those harms are being inflated while benefits are deflated? Today, successful studies of informed consent for screening will attempt to show how the educated woman will screen less, or not at all, after discovering the "true" harm-to-benefit ratio, as portrayed by the researchers. The idea is to re-program women who have previously decided to screen.

But why are there no studies with the goal of properly informing women who have already opted out of mammography based on false assumptions? The rationale that some women use in the rejection of mammography is often erroneous, to a far greater degree than the opposite error of overestimating benefit. Yet no one seems to be targeting this group to bring them into the mammographic fold. "I don't get mammograms because breast cancer doesn't run in my family" or "I do a thorough self-exam instead of mammography" are common reasons to avoid mammography where there is scant scientific basis. Yet you'll have trouble finding current research on how to identify these women and enlighten them with a proper informed consent that prompts screening. Instead, modern efforts to inform the public are *unidirectional*—how to inform women as to the minuscule benefit of mammography when

1

compared to the many harms, an example of the latter being lifetime psychological damage due to an "unnecessary" benign biopsy, a fashionable position. And the reason for these unidirectional efforts is because there is a singular goal—less is more.

Unfortunately, breast cancer doesn't give a flip about our fashions. This book is intended to depict the true and unchanging nature of breast cancer. We will first take a look at why, theoretically, lives *should* be saved through screening, and then, we'll learn why this theory means so much more to the future of early detection than simply getting regular mammograms.

My approach is not a dry recitation of medical studies and their outcomes that culminate in marching orders. Instead, I've written a narrative—from the bizarre introduction of mammography to the world, or at least to the streets of Manhattan, when Dr. Philip Strax parked his mammomobile alongside the hot dog and ice cream vendors in 1963, continuing to modern-day mammography, then onward to imaging methods that are the stuff of science fiction. It's about the past, present and future, with the past as prologue. Along the way, it's also about warring egos, smoke-filled consensus rooms, irregularities in scientific conduct, and most of all, an explanation as to why we're in the fix that we're in today—where few agree on screening recommendations.

Human nature drives us to support and strengthen our positions using the weaponry of words and numbers. Indeed, both sides of the screening controversies are prone to go overboard to make their case. Accepting that premise, when dealing with the results of clinical studies in this book, I've attempted to present the data and conclusions using both ends of the telescope, explaining how interventions can look different when considering the whole population vs. an individual. Furthermore, in discussing guidelines issued for screening mammography, it is important to know which end of the telescope was in use at the time. Indeed, I've devoted an entire chapter to the techniques used to churn data, win friends and influence people. By the time you've finished this book, it is my intent that you will not only understand the constant barrage of conflicting headlines, but you will also be able to make the right decision about screening for yourself or your patients.

I've had to walk a tightrope of terminology and semantics in this book, attempting to appeal both to an interested lay audience and health care providers. At times, the reader is likely to feel I'm falling one direction or the other, or perhaps falling off the wire entirely, but it has been my intent to appeal to both audiences, lay and professional.

Another challenge in a book of this sort is timeliness of information. Fortunately, for our purposes here, the core evidence for screening mammography was generated by clinical trials that are already 40 years old, so what's another decade going to matter? Yet when we come to current recommendations for screening, these are constantly changing. For instance, the guidelines for screening high-risk women using MRI that were issued in 2007 by the American Cancer Society still prevailed when my manuscript was complete, but were due to be updated about the same time as the book's release. While second editions are certainly possible, some references will be outdated in short order. Again, the critical data was generated by the historical trials, so the gist of the book will remain timeless, more or less. For those who desire regular updates on new developments in the early detection of breast cancer, let me invite you to read my blogatorials at www.alanhollingsworth.com.

References are provided in two ways, without the rigidity that would ordinarily be seen in a textbook. For direct quotes from newspapers, lay texts, online news outlets, or editorials, I have embedded the references as part of the narrative. However, if a quote focuses on specific

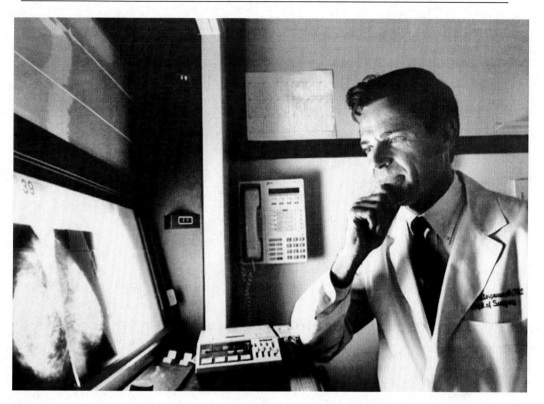

In 1990, I began studying why so many cancers were invisible on mammography, especially when the background pattern was dense. In 1993, I published one of the early papers that analyzed the reasons for false-negative mammograms, predicting the need for adjunct forms of breast imaging. In 2006, I became the first non-radiologist in the country to present screening outcomes using breast MRI in high-risk patients at the general assembly of the American Society of Breast Disease.

results of a scientific study, the complete reference is listed as a note. Also in the chapter notes are anecdotes of personal experience, editorial comments, or particular curiosities that depart from the narrative, but still may be of interest.

At a minimum, this book should serve as a comprehensive informed consent for breast cancer screening, beyond the wildest imagination of the critics who currently complain about the lack of said information. But more than that, I intend the book to be, quite simply, an enjoyable read. It doesn't matter whether one is attending a breast cancer guideline committee or is in the boardroom of corporate America, the dynamics of debate are both enduring and predictable. In the case of screening mammography, the arguments have been raging for more than 50 years.

Remarkably few books are available to support the majority opinion of the public that early detection is of paramount importance. In contrast, one has no trouble finding volumes written by anti-screening experts, or cautionary accounts that reveal hidden harms, or books by individualists who have identified a massive radiologic-industrial-government conspiracy to cause breast cancers by irradiating all women. "Man bites dog," or more aptly, "Mammography bites women" might be the attraction of these books, while pro-screeners have been complacent, basking in the majority opinion.

But the day when pro-screeners can sit back and say, "Everyone knows that early detection is the key" are drawing to a close. Indeed, an increasing number of experts claim this is not the case at all—that is, breast cancers are each predestined to behave in a certain way and that the benefits of screening mammography are artificially derived. Furthermore, critics indirectly calculate high probabilities for "overdiagnosis," often called "fake cancers that prompt over-treatment." Yet, if a patient is diagnosed with a very real cancer through screening, but she succumbs to an unrelated illness or accident before the natural history of that cancer unfolds, well, guess what—she will be tallied in the epidemiologist's ledger as "overdiagnosis."

Thus, my motivation in writing this book is the need for a work that explains and confirms what virtually all breast radiologists believe already, but what fewer and fewer physicians in other specialties believe—that is, that mammography saves lives through early detection, and that the benefits outweigh the harms.

"Discuss screening with your doctor" is seen by many as a cop-out. Very likely, your doctor would rather defer to an authoritative source, an organization that issues guidelines. But these sources have been in conflict, long before recent headlines and social media have made them widely known. In fact, the conflict dates back to 1963 and that very first clinical trial where Dr. Strax introduced his mobile mammography unit. When that study had concluded—oops—the researchers had forgotten to exclude women who had previously been diagnosed with breast cancer, so delayed deaths from those breast cancers that had occurred *prior* to the study ended up contaminating the benefit of screening. Even the study's organizers disagreed on what they had discovered, or not.

We are rapidly approaching the time when those of us who once performed radical mastectomies in the pre-mammography era will no longer be around to provide historical perspective. While history can easily be manipulated each day before the sun sets, it is no problem at all to re-write history once its participants are gone. Historical perspective through direct experience is both unique and fleeting. As the French composer Berlioz said, "Time is a good teacher, but unfortunately it kills all its pupils."

That said, my personal experience is woven into the narrative, explaining how, as a general surgeon with little interest in breast cancer, I became so consumed by all things related to prediction, prevention and early detection of breast cancer that I eventually abandoned surgery altogether in order to devote full efforts to improving how we do things up front, before ever crossing the threshold of the operating room. As the guide on this journey, I intend the reader to appreciate the same revelatory idea that grabbed me many years ago—mammography is saving lives with one hand tied behind its back. Therefore, imagine what we could accomplish if we freed that hand, not through a mirage of imagined breakthroughs, but by efficiently using technology that is available today.

# 1

# Last Word vs. Final Word

Mammograms? Yes. Mammograms? No.

Mammograms every year? Every other? Not at all?

Start at 40? 45? 50? Pick a number. Any number. It probably won't matter ... unless you're in the 1% where it does.

Stop at 75? Don't stop. Go. Stop.

Do you feel like a ping-pong ball?

You should. Of all the controversies in breast cancer today, none is more contentious and enduring than mammographic screening. Yet we are not even close to a resolution. In fact, the line in the sand is getting deeper and deeper. This debate has been raging for 50 years, and there is very little in the way of new data. New spins on old data, yes, but when it comes to direct measurements of lives saved through screening, we're chained to the past.

How is a woman supposed to decide what is best for her situation? How is a primary care physician supposed to counsel patients if the experts are at war?

Understand, these ping-pong recommendations are *not*, as many claim, the routine airing of dirty laundry as the natural backdrop of the so-called "scientific method." Instead, when it comes to this controversy, scientific method has been beaten and brutalized. The incessant flip-flopping of screening recommendations as reflected in the media, not to mention professional organizations, is testimony to the torture.

When you see media coverage of a "new study," either supporting or bashing mammographic screening, most of the time it will be what is called an "observational" study, considered to be low quality evidence. Anti-screening epidemiologists like to pretend that these studies don't even exist, opting for "high quality evidence" generated by prospective randomized trials. One problem—these randomized trials, and the technology that went with them, are ancient, bearing little relationship to what we do today. Usually, the only thing "new" is the commentators themselves who are new to the controversy.

What we have is a smelly brew of corrupted randomization, primeval mammograms, twisted statistics, bombastic personalities and back door politics where subjective opinion is couched as pure science. But that doesn't stop some experts from dipping your cup into a meatless stew and recommending which vegetables are going to be good for you while, at the same time, asking you to ignore those nearby who are choking.

There is nothing good about the current state of affairs. It's not healthy, and it's *not* the scientific method working its way toward truth, any more than the Republicans and Democrats are working toward a one-party system. It's one half avoidable and the other half absurdity. Women and their physicians need a last word on this issue—they don't need slants and slopes, nor do they need heart-felt testimonials. They need an unbiased presentation of the facts … *because the facts speak for themselves.* They may speak pro or con to you, but nevertheless, one can't make a decision without the facts. Unfortunately, it is very difficult to assemble the facts. I've been at it for 25 years.

If you are age 40 or older, you'll probably not live long enough to witness the end of the controversy. This threadbare debate began in 1963 with the very first clinical trial that evaluated mammographic screening, the Health Insurance Plan of Greater New York. And today, long after the major mammography screening trials have been completed, the warring parties are more deeply entrenched than ever, dragging the argument into the sunlight periodically for a miraculous vision of "new data."

The American College of Radiology and the Society of Breast Imaging keep it simple— *yearly mammograms starting at age 40, continuing as long as good health prevails.* At the other extreme, a merry band of iconoclasts has been making the claim that mammograms don't save lives at all. And, while some may call the 2009 recommendations from the U.S. Preventive Services Task Force (and its 2016 regurgitation) a reasonable compromise, their dictum to delay screening mammograms until age 50, then every 2 years after that, is believed by many to be a prime example of a death panel.

To be sure, if mammograms are truly saving lives, these questions arise: Why would we want to compromise? Who benefits by doing *less*? Is *less* screening going to drive the curious axiom "less is more" to a potentially fatal extreme?

Perhaps the "no screening" position is easier to defend than the "do less" position. After all, if we follow the "first, do no harm" injunction, then the rote counting of potential harms will add up, perhaps seeming to outweigh benefits in mammographic screening. But just how many "unnecessary" benign biopsies add up to a life saved? A ridiculous question? Not at all. At least, not ridiculous to the bean-counters who weigh these things in a balance scale, then announce to the world that harms exceed benefits. It's very clear-cut in their minds, complete with back-up statistical analyses that include things like measurable psychological damage from false-positive findings on mammography.

The "against routine screening" position for women in their 40s was advocated by the 2009 U.S. Preventive Services Task Force. Now forget for a moment that 2009 was not the first time the Task Force met to evaluate breast cancer screening—it was the fourth time they had issued recommendations since 1989 (ignored by mainstream media the first 3 times at bat), and their rotating membership also rotates recommendations, sometimes yes, sometimes no, when it comes to screening women in their 40s. But ignore the flip-flopping for now.

Instead, consider this: when we follow the aggressive "begin at 40" policy, we are already disenfranchising women *under* 40 who will be diagnosed with breast cancer. We offer the under-40 group nothing more than *self-exam*, an exercise with even less evidence than mammography to indicate that lives can be saved (though remarkably inexpensive). How many breast cancer victims are thus ignored? The answer: 5% of eventual cancer patients are excluded from screening. Or nearly 11,000 women a year[1] who will be diagnosed with breast cancer in their 20s and 30s are effectively told, "you're on your own." Their self-discovered cancers, by the way, are usually Stage II or worse.

The only hope for an early diagnosis through screening in this age group comes through a different set of recommendations customized for women at very high risk for breast cancer. Ah, if only risk factors predicted future victims. But risk factors for breast cancer are not very good at forecasting. Only 20% of eventual breast cancer patients have a positive family history for the disease. Even if we identify the 2,000 women in their 20s and 30s destined for cancer based on high risk status, enough to warrant aggressive, early age screening, we still leave 9,000 eventual victims every year, *out in the cold*, in their prime of life, knowing full well that cancer in this age group is often deadly.

But what would happen if we were to start screening at age 50, according to Task Force guidelines? Now, instead of leaving 11,000 women to the deceptive hope of self-exams, we'll be leaving an additional 49,000, bringing our total of "out in the cold" women to nearly 60,000, or roughly one-fourth of all eventual breast cancer patients. And, finally, if we stop screening at 75 (the next cut-off being monitored by screening minimalists), the total number keeps climbing, and we will succeed in excluding *50% of eventual breast cancer patients*, or approximately 120,000 women per year (not including ductal carcinoma in situ where an additional 30,000 would be excluded).

This same nugget of 50% exclusion will be viewed from many angles in this book, but the inescapable conclusion, if you believe screening saves lives, is that "compromise" may be the least acceptable position. Maybe you see now why I said that it might be more intellectually honest—if you believe that mammograms have little or no impact—to avoid mammography entirely. How does the Task Force justify cutting out *one-fourth to one-half* of the population who very likely benefit from a screening tool? Instead, witness Switzerland where, in 2014, experts weighed the evidence as they saw it, and recommended that mammographic screening for their entire population be completely abolished. Wow. And don't think for a minute that those same voices aren't echoing in the United States.

Many blame media in its various forms for the ping-pong coverage of breast cancer screening. But let's be real—*the media has no intent to sort out the controversy*. Conflict pumps the headlines to larger and larger fonts. Media are the mirrors reflecting bickering experts. Like reeds blowing in the wind, the journalists of today catch the puff and add the fluff with every new publication. Back and forth, back and forth—start at 40, no, 50, no, back to 45, every year, no, every other year, stop at 75, no, keep going as long you are healthy, no, no, no—mammograms don't help at all!

We need the last word on this controversy now. Why? Because what we see is what we are going to get for the next 30 to 50 years. Oh, yes, there are some new bells and whistles for mammography, and other types of imaging, and we'll cover those later. But the true ending to this controversy will happen only when screening is no longer needed.

Someday, a woman will feel a breast lump that is diagnosed as malignant, then she will receive a sophisticated, personalized treatment of some sort based on tumor biology, and the breast cancer will be gone for good, even if it has already spread outside the breast. Or perhaps all women will be immunized against breast cancer early in life. When that day comes, there will be no need to screen for early detection. Until then, however, we are faced with early diagnosis as one of the ways to lower the number of deaths due to breast cancer. And to be clear, early detection is not necessarily limited to, or synonymous with, screening mammography.

To whom do you turn in order to get the facts about breast cancer screening? "10 Myths About Breast Cancer" found online will sometimes include new myths to replace the old.

TV doctors and syndicated columnists may claim expertise on every health issue under the sun, but they routinely stumble with mixed messages on this topic. And the greatest cop-out of all is "Discuss breast cancer screening with your doctor." Most primary care physicians depend on guidance from the experts. Yet the experts are locked in an ugly, sometimes profane, battle. To whom does the primary care physician turn? Even respected medical journals and researchers have stoked the fires of controversy, fully realizing that the more often a journal or an author is cited by others, their "impact score" (for the journal), or the "h-index" (for the researcher), i.e., digitalized indicators of self-worth, are going to rocket.

Forget TV doctors. Forget talking heads and YouTube stars who are discovering this controversy for the first time. The premise of this book is that *you* have the responsibility, not YouTube. If you have taken the position "I'll just follow what so-and-so organization says," then fine. Or, if you want to follow what your doctor recommends, fine. A survey of women under 50 revealed that only 7% want to completely yield the decision-making process to their doctors, while 44% want to make the decision themselves and 49% want to share in the decision-making process about mammography with their doctors.[2] We all carry too much clutter in our brains, so if you're in the 7% who yield entirely to physician direction, you can stop reading right now. Read on, however, if you are a woman or a health care professional who is grumbling, "Stop the madness. I'm sick and tired of conflicting information being thrown at us. I want to know what the controversy is all about so that I can discuss this intelligently with my doctor (or my patients) and/or make my own decision."

When you are finished with this book, you will never look at this controversy again in the same light. First of all, you will have a more profound understanding of the debate than any TV doctor alive today. The key to understanding is not the "latest study" or what "this group says" or what "that doctor does." The troublesome issues about screening may seem complex when placed in the hands of researchers who use fancy words and shifty statistics, but it's remarkably straightforward when explained by an unbiased expert.

But where do you find an unbiased expert? While I can claim expertise, I'm no longer unbiased. Once, I was. My training was in surgery, and I had no abiding interest in breast cancer, nor in the screening that went with it. The journey I'm going to take you on begins with the single step I took in the 1980s when I asked a very simple question: "What percentage of breast cancers are missed by mammography?" I remember where I was at the time (a breast radiologist's office), as clearly as I remember being in ninth grade biology class when Kennedy was assassinated. And then, the related question: "How do you count these missed cancers if you don't even know when you've missed them?" (Mammography was the only accepted imaging tool at the time.) From that point on, with those questions unanswered, I experienced a long and agonizing metamorphosis, shedding two exoskeletons, from general surgeon to breast surgeon, and then to a breast disease specialist focusing entirely on risk stratification and screening, *and how to improve the current state of affairs.*

Reaching true expertise is akin to reaching nirvana, so let me abbreviate my definition as it applies here—to be an expert in breast cancer screening, one must know the anti-screening position as well as the pro-screening position. This is a simple concept, a holdover from high school debate. Or, if you prefer, it's the dialectical method of the ancient Greeks. It's easy for either side to sling mud against your window, but it's going to take the length of this book to clean it off.

Today, I can argue the *anti-screening* position with as much zeal as the Swiss Medical

Board hell-bent on abolishing mammography and all the pain that goes with it. Perhaps that's why, by the final pages of this book, I'll propose that the approach to screening needs to be overhauled, while at the same time arguing against a jump into the pit of compromise, i.e., *less* screening.

One more word about the semantics of "last word" as distinguished from the "final word." Whereas "last" can imply "most recent," the word "final" has a stronger temporal ring, implying no further modifications. The Final Word on screening will come when breast cancer is curable 100% of the time after diagnosis at any stage. We're not there yet.

Even though many anti-screening visionaries like to wallow in the future of curative systemic therapies as if it's already arrived, it hasn't. Others, including some breast cancer activists and their organizations, believe "we're very close to a cure," so we can begin to de-emphasize screening now and focus instead on our new and exciting therapies. I still disagree. We're not that close, and efforts to throttle screening are decidedly premature. In 1995, approximately 46,000 women in the U.S. died of breast cancer[3]; 20 years later, in 2015, the number was still 40,000 (not fully reflecting the progress if one considers the population increase). Since this decline in breast cancer mortality is partly due to the impact of screening, does it make sense to back off now?

Furthermore, the two approaches that can improve cure rates—systemic therapies and screening—do not necessarily target the same women. For a given patient, early detection might have made the difference without systemic treatment being used at all. And, for another, early detection might have failed, but systemic therapy made the difference. Overall, it's felt that both approaches have contributed equally to the modest decline in breast cancer mortality—but we're still looking at 40,000 deaths per year, which happens to be 40,000 too many. And that's in the U.S. alone. This is no time to scale back on either screening or systemic therapies. There are mind-boggling biotherapies being developed and introduced, such that we may one day look upon our current era as the turning point in cancer control. However, early diagnosis through screening will be a mainstay for the next several decades, and probably longer.

# 2

# Early Diagnosis May Be the Key, but It's Not a Lock

On November 8, 1895, Bavarian physicist Wilhelm Roentgen[1] asked his wife Bertha to place her left hand on a photographic plate where, for the first time, the mysterious rays that he had previously discovered were focused on a human being. The resulting X-ray image showed the bones of Bertha's hand as distinct from the soft tissue, while her wedding ring stood out most prominently, today a matrimonial symbol reproduced in many radiology texts. Other experiments followed before Roentgen made the startling announcement about his discovery to the world in January 1896 at the Wurzburg Physico-Medical Society.

The medical implications were staggering, not only for diagnosis, but for therapy. Within a few *days* of Roentgen's notice, an "electrotherapist" in Chicago, whose equipment happened to generate X-rays, aimed these "Roentgen Rays" onto the chest wall of a woman in order to treat her recurrent breast cancer. These "surface cancers," and later, deep cancers, that were exposed to high dose X-rays responded remarkably well, so the field of radiation oncology emerged in tandem with diagnostic radiology, not to mention the miscellaneous uses of Roentgen Rays as a cure-all.[2]

The first recorded diagnostic X-ray of the human breast was performed on a mastectomy specimen. In fact, 3,000 mastectomy specimens were X-rayed by Albert Salomon,[3] a surgeon in Berlin who first published his findings in 1913, offering exquisite detail of various growth patterns of cancer, and how cancerous tissue differed from benign tissue. Yet he never attempted a diagnostic X-ray of a breast while it was still attached to one of his patients.

When a host of pioneers began primitive mammography on living patients, the novelty was neither appreciated nor widely adopted. Even with Dr. Robert Egan's 1960 landmark study of 1,000 mammograms at what was then called the M.D. Anderson Hospital and Tumor Institute, the focus was on distinguishing benign changes from malignant ones and how these findings could assist in diagnosis and treatment. The idea of *mass screening* for breast cancer in a healthy population was still a few years away.

Importantly, the definition of breast cancer screening deals with the patient's status, not the X-ray technique. A "screening mammogram" is the same as the first step in a "diagnostic mammogram," though extra views follow in the latter. The point is that the definition of screening today means that the patient has no symptoms—no lumps, no pain, no concerns. Screening healthy women is where the controversy lies, not with diagnostic mammography.

Age guidelines, too, apply only to screening. The following discourse played out all too often in the early days of mammography: "Why didn't you order a mammogram?" the malpractice attorney asks the doctor-defendant. "Because the patient was only 33 and too young for mammograms." "But she had a lump," the attorney responds, "and there are no age restrictions for a diagnostic study, nor are there age restrictions on cancer."

This definition of screening, where the patient is asymptomatic, was not always the case. This made it very difficult to tease out the impact of the clinical exam from mammography. The much-publicized Canadian trial violated this premise for pure mammographic screening, as it accepted women with palpable lumps. By today's definition of screening, this trial should not be considered part of the pack. Yet, when we discuss the historical trials for screening mammography, we'll see how enthusiastic endorsement of the Canadian trial by epidemiologists forms the very core of the controversy we face today.

Many people, if not most, have an exaggerated sense of benefit that comes through early detection for all types of cancer. The propaganda is everywhere: "Early detection is the key," "The sooner the better," "We are all aware that the most important thing is early detection," and so forth.

In survey after survey, the finding is always the same—when asked to *quantify the benefit* of screening in terms of lives saved, the public perception about the impact of early diagnosis is grossly overblown. A surprising number believe that mammograms actually prevent cancer, that the X-rays have a therapeutic benefit. It is these very surveys that the anti-screeners use to gather their stones in preparation for casting.

Picture a tumor the size of a match head (1mm), so small that it cannot be detected clinically. This micro-tumor, perhaps 5 years away from becoming detectable, already contains 1,000,000 (one million) cells, any one of which can jump into the bloodstream and spread elsewhere in the body as a future metastatic site. Allow that tumor a few years to grow to 1.0cm, the size of a shelled peanut, and it is now composed of one *billion* cells. This is the average size of an invasive cancer discovered on mammographic screening, the goal where we pat ourselves on the back and cheer an early diagnosis—1,000,000,000 malignant cells. But are we to believe that millions upon millions of cells sat quietly in the breast for several years and behaved themselves until a mammogram caught them "in the nick of time"?

Well, it's more complicated than that. First of all, no one knows how long tumors are present before detection, and the "5 to 7 years from first malignant cell to detection" that we often hear as gospel is based on one model that oversimplifies what is actually a wide range of growth rates.

Next, tumor cells have been known to shed routinely from primary cancer sites into the bloodstream for well over 100 years, but this clearly does not equate to those cells surviving and thriving. The overwhelming majority of these traveling cells, officially called CTCs for "circulating tumor cells," are kept at bay or are destroyed by the immune system. CTCs don't evolve into clinically evident metastatic tumors unless these circulating cells figure out how to get back *out* of the blood stream, how to dive into a new and receptive environment, and then how to recruit their own blood supply in order to grow larger than 1mm before they go on auto-pilot.

Nevertheless, the point of this exercise is to explain that "early" does not mean "by the calendar." That is, "early" is only loosely correlated to the amount of time malignant cells have been present. Furthermore, if we use tumor size and stage instead of the calendar in our definition of "early," we must deal with the sobering fact that some women die after an "early" diagnosis, when their cancers were no bigger than a peanut.

So let's add some biology (behavior) to the mix as we confess that tumor size is not the end-all. An aggressive tumor might send out lethal cells, capable of developing into metastases, very early in its course when the primary is still tiny, whereas a slow-growing tumor might expand to a very large size without shedding viable cells into the bloodstream. This makes our definition of "early" even more difficult to nail down. With biology added to the picture, size may or may not correlate to outcomes.

As it turns out, breast cancer has a wide array of "biologies," making it very difficult to generalize. And, in the current era of molecular sub-types that are dictating the future of systemic therapies, it seems almost reactionary to discuss *the* singular biology of breast cancer. Yet it is the *general biology* that guides current screening as we don't get to pick and choose which types we are going to see on imaging studies (not yet, anyway). And that's not all— *general biology* also drives local therapy (surgery and radiation), locking mammographic screening and safe lumpectomy at the hip whether clinicians realize it or not.

The Halsted radical mastectomy was not invented in a vacuum. In the late 1800s, William Stewart Halsted[4] formalized a biologic theory for breast cancer that drove the believer to accept the need for a highly regimented surgical procedure customized to address each point in that theory. In brief summary, Halsted espoused a theory that fits what the casual observer of untreated breast cancer might still see today—a predictable and orderly spread of cancer from its initial site in the breast, to the lymph nodes in the armpit where it is held in check for a while, then finally to the rest of the body. Untreated breast cancer displays this sequence quite often—breast mass, enlarged axillary nodes later, with systemic metastases and death later still. This "anatomic" basis for cancer's behavior prompted an "anatomic" solution, the radical mastectomy, removing the entire breast and underlying muscles down to the ribs, as well as a thorough evacuation of axillary lymph nodes to levels not seen by most surgeons today.

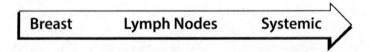

Breast　　　　Lymph Nodes　　　　Systemic

Halsted Theory. This schematic represents a sequence over many years with breast cancer spreading in a predictable, orderly fashion, first to lymph nodes, then distant metastases to other organs.

At the turn of the century, Halsted's results were vastly superior to his colleagues, and his theory was widely accepted, unshakeable for the next 75 years. Because the standard of the day for reporting surgical results in cancer treatment was 3-year follow-up focusing mostly on local control rather than survival, not many clinicians seemed to notice that, as time went on, Halsted's mastectomy was no better than other available options. Nevertheless, due to Halsted's near-total dominance of American surgery at the time, few chose to challenge the king.

While a number of innovators eventually did make the challenge, the prize for top iconoclast goes to Dr. Bernard Fisher, a surgeon who re-wrote the textbooks, along with his brother, pathologist Edwin Fisher, both men working at the University of Pittsburgh. During the same years when mammography was under development, leading up to Egan's 1960 landmark paper, the Fisher brothers were busy in their laboratory systematically destroying the Gospel According to Halsted.

Through a series of some 50 scientific papers, the Fisher brothers charted the behavior of breast cancer using experiments that were both novel and ingenious at the time, albeit crude by today's standards. From this experience, Dr. Bernard Fisher proposed the Alternative Theory of breast cancer, re-christened by clinicians as Fisher Theory, a system that was diametrically opposed to Halsted on every major point. Bernard Fisher, M.D., would subsequently become chairman of the National Surgical Adjuvant Breast and Bowel Project (NSABP), a large cooperative research group that sponsors clinical trials to this day (albeit folded into NRG Oncology). The NSABP B-04 and B-06 clinical trials begun in the 1970s dismantled Halsted Theory and supported Fisher Theory, introducing the option of breast conservation (lumpectomy) and radiation therapy as equal to mastectomy. It is difficult to overstate the revolutionary consequences of Fisher Theory, and many today wonder why Bernard Fisher has *not* won the Nobel Prize.[5]

While Fisher Theory completely revamped the local management of breast cancer by introducing the safety of lumpectomy, it had implications for screening as well. As far as the Fisher brothers were concerned, however, they did not need to consider screening mammography when they were working on their lab rats. Mammographic screening did not exist in the 1950s. As today's insurance companies would say, mammography was "investigational."

So how does Fisher Theory, and the lumpectomy option that it canonized, relate to screening mammography?

For cancer screening to work, there are only two factors at play: (1) tumor biology, and (2) sensitivity of the screening tool.

First, the tumor biology must be vulnerable to early detection. "Biology" is the *built-in set of instructions* at the molecular level that are going to drive the behavior of the tumor. "Vulnerable" biology implies the presence of a clinical window during which detection alters the natural history. The biology can't be "too hot" and it can't be "too cold" for screening to work. At least some of the cancers must have "Goldilocks" biology—that is, "just right." When cancer biology is "too hot," it will spread *prior* to early detection. When biology is "too cold," it will *not* have spread even after a delay of one or more years when it is finally detectable as a lump on exam. But when it's Goldilocks biology, cancer is vulnerable to early detection— that is, it can spread during the clinical window of opportunity.

We have no control over the inherent biology, but there is one variable that can be used to negotiate with biology—the *interval* at which screening is performed. Biology dictates the interval. So how do we address the wide range of breast cancer biologies? Therein lies one of the problems in trying to get experts to agree. If you extend the interval to 2 or even 3 years between screenings, you are "giving up," so to speak, on the aggressive cancers (too hot), and instead, you will skew outcomes toward identifying the slow-growers (too cold). However, the greater danger is giving Goldilocks tumors, the ones that are vulnerable to early detection, a longer time frame to transition from local to systemic.

In theory, it is impossible to extend the interval between screens without losing benefit. Even the U.S. Preventive Services Task Force in their recommendation to switch screening from annual to biennial (every 2 years) acknowledges this. The controversy surrounds quantifying that loss of benefit, as well as agreeing upon a harms-to-benefit ratio. We will eventually address the many implications here, but for now, be aware that the interval is not a number that is drawn from a hat. Because of the diverse biologies seen in breast cancer, there are no straightforward answers. Unfortunately, the latest trend is "How little screening can we get away with, without a huge negative impact?"

Second, sensitivity. The screening tool must be able to detect a good percentage of these Goldilocks tumors, earlier than what would have happened naturally without screening. This detection ability is referred to as Sensitivity, a word to be capitalized from here on to stress its importance. A Sensitivity of 90% is highly desirable for most medical testing. For mammography and its historical claim of 90% Sensitivity, this would mean that if 100 asymptomatic women with undiagnosed breast cancer undergo screening mammography, 90 of them would be visualized and diagnosed from the X-ray.

**Biology (interval) + Sensitivity = Screening Benefit**
**(X + Y = Z)**

"But what about false-positive call-backs, unnecessary biopsies, cost, disease prevalence, patient anxiety, radiation exposure, radiologist skills, overdiagnosis prompting overtreatment, and so forth? Don't those things matter?"

Yes, they matter enormously when it comes to the *practicality* and *acceptance* of screening, but they don't matter one twit when it comes to *effectiveness*. When it comes to screening benefit, i.e., *saving lives*, only two things matter—Biology and Sensitivity. This will be a repetitive theme throughout this book, given that its simple subtlety seems to have been lost. In addition, using simple math, the implications will be huge if we change X (interval) and/or Y (Sensitivity) in the equation above.

To jump start your thinking, though, consider this: What if Sensitivity (Y) isn't anywhere near what we've been told? What if the Sensitivity of mammography is only 50%, rather than 90%? What does that do to our formula, given that we already know Z (Effectiveness) to be a 20–30% relative risk reduction in mortality with screening mammography?

Well, if Z (Screening Benefit) is held steady, and we lower Y (Sensitivity), then X (Biology) must be "greater" to maintain the same Z. Converting to plain English, if mammographic Sensitivity is only 50%, then the general biology of breast cancer must be *more vulnerable* to early detection than we ever imagined. Are we really saving lives with only a 50% detection rate? If so, Goldilocks must rule! And if Goldilocks rules, the last thing we should be considering is cut-backs on screening. Thus, a great deal hinges on the true Sensitivity of mammography.

**Biology + Sensitivity (90%) = Screening Benefit**
**Biology** + Sensitivity (50%) = Screening Benefit

One other key point about our algebraic experience (a.k.a. "logic"): if Sensitivity (Y) is far less than what we've been told (let's say 50%), not only are we facing a Goldilocks Biology (X) exquisitely vulnerable to early detection, but also there's plenty of room for improvement in Sensitivity. This is not a pipe dream—mammographic Sensitivity is improving with new technologies, and multi-modality imaging offers even more improvement.

On the other hand, if we cling to inflated values of mammographic Sensitivity (Y), then we're stuck with the same X, Y, and Z, with very little wiggle room for improvement. We could alter X in a beneficial direction by increasing the frequency of screens to every 6 months, but you can imagine the reception to that idea. This leaves us with our only chance for improvement being Y, or Sensitivity, i.e., increasing the percentage of detected cancers.

A point I will make again and again—*neither side of the warring parties will admit to inflated values for Sensitivity*. Over the years, "90%" has gradually given way to "80%," while also admitting that certain sub-groups, e.g., women with dense tissue, might be as low as "50%." But I maintain the true numbers are lower still, and I'll back that claim with evidence that is remarkably straightforward. It will become increasingly clear (1) why neither side of the debate is willing to budge on Sensitivity numbers, and (2) that true Sensitivity levels are the keystone for my construct, the core principle behind this book.

These two key components (Biology and Sensitivity) for effective screening are *not* either/or. You must have both. A tool that finds 100% of cancers cannot save lives if the biology of the cancer offers no window of vulnerability. Likewise, there's no benefit to a cancer biology with a wide-open window of clinical vulnerability (Goldilocks 100%) if your screening tool fails to detect the cancers earlier than what would occur naturally. You must have both X and Y.

We will eventually dwell more on Sensitivity than Biology, but to understand what is to come, we must examine the biology at the root of the controversy, whether pro-screeners and anti-screeners realize it or not. Why? Because strict Fisher Theory, at the very core of breast conservation surgery today, would predict *no benefit* to early detection through screening mammography. None.

# 3

# Biology Can Trump, but Size Matters

Put yourself in the University of Pittsburgh laboratory in the 1950s where surgeon Bernard Fisher and his pathologist brother Edwin are fiddling around with rats and cell lines, trying to get a handle on the biology of cancer. Now imagine the excitement they must have felt when every experiment they performed yielded results opposite to what Halsted would have predicted. The implications were staggering, almost beyond comprehension. The Halsted radical mastectomy was not simply the "standard of care" at the time—it was a mandate. Anything less, and the errant surgeon might be accused of "murdering" his or her patient. Yet, to the Fisher brothers, it was looking more and more like Halsted was dead wrong.

While I might be tempted to make the claim that I'm the last living human who has read the 50-plus publications from that laboratory, some of the authors of those papers are still alive at the time of this writing. Edwin Fisher died at age 84 in 2008, but Bernie Fisher is in his 90s, as are others who were involved in that research. Although these basic science reports were a tedious reading chore, I took the task to heart when I made the decision in the 1980s to leave my original area of training and become a "breast surgeon," returning to academic medicine to organize a multidisciplinary breast cancer program. If I were going to be teaching this fledgling concept of lumpectomy to surgery residents, and performing the surgery myself, I wanted to know everything about it.

In those days, at the relatively few breast cancer meetings, Bernie Fisher was often the headliner, an imposing figure at the podium, bellowing out the background of his theory for breast cancer biology. He never failed to remind the audience that breast conservation surgery was based in a theory of biology, not the random decision to start doing less.[1] He would point out that Fisher Theory was composed of several sub-theories, e.g., common vascular channel theory, dormant cell theory, etc., but when combined, his theory was stated succinctly and mysteriously as "All breast cancer is systemic at its inception." At least, that was the first incarnation.

True or not, this turned out to be a poor way to communicate a new concept to surgeons who rattled off countless reasons why this was impossible. The next version made more sense, paraphrased as "Breast cancer is either local or systemic at the time of its discovery, and does not progress from local to systemic during its brief clinical window." The surgical implication was still huge no matter how it was stated in Fisher Theory: "Variations in the manner of local control are *unlikely* to have a *substantial* impact on survival." It is those qualifying words— unlikely and substantial—that keep Fisher Theory humming today.

Although Dr. Fisher did not use the word "predestination" (as far as I ever heard or read), he was describing a built-in set of instructions that drove tumors to their endpoint, regardless of the type of surgical intervention, just as long as the tumor was removed. Importantly, the host response to the tumor was every bit as important as the built-in instructions, which is probably why he shied away from the idea that tumor biology alone had a predestined outcome. Fisher Theory would sometimes be explained in terms of A and B. There are A tumors that are local in the breast, and there are B tumors that are systemic long before diagnosed. And, key to Fisher Theory, A tumors *do not progress* to B during what is a very brief clinical window, given the long life of tumors from start to finish.

| Biologic A | **Local** | Biologic B | **Systemic** |
| --- | --- |

**Fisher Theory. Breast cancer is either local or systemic at the time of discovery, and progression from Biologic A to Biologic B does not occur during the clinical window. Thus, variations in the manner of local control are unlikely to have a substantial impact on survival.** *NOTE: Unlike Halsted Theory, there are no arrows in this schematic.*

The Fisher brothers didn't dream up their theory out of the clear blue. There was existing evidence at the time that lumpectomy worked fairly well. Iconoclastic physicians (e.g., George Crile, Jr.) and pioneer radiation oncologists (e.g., Geoffrey Keynes) theorized breast cancer to be primarily a systemic disease, as had medical theorists more than a century earlier. Adding support to the idea that breast conservation could be successful were those women who flatly refused mastectomy after diagnosis, with respectable outcomes in spite of their unwillingness to abide by surgical standards of the day.

With equivalent survival no matter what was done locally, it seemed from the historical data that breast cancer (and the host response) had already "made up its mind" as to what it was going to do before local therapy was performed. For Fisher, the cure would not come through perfecting a local treatment. Instead, the *only way* to eradicate deaths from breast cancer would be through the development of effective systemic treatments. (Note here for future reference that screening minimalists are grounding themselves in Fisher Theory when they claim that current systemic therapies are finally to the point that we can back off from screening.)

With screening mammography not yet on the radar during the laboratory development of Fisher Theory, there was no need to consider the impact of a larger clinical window. The clinical window Fisher was concerned about was not *before* diagnosis, as we have with screening; it was the very short period of the treatment itself, and then—oh yes—the window *after* treatment in those few patients who recurred in the breast a few years later. For those women, the window had to be measured in years.

Dr. Fisher didn't ignore those women who recurred at the lumpectomy site, but he noted no real changes in tumor biology (based on techniques of the day) when comparing the recurrent tumor to the original. In fact, his position was so strong on this issue that in the early days of the B-06 trial where two of three randomized groups underwent lumpectomy (the third group underwent mastectomy), these in-breast recurrences were simply called "cosmetic failures," and the patients proceeded to mastectomy. As data and controversy emerged, beyond our scope here, the terminology was adjusted to IBTR—that is, ipsilateral breast tumor recurrence, today often called "in-breast recurrence," "breast only recurrence," or "breast parenchymal recurrence."

It should be apparent by now that if tumors have built-in instructions that predestine them as to final outcome, long before clinical detectability, that our goal of early detection is doomed. If a relatively long *post*-treatment window, during which in-breast recurrences take place, does not alter survival, then the pre-diagnosis window of screening mammography won't alter survival either. Breast cancer screening and breast conservation are inexorably linked by their windows, the former being a pre-treatment window, the latter a post-treatment window.

Breast conservation surgery was gradually accepted during the late 1980s and early 1990s and is, today, the most common approach for the local treatment of breast cancer. Although several clinical trials proved the equivalency of conservation to mastectomy, every woman who undergoes lumpectomy for her breast cancer has Bernie Fisher and his disciples to thank, not to mention the courageous participants in those early clinical trials when, in contrast, the majority of surgeons in the U.S. considered the NSABP to be treading on thin ice, if not already cracking through to chilly depths.

If biology trumps everything in the surgical management of breast cancer, as stated by Fisher Theory, we are facing a difficult task. The clinical window post-lumpectomy with in-breast recurrence was deemed harmless, distinct from those breast cancers that recurred elsewhere in the body. If a *post-lumpectomy window* was harmless, wherein tumor remained in the breast only to emerge later, then a *pre-diagnosis window*, opened widely through the use of screening mammography, should be a losing proposition.

However, the mammographic screening trials were well underway based on Halsted's basic principles by the time Fisher Theory took hold. Had mammography been introduced 20 years later, it would have had a hard time emerging as a screening tool, likely floundering to an early death. Its very premise would have been suspect, in violation of the newly dominant Fisher Theory. Instead, the impossible happened—screening mammography worked, or apparently so. It saved lives. And this discovery occurred *in tandem* with the emerging Fisher Theory, recalling that Halsted and Fisher theories are mutually exclusive. How is this possible?

Today, clinicians and scientists don't worry much about these over-arching "biologies." Researchers are so consumed by newer classifications of cancer biology based on genetic profiling of tumor cells, Halsted and Fisher are rarely discussed. However, in the world of screening, we don't know which tumor biologies we are going to encounter—Luminal A, Luminal B, basal-like, HER2 positive, or other designations from 25,000 gene arrays that are creating additional sub-groups. Therefore, the appreciation of an overarching biology is still important when analyzing how screening works up front, before details emerge regarding biologic sub-groups.

For many years, dating back to 35mm slides, I would show a diagram with breast conservation trials overlapping screening trials during the 1970s and 1980s, based on two competing theories—Halsted and Fisher—diametrically opposed on each component. Yet both the Fisher-based surgical trials and the Halsted-based screening trials were successful!

Cognitive dissonance is supposed to describe the anxiety that one feels when holding two mutually exclusive theories in the brain at the same time. But in this case, there was no dissonance at all. No one seemed to care about mutually exclusive over-arching biologies. If it works, it works. After all, Ptolemy's theory of an Earth-centered universe was highly developed and made very accurate predictions of what would occur in the night sky.

But Ptolemy was flatly wrong. In the case of breast cancer screening, it seemed we should be more attentive to this question of a general over-arching biology, especially since X + Y = Z. Again, two things make screening work—*biology* and Sensitivity. We are impelled to understand the general biology of breast cancer, all sub-types combined, when it comes to the justification for screening.

Meanwhile, an astute observer and logical thinker looked at these impossible outcomes from Mars and Venus, and argued a middle-ground biologic theory upon which most clinicians base their practice today, whether they realize it or not. Apparently struggling with cognitive dissonance, a prominent radiation oncologist from the University of Chicago proposed Spectrum Theory, best summarized in his Karnofsky Memorial Lecture and published in the *Journal of Clinical Oncology* in 1994.[2] The title of Dr. Samuel Hellman's lecture was "Natural History of Small Breast Cancers," and it is as applicable today as when it was delivered more than two decades ago.

The four key points that Dr. Hellman made to combat strict Fisher Theory were (1) tumor size, (2) tumor progression, (3) impact of radiation therapy on survival, and (4) the successful outcomes of the mammography screening trials.

As for *tumor size*, Dr. Hellman presented published outcomes based on tumor sizes prior to the era of mammographic screening. Even small increments in size showed a direct correlation to both the degree of lymph node involvement and survival. This would not be expected if predestined biology totally trumped anatomic stage. Volumes of research have confirmed the tight correlation of size to survival, with one recent attempt at precision indicating that the "death rate increases by 1.3% per millimeter increase in size.[3]

As for *tumor progression*, the word "progression" is not used in the common lay sense, or even the clinical term that implies tumor has grown or moved to a new spot. No, for basic scientists, cancers occur through "initiation and promotion," but even after a malignancy develops, tumors undergo further mutations, making them even "more malignant," a well-known phenomenon that, when applied to Fisher Theory, implies that Biologic A can sometimes progress to Biologic B. In other words, predestination has its limits.

We actually see this clinically, whether it is appreciated or not. For example, there are fewer Grade 1 (less aggressive) breast cancers that grow to a large size.[4] This is especially true for invasive tubular cancers that can be considered Grade one-half. There are very few pure tubular cancers larger than 3.0cm. How can that be? What happens to them as they grow? The answer is quite simple: as tumors grow, they *de-differentiate*, changing to a higher grade as the "more malignant" cells divide quicker. Thus, basic science "progression" is reflected clinically. Increasing size correlates to higher grade. And this is what led to the "sweet spot" that was theorized for mammography—the transition from A to B, local to systemic, seems to pick up speed once tumors grow larger than the 1.0 to 1.5cm range. Size and progression are thus related, and there seems to be a watershed size that matches nicely with the average size of screen-detected cancers.

As for the *impact of radiation therapy* on survival, if Fisher Theory has its feet held to the fire, then radiation should be in the same category as surgery—that is, it's another means for locoregional control, and should not substantially alter survival. Yet Dr. Hellman provided natural history data from the era prior to chemotherapy where the addition of radiation to mastectomy improved survival. Two decades would pass subsequent to the lumpectomy trials before a consensus was reached that radiation, added either to mastectomy or lumpectomy, improves survival in some patients. The effect was small, but measureable, and for those of us who followed these developments closely, this benefit has been suggested all along.[5] When a recent meta-analysis confirming the benefit of radiation therapy on survival was announced, I heard a "talking head" physician online describe how he was going to have to re-think his position on local control not having a survival impact. If he had been paying attention, Sam Hellman, M.D., not only told us this was the case long ago, but also used it as one of his reasons to forge a crack in Fisher Theory.

When it comes to the *successful mammography screening trials*, one can claim Dr. Hellman was using circular reasoning, i.e., using the conclusion as a premise. But at this point in time, the early 1990s, the mammography screening trials were so successful that thinkers had to come to the conclusion that Fisher Theory could not be completely valid. If breast cancer were predestined as to outcomes, then early detection would not matter. (The Canadian trial, however, is about to burst on the scene here, reinforcing Fisher Theory.)

Dr. Hellman ended his lecture with this cautionary statement: "Halsted became dogma and, more recently, the notion of breast cancer always being systemic has become dogma. Like all dogma in science, both are too restricting. They tend to limit our inquiries and deny the conditional and approximate nature of our scientific knowledge."

In personal testimony, I heard Dr. Hellman deliver his message more than 20 years ago, and it put an end to my cognitive dissonance. Maybe it's like Copernicus and his new concept of a sun-centered solar system, which still didn't have it nailed down perfectly, but it was a whole lot closer to the truth than Ptolemy. Nevertheless, Spectrum Theory explained what we see clinically and took away the screening nihilism as a by-product of Fisher Theory, yet without casting us back into the flames of Halsted.

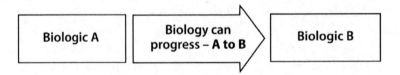

Biologic A    Biology can progress – A to B    Biologic B

**Spectrum Theory. While there are several ways to explain Spectrum Theory schematically, this approach helps one visualize a "middle group" of tumors that might progress from local (A) to systemic (B) during the clinical window. The majority of breast cancers are likely A or B, explaining the success of the Fisher Theory, but the middle group would be responsible for gains made in screening. Simply being in this middle group and being screened is not enough to alter outcomes, though. The screening tool still has to be Sensitive, and the frequency of the screen has to be such that these tumors can be caught while still Biologic A.**

While we don't know the exact numbers as to how many cancers are A, B or in the middle, we can calculate a very disturbing truth: in spite of the fact that nearly all women with cancer discovered on mammography might initially claim, "Mammograms saved my life," this is not the case for the *majority*. If mammograms saved the lives of everyone diagnosed by screening, we would see more dramatic mortality reductions in the prospective, randomized trials for those in the mammography group. And we would see a much greater reduction in breast cancer deaths in our population statistics. Even the most radical pro-screening enthusiast, one of the "fathers of screening mammography," László Tabár, calculated in the late 1980s that only *1 in 7* women with cancers discovered on mammography actually had her life saved.

Recent modifications are more optimistic. Lives saved through screening mammography might be as high as "1 in 3" of cancers detected when women are compliant with annual screening using modern technology, but there's no possible way that the majority of women have their life saved when breast cancer is discovered on screening mammography. I don't say this to deflate the rock star status of breast radiologists who, as some "poisoning medical oncologists" point out, are given more credit than they deserve. I state it so that we can stick to the facts.

In today's era of DNA microarray classification of cancers that dictate therapies and the design of clinical trials, these buzz-word classifications have not yet impacted screening recommendations. They might. Picture a day when we don't use radiologic images to screen for cancer. Instead, we use a blood test designed to pick up only those cancers that are potentially deadly, and in which targeted therapy improves survival. Then, if positive on the blood test, the patient would have radiologic imaging performed, not to screen, but for diagnosis—that is, localization of the tumor and biopsy.

Some visionary researchers are thinking way beyond even my futuristic scenario. They have combined radiologic imaging and therapy all in one step. The very tracer that makes cancer cells light up for the radiologist will simultaneously kill those same cells. Diagnosis and therapy rolled into one step. Science fiction? Actually, the preliminary work is underway for a variety of cancer types, and the only limiting factor is time.

In our world of screening, in the meantime, we don't get to pick and choose specific biologies. We can only deal in terms of an overarching biology that explains breast cancer in general. For those who have remained firm in Fisher Theory, the mortality reductions seen with screening seem implausible. But for those who have adopted Spectrum Theory, screening remains strong in its foundation.

For breast cancer, at present, mammographic discovery is stage-based. In contrast to the critical importance of (Goldilocks) biology when it comes to the final tally in terms of lives saved, when it comes to the mechanics of mammographic screening, biology takes a back seat to tumor stage. That is, size matters.

This is not true for all types of cancer. In the next chapter, we will visit the biologic test used for prostate cancer screening (PSA), which is *not* based on anatomy. Tumor size and/or stage are *not* an integral part of the detection process for prostate cancer. The evidence for lives saved through PSA screening is less convincing than what we know about mammographic screening, yet the anti-screening crowd is salivating in the hope that mammography guidelines will suffer the same fate as PSA where recommendations have been curtailed. To that end, distortions and gyrations are being used to link the two cancers as two sides of a zipper. Or, in a different metaphor, the ball and chain of PSA screening is being tied to screening mammography, with the intent to throw both overboard.

# 4

# Prostate Is Not Breast, So Give It a Rest

Charles B. Huggins, M.D. (1901–1997), a Canadian-born American surgeon, working at the University of Chicago, won the 1966 Nobel Prize for Physiology and Medicine. Or, more accurately, he won half of the Nobel Prize[1] for his discoveries that revealed the effectiveness of hormonal treatments for prostate cancer. Unlike many Nobel Prize winners whose names have been lost to history, Dr. Huggins' contribution is perpetuated as the answer to a trivia question designed to inflict suffering on medical students: "Name the Nobel Prize winners who were surgeons." (At last count, there were nine Nobel Laureate surgeons.[2])

Dr. Huggins discovered that prostate cancer responded to endocrine manipulation, either through bilateral orchiectomy (a.k.a. "castration") or estrogen therapy. Alternatively stated, prostate cancer was often a hormone-dependent tumor, using circulating androgens as "fertilizer" for faster growth. Cutting off the fertilizer supply helped. A lesser known fact about Dr. Huggins is that he also studied breast cancer in the same light—that is, a cancer type that can also be tricked into submission through hormonal leverage.

The idea did not originate with Huggins, dating back to at least 1882 when Dr. T.W. Nunn observed an advanced breast cancer regress spontaneously six months after his patient entered menopause. Others toyed with the idea of intentionally removing the ovaries in premenopausal women with breast cancer, but held back out of ethical concerns, demonstrating unusual restraint for that era. Dr. G.T. Beatson from Scotland forged ahead, however, and in 1895, reported that his first patient, thought to be "terminal" with extensive breast cancer metastases, had a complete remission followed by 4 years of survival after bilateral oophorectomy. He went on to report a series of his first three patients in *The Lancet* in 1896.

Concurrent with his endocrine studies on prostate cancer, Dr. Huggins was assisted in the laboratory by Ling Yuan Dao, the latter more focused on the endocrine treatments that might starve breast cancer. In the 1950s, Huggins and Dao added much weight to the notion that the same processes were at work in both types of cancer, and that manipulation could result in disease regression. Endocrine ablation to treat breast cancer through oophorectomy, and sometimes adrenalectomy, subsequently became standard clinical practice, later replaced by the hormone-blocking drug tamoxifen for the majority of patients. Dr. Tom Dao[3] went on to his own illustrious career as director of the breast surgery department at Roswell Park Cancer Institute from 1957 to 1988.

The two types of cancer—breast and prostate—have been linked ever since.

22

Yes, both types of cancer are quite common. In fact, each type is the most common cancer for the respective gender. Both types are currently pushing the 250,000 mark in the number of affected patients in the U.S. This is excluding the controversial Stage 0 breast cancer, a.k.a. DCIS (ductal carcinoma in situ), a generous number in its own right, with more than 60,000 patients diagnosed with DCIS in the U.S. in 2015. Breast cancer has a slightly higher number of women dying of the disease, with current numbers running around 40,000 per year, while less than 30,000 die from prostate cancer each year in the U.S. If one includes breast DCIS, however, both types of cancer have a ratio of *disease incidence-to-mortality* of 8:1. For every 8 cases diagnosed, 1 patient will die of the disease.

Other similarities have been drawn in pathology and epidemiology, in addition to anti-hormonal treatments still regarded as a mainstay of treatment for both types, today accomplished with drugs far more often than surgery. But there are differences, too. For instance, the anti-hormonal drugs used to lower the risk of developing breast cancer have an anti-androgen counterpart for prostate cancer. Yet those prevention trials for reducing the risk of prostate cancer were not nearly the success as was seen in breast cancer. And then, of course, there is screening, where PSA doesn't get the same nod as mammography.

This is rarely discussed, but here's why screening with PSA and mammography are worlds apart. Breast cancer prognosis is accurate using the *anatomic* staging system known as TNM (Tumor size—Nodal status—distant Metastases). Mammography is 100% *anatomic-based*, and detects earlier stage disease. The screening tool matches the staging system. Thus, the default position, based on logic alone, without any supporting data whatsoever, ought to be that anatomic screening *should* save lives. Mammography clearly finds earlier stage disease (no debate about this at all), but there's plenty of debate as to whether lives are saved, coming from those who believe that biology trumps stage.

Indeed, this "early detection" is how the vast majority of people think about screening anyway, whether they use anatomic vs. biologic terms or not. In fact, most think in terms of anatomic stage exclusively. Stage I prognosis is better than Stage II, so find the Stage I cancers through screening. It's deceptively simple. Here's a schematic representation to illustrate the remarkable reliability of anatomic stage in breast cancer prognosis, even when Stages are subdivided into A, B and C:

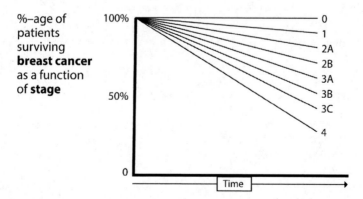

Classical anatomic staging is unusually accurate in determining breast cancer prognosis. While additional tumor markers refine prognosis, it is these clear distinctions between stages that allow a screening strategy to succeed when the screening tool itself is based on anatomic stage. Earlier stage discoveries *ought* to translate to improved survival.

In contrast to breast cancer, the TNM system based on anatomy alone doesn't help much in prostate cancer. That's why you will hear friends, relatives, and patients with prostate cancer discuss their "Gleason score." Gleason score is a grading system that addresses *biology*, not *anatomy*. "Grade" reflects how "aggressive" cells look under the microscope, whereas "Stage" is a system that involves *Tumor* size, *Nodal* status, and *Metastases*. In order to achieve a prognostic staging system useful in prostate cancer, both Gleason score and the PSA value are combined with TNM status into Groups.

All types of cancer diagnoses and management are gradually migrating toward more and more dependence on biology for predicting therapeutic response and long-term outcomes, rather than anatomy. Someday, cancers will likely be staged exclusively by their biology. But we're not there yet. The prognosis for each type of cancer is accomplished by blending anatomy and biology, with the weight distribution different for each cancer type. Breast cancer is still in the transition process. We are slow to leave anatomic staging because it remains remarkably helpful in breast cancer. Whether or not biology trumps Stage (anatomic extent) is what we've been discussing in this book so far, and it is at the very heart of the controversy about screening.

This is where prostate cancer refuses to hold hands with its sister cancer. The classic TNM system of anatomic staging alone is not very helpful in predicting outcomes in prostate cancer. Here is the 5-year unadjusted (not cause-specific) survival data for prostate cancer in nearly a half million patients diagnosed between 1998 and 2002, drawn from 1,406 cancer programs that participate in the Commission on Cancer, sponsored by the American College of Surgeons and the American Cancer Society:

Stage 0   — 76% survival at 5 years
Stage I   — 80.5% survival at 5 years
Stage II  — 89.1% survival at 5 years
Stage III — 89.7% survival at 5 years
Stage IV  — 39.8% survival at 5 years

A schematic representation of these numbers would look like this, a stark contrast to the orderly breast cancer diagram above, with the classic TNM Stage bearing no relation to outcome, with the exception of Stage 4 (distant metastases).

Surprised? You should be. The Stage 0, I, II, and III curves are upside down! Is it really better to have Stage III disease than Stage I? And how about that Stage 0, which for breast

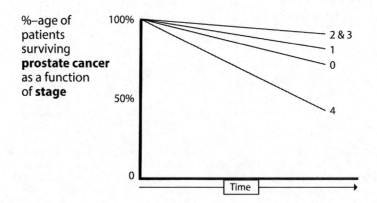

cancer means a near-100% survival? Granted, not many patients were in that category (134 out of 474,301 total), but it still screams for an explanation. It should be clear that TNM staging for prostate cancer is worlds apart from the anatomic staging of breast cancer. To that end, the American Joint Committee on Cancer has adopted groupings for prostate cancer, analogous to Stage, but with Gleason's score and PSA levels added to traditional TNM anatomic stage. When "biology" is added to Stage, the survival curves separate quite nicely, as seen with breast cancer. The point is that, in *breast cancer*, the survival curves are quite distinct even *before* "biology" (Grade, ER, PR, HER2, Ki67, etc.) is added to the mix.

Given that biology in prostate cancer gives more prognostic information than anatomic stage, an anatomic-based screening method (radiologic imaging) as a single tool would not help much, if at all. Rightly so, prostate cancer screening is done through a biologic tool (PSA blood test) augmented by the digital exam. Unfortunately, the cancers detected by PSA tend to be the low grade biologies, i.e., "Biology A" if we draw from our earlier terminology in breast cancer, rather than the ideal Goldilocks biology where clinical intervention makes a difference. That is, PSA favors detection of the cancers less likely to be lethal.

As a result, a prostate cancer mortality reduction through widespread PSA screening is even more difficult to demonstrate than mammographic screening. Only two major studies provide the evidence for prostate cancer screening guidelines using PSA—the PLCO study in the U.S. showing no benefit at all, while the ERSPC trial in Europe initially reported a marginal mortality reduction that failed to show statistical significance.[4] However, as occurs with long natural histories in sub-types of certain cancers, the benefit may not be evident for many years subsequent to the screen-detected tumor. Indeed, a recent update of the ERSPC trial with 13 years of follow-up, published in the December 6, 2014, issue of *The Lancet,* revealed a statistically significant relative mortality reduction of 21% with PSA screening. As with the mammography trials, of course, there is considerable controversy about confounding variables and interpretation of results.

Both the American Cancer Society and the U.S. Preventive Services Task Force have withdrawn support for routine PSA screening. To be exact, the U.S. Preventive Services Task Force gave PSA a worse grade (D) than it gave screening mammography in women aged 40–49 where mammography scores a "C." The official explanation of "C" changes with each incarnation of the Task Force, though in 2009, it meant "against *routine* screening," but if circumstances warrant, and if you discuss it with your doctor, and if you have risk factors, and if you want to open yourself up to possible overdiagnosis with unnecessary biopsies and treatments, and if you realize your breast density may preclude detection, then "Sure, go ahead and screen, but do so at your own risk." In 2016, the Task Force kept the "C" rating, but softened the definition of "C" by removing the word "against."

*Opposite* **In contrast to breast cancer, traditional anatomic staging is of little benefit in predicting prostate cancer outcomes. When "biology" (PSA level and Gleason score) is added to the TNM stage, however, the survival curves separate nicely into Groups. In this illustration of unadjusted (not cause-specific) survival based solely on TNM anatomic stage, the curves do not prompt one to think anatomic screening would be a wise approach. Thus, biologic-based screening is the goal, using PSA and its newer modifications. Unfortunately, basic PSA tends to identify lower grade tumors, prompting overdiagnosis controversies much more substantial than seen in breast cancer. However, new approaches to PSA are now available that could bring widespread prostate screening back into favor—e.g., the 4Kscore™ has recently been added to guidelines from the NCCN, a PSA-plus approach that identifies cancers that are more biologically significant.**

By the way, the Affordable Care Act only provides preventive health coverage for A and B recommendations from the Task Force, and this little tidbit might help you understand what goes on in the smoke-filled rooms where public health experts and epidemiologists decide what's best for you—no, let me re-phrase that—where they decide what's best for society.

"D," by the way, means "stop it."

Part of the difference between breast and prostate screening recommendations, admittedly, is that "harms" are more easily identified after a high PSA. As one example of the differences, even a routine prostate needle biopsy can send men to the ICU in septic shock, and rarely, death—a very small number in percentage terms, sure, but there's nothing comparable for breast biopsies.

This "D" recommendation for PSA is unfortunate in many respects because few urologists use the original PSA test by itself anymore. "Free" PSA, PSA velocity, PSA doubling times are already in clinical use, and a new test that expands PSA to 4 markers, called the 4Kscore®, is much more accurate than PSA alone in the detection of biologically aggressive prostate cancer. In 2015, the 4Kscore® was added to NCCN (National Comprehensive Cancer Network) guidelines, one of the mainstay references for cancer care, once again forcing the U.S. Preventive Services Task Force to play catch-up.

The point of all this is to demonstrate that screening for the two cancers is different, as is their anatomic-biologic basis. Conceptually, prostate cancer screening is more suited for the future, based on biology rather than anatomy, but the reality needs to play catch-up to the ideal. As for breast cancer, screening is based on anatomic extent of disease that is exceptionally reliable in the prediction of outcomes, thus providing a solid default position—image-based screening for breast cancer *ought* to work.

Everything seems so straightforward for breast cancer in this regard, at least for now. If breast cancer that is discovered at Stage IIA is reliably going to have a 10-year survival of 80%, while Stage I is 90%, then let's find Stage I breast cancers more often. It's so simple, why bother describing all this detail for something so obvious to begin with?

Why? In order to nix what the anti-screeners are attempting to do when they lump breast and prostate screening together, then declaring both ineffective. Anti-screeners love to drag mammography into the pit of PSA. Don't be fooled. Furthermore, the jury is still out on PSA screening, and the Task Force may eventually have to swallow its pride and give it some grade inflation from D to C.

At this point, let me introduce one of the most popular words today when it comes to discrediting cancer screening—*overdiagnosis*. Yes, it's real, but how common is it? Well, in prostate, it appears to be rather common, as evidenced by the higher number of cancers discovered by PSA in the PLCO Trial, without a concomitant mortality reduction. This phenomenon is respected by urologists and medical oncologists who sometimes offer "no treatment" or "simple observation" as an option to some men newly diagnosed.

Breast screening critics are shouting the same song, but the two cancers have different melodies. We will circle back to overdiagnosis later on, but for now consider one of the oft-forgotten ways in which we can actually measure overdiagnosis—autopsy studies. Here, we can directly observe occult cancers that sat idly in the body until death, then compare those numbers to what we see emerge in the living.

If cancers just "fester" throughout life without emerging clinically, then they pile up—

that is, they can be found in autopsy studies at a much higher rate than what would be anticipated. Or they must regress (disappear), a phenomenon that only epidemiologists believe in, given that those of us in the business have never seen a single case of invasive breast cancer disappear naturally. For prostate cancer, the evidence for overdiagnosis is firm (not to detract from very real killer-forms of the disease), *not because they regress,* but because they can "fester."

This topic has been covered in both the scientific and lay literature, but a good example of "festering" was published in the February 2008 issue of the *Canadian Journal of Urology* where worldwide statistics were reviewed.[5] In the United States, both in white and black populations, the autopsy prevalence of prostate cancer was found to be roughly proportional to age. This means that, by age 30, 31% of men have focal areas of prostate adenocarcinoma. By age 80 the number has risen to 83% in whites, 81% in blacks, prompting some to assume that by age 100, 100% of men will have prostate cancer if they live that long. There is no better demonstration of a mismatch between microscope findings of "cancer" and clinical behavior than we have here. This is strong evidence that prostate cancer can "fester," so it should be no surprise that it is frequently diagnosed from PSA elevations and biopsies.

But the real test of subclinical disease festering quietly in the body would be if you performed prostate biopsies on living men with *normal* PSAs and *normal* exam. Is that even ethical?

In fact, it has been done, as part of a large prevention trial and published in the *New England Journal of Medicine*.[6] Using random prostate biopsies in men with normal PSA and normal digital exam, *15% had prostate cancer,* and this was only very limited sampling of the prostate, as opposed to the entire gland in autopsy studies. This means we have a very high disease reservoir in prostate cancer, many cases never emerging during the average lifetime.

In an effort to prove that Stage 0 breast cancer (a.k.a. ductal carcinoma in situ or DCIS) acts similar to festering prostate cancer, a review of autopsy studies was performed with the intent of showing the same large reservoir of undiagnosed disease. This was back in the day when many of us thought that stopping breast cancer in its tracks was perfecting the science of DCIS detection and treatment. (In the kinder, gentler world of today, the fact that some DCIS can be considered "overdiagnosis" has come to the point where we're nearly apologizing for detecting it.) Regardless, the autopsy review was performed with the express purpose of demonstrating a large reservoir of undiagnosed DCIS and thus its demotion from "cancer" to "non-obligated precursor" or perhaps a term even more bland so as not to frighten the public.

The autopsy review was commandeered by a prominent anti-screening crusader, H. Gilbert Welch, M.D., MPH, from Dartmouth. One weakness inherent to all studies of occult disease in pathology, perhaps more so in breast than prostate, is sampling error. A pathologist takes random tissue samples to be converted into microscope slides, based on visual and palpable clues. Because DCIS can be non-palpable, it's likely that the actual numbers in this study would have been higher if comprehensive sampling had been performed. So what did the study show?

Drawing from articles published between 1966 and 1996, in this autopsy review,[7] the median prevalence of DCIS was 8.9%, with a range from 0% to 14.7%. The number of microscope slides examined (samples taken) in the 7 studies that they reviewed ranged from 9 to 275, with the higher numbers for detecting DCIS in those studies where more slides were made and reviewed. Two hundred seventy-five is generous sampling, yet DCIS never exceeded

15% in any study. While this was called a "substantial reservoir of DCIS" that went undetected during life, and thus supported the notion of overdiagnosis of DCIS, the numbers are not even in the same ballpark with the aforementioned autopsy data on prostate cancer. Compare the 0-to-14.7% incidence of DCIS in all women who underwent autopsy to the 80% incidence of prostate cancer at autopsy in men aged 80 or over.

The study confirmed the authors' bias, both authors (Welch and Black) already having established themselves as anti-screeners by the time of this 1997 publication, which by the way, was entitled "Using Autopsy Series to Estimate the Disease 'Reservoir' for Ductal Carcinoma in Situ of the Breast: How Much More Breast Cancer Can We Find?" (And they didn't mean "How Much More Can We Find?" in a positive sense.) The message was clear: we are diagnosing and treating women for a disease process that they would carry silently to the grave if we would just leave them alone. This is overdiagnosis.

This article was published during the Mammography Civil War of the 1990s, when Dr. Welch was still gathering ammunition for his position that breast cancer screening does more harm than good. However, in recent years, the anti-screening argument of overdiagnosis moved beyond the realm of DCIS, where nearly everyone agreed it occurred to some degree, and entered the world of *invasive* breast cancer.

With this expansion from overdiagnosis in DCIS, now to include invasive cancer, Dr. Welch and others wrote books and hit the lecture circuit, announcing rampant overdiagnosis of invasive breast cancer, with an indirectly calculated 70,000 invasive cancers overdiagnosed per year in the U.S. alone. Since most of us have never seen a case of invasive breast cancer that "stabilizes" or "regresses" without treatment, we have to wonder—"Where are these women hiding their disease?" In their 2012 article in the *New England Journal of Medicine*,[8] Drs. Archie Bleyer and H. Gilbert Welch, using a large database, determined that 31% of invasive breast cancers were overdiagnosed in 2008, and that 1,300,000 women over the past 30 years have been diagnosed and treated with cancers that never would have killed them if they had just avoided mammography like the plague.

With no retort to such claims, and no motivation to seek alternative explanations, the minions who convert half-truths into truthiness adopted the "one-third" overdiagnosis of invasive cancer as a proven fact, and many now believe it is a critical component of an informed consent before a woman gets a mammogram.

I'm not talking about lunatic claims of overdiagnosis here. Dr. Welch is very bright and a skilled communicator (a.k.a. rhetorician). His presentations are captivating. Having served with him on an ad hoc committee for screening guidelines, orchestrated by the American Society of Breast Surgeons in 2014, I found him both humble and responsive to other opinions (perhaps on guard because of the palpable antipathy by some in the room). Today, he has easier access to the podiums at breast cancer conferences than the pro-screening radiologists, and his calculations can be convincing ... until your reach the endgame—70,000 per year? Where are they?

Well, the epidemiologist's response would be "You don't recognize them because you took them all out. We public health specialists are comparing the increase in cancer rates after the institution of mammographic screening, and there is not an equivalent decrease in the number of advanced stage cancers, as we have historically seen, for instance, with Pap screening."

Unfortunately, it takes the skill of a pro-screening epidemiologist to recognize all the flaws in the deductive reasoning process, most notably the failure to correct for lead time, to which we will return. Thus, many practicing clinicians are bowled over by the Welch argument, becoming instant converts to a belief in massive overdiagnosis *just like prostate cancer*. This is a surprising development in light of what we know about breast cancer biology and disease progression.

As it turns out, 70,000 may be an appropriate number to use if we define overdiagnosis to mean those patients with Biologic A tumors. But if we stick to the strict definition of overdiagnosis, that being cancers that would *never* kill the patient even if untreated (as we see in some prostate cancers and some DCIS), then 70,000 is inconceivable. If this were true, we should see cancers "stabilize" or "regress" in women who refuse treatment after biopsy and in cases where there was a delayed diagnosis. We simply don't see it. But one way to measure "going to the grave" with non-life-threatening cancers is to literally go to the grave—that is, as we have seen with DCIS—autopsy studies. At 70,000 harmless cancers per year, there should be a staggering reservoir of invasive disease in the autopsy studies of unscreened women, comparable to prostate, or at least to DCIS.

Recently, as I dusted off my Civil War files, preparing for this book, I recalled the old autopsy article by Welch and Black, and pulled it out for review. Pages had yellowed with time after nearly 20 years, but I re-read the exposé that had targeted DCIS. Much to my surprise, the authors had included something else in their review—invasive breast cancer. It had not been their target at the time, which was only DCIS in 1997, but they reported results anyway. No one really dreamed that charges of overdiagnosis would someday be levied against invasive cancer as well.

Remembering that prostate cancer incidence at autopsy matches up with age, up to *80%* incidence, and that DCIS has a range from *0 to 14.7%* (the higher numbers when more sections were taken), what would you imagine for invasive breast cancer? How large was the reservoir for invasive disease in these old studies, largely from the pre-mammography era?

The answer: *1.3%* (full range in the 7 studies reviewed—0 to 1.8%).

To put that number in perspective, if we randomly pick 100 women to undergo mammographic screening, on their first study, we would find cancer in one patient (1.0%). If we then take the remaining 99 and perform one MRI (essentially looking for "next year's cancer" to be seen on mammos), we will find one additional cancer (another 1.0%). If we perform a breast MRI for a problem that turns out to be nothing, there is still a 1.0% chance we'll find a cancer unrelated to the problem that prompted the MRI. If, during a reduction mammoplasty, the plastic surgeon removes 50% of the breast tissue, the chance that an occult invasive cancer will be found on pathology is 0.5%. Do you see the obvious? The disease reservoir for invasive breast cancer is 1%, dead or alive. *Nothing* to support overdiagnosis under its strict definition. This autopsy review, performed no less by the chief architect of overdiagnosis in the U.S., negates most of the "one-third" rhetoric being tossed about today, based on presumptions and indirect calculations. The autopsy reservoir for disease is the closest thing we have to a direct measurement of overdiagnosis.

Prostate is not breast, so give it a rest.

Sometimes, stories can come to a happy ending, only to be derailed by another act where disaster waits to strike. Think of the disappointment you might have felt with *The Fantastiks* or *Into the Woods* when the neatly packaged finale was merely the calm before the storm.

Oh, how I would like to stop right here, and wallow in the certainty of anatomic screening applied to anatomic staging. It's a perfect fit. Find Stage I instead of Stage II, and you will save some lives. Find Stage I instead of III and you will save more lives.

Sadly, strange and mysterious forces are about to descend. A malevolent trickster is at work. And here's how it plays out.

Let's take 200 women of comparable age, ethnicity, risk factors, etc. And all of them are newly diagnosed with breast cancers of identical size (1.5cm), identical grade and negative nodes. Accordingly, they should all have identical outcomes. But there's one point of distinction—100 women had their cancer discovered by mammography while the other 100 felt their cancers on self-exam. At the end of 10 years, *the number of survivors will not be equal.* Those diagnosed through screening might have 95% survival, while those who palpated their tumors on self-exam will have 85% survival, all other factors being equal—the only difference being *mode of detection.*

While my 200-patient example above is theoretical, the studies have actually been done, so the differential outcomes are not theoretical. They are real.

What gives? This explodes the entire concept of anatomic stage-based screening. It is counterintuitive. How can the method of detection make a difference?

In the next chapter, we will visit the Four Horsemen of the Screening Apocalypse—the 4 epidemiologic biases that make mammography appear to work even if it doesn't.

# 5

# The Four Horsemen That Inflate the Power of Mammography

Maybe I cut class that day in medical school. More likely, the topic was never covered in the 1970s brand of medical education where we were trained to treat people rather than populations. Nevertheless, there are 4 primary biases that can exaggerate the power of a screening tool. Note: these biases are not limited to mammography. And this list of 4 is not exhaustive, as there are minor biases as well. They apply to any screening tool proposed as public health policy, examples including colonoscopy, Pap smears, PSA, lung CT, and CA-125 for ovarian cancer, the common feature here being the application of the tool to a healthy, asymptomatic population. And these potential biases were well known (to an inner circle) prior to the initiation of the first mammography screening trial in the 1960s.

I first learned about these tricksters when I switched from general surgery to breast surgery in the late 1980s and heard mutterings that mammographic screening was controversial. How could that be? The buzz phrase at the time was "Breast cancer survival is 60% overall, but it's 90% if your cancer is discovered on mammography" (or variations thereof). How could there be an argument with statistics like that?

Amazingly, the above statement can be true, without mammographic screening making one bit of difference. How? Through the power of the Four Horsemen. Instead of War, Famine, Pestilence, and Death, we have Selection Bias, Lead Time Bias, Length Bias, and Overdiagnosis Bias.

It should go without saying that biases are not the same thing as "harms" of screening. Certainly, overdiagnosis has a dual role, as both a bias and potential harm, by virtue of accompanying overtreatment. But the other three should be held harmless. Yes, they can inflate the power of screening, as we will see, but they result in no direct harm to patients. Why mention this? As you might imagine, anti-screeners and screening minimalists have no remorse as they rechristen these biases as harms. If lead time bias is to be called a screening "harm," as was recently claimed,[1] then nothing is too far-fetched to build the case against screening.

Returning to substantive issues, here are the four primary biases that inflate the power of screening:

*Selection Bias:* Let's say you study 10,000 women who complied with yearly mammography and 10,000 who did not have mammograms. In this retrospective analysis, you find that the women who underwent mammography were less likely to die of breast cancer, even to the point of reaching statistical significance. As it turns out, the 10,000 who complied with

31

mammography might also have been compliant with other health measures that lowered their breast cancer risk and mortality, such as exercise, healthy diet, minimal alcohol intake, etc. Their benefit may not be due to early detection with mammography, but the other healthy habits they adopted. Mammography went along for the ride.

This bias is the easiest to understand, and the easiest to eradicate through prospective, randomized trials. (It can also be an avenue for manipulating the data, even in prospective randomized controlled trials [RCTs]—if you don't like your results, then "correct for possible selection bias.") Selection bias is always an issue in observational studies, though some believe that the effect can minimized. Today, we have observational studies with mammography that include millions of women. And when the benefits are consistent with outcomes from prospective, randomized trials, one has to consider that these studies are providing valid information.

*Lead Time Bias*: Suppose identical twins develop their first malignant breast cell on the same day, with the biology dictating very aggressive disease that will result in the death of both women 10 years down the road. At 5 years, however, the tumor is large enough to be detected on mammography, and one twin believes in annual mammograms but the other doesn't. The mammography twin has her cancer discovered at the 5-year point, while the twin who feels her lump on self-exam discovers her cancer at the 7-year point. Both twins die of breast cancer at the same 10-year interval following the very first malignant cell, but it *appears* that the twin who was undergoing annual mammography lived longer thanks to her early detection. Her survival was 5 years after the mammogram, while her twin's survival was only 3 years from the time she felt the tumor.

This is lead time bias, and it's not merely theoretical. In this instance, mammograms had no impact on survival at all, but there is the *illusion* of benefit. This is why "survival years" after a screening study is a statistic held with caution. In the end, to prove the benefit of screening, we will be using "mortality reduction," which on the surface sounds like it ought to be the same thing, but it's not. And again, there's no "harm" with this bias. It's merely an observable phenomenon that must be held accountable.

*Length Bias (or Length Time Bias)*: All screening recommendations come with an "interval" that describes how much time should elapse between screens. The longer the interval, the more likely a cancer will appear in between screening visits. These "interval" cancers are classically described as more aggressive, in that they were not present on the prior screen and therefore must have grown quickly during the interval. The implication here is that the more deadly cancers emerge in between screenings, while the low grade cancers that are less likely to kill the patient grow slowly and are plucked like low-hanging fruit at the screening session.

By selectively picking the slow-growers, mammography appears to be a doing a better job than it really is. As with lead time bias, the presence of length bias is not theoretical, it is at work to some degree in population screening, and must be dealt with. Like the other biases, the only tool that can keep it at bay is a prospective, randomized trial that has mortality reduction as its endpoint. A mortality reduction is mandatory to rule out length bias or, at a minimum, to show that the benefit overpowers the length bias.

Length bias will keep popping up in our discussions. If a prospective, randomized clinical trial shows no mortality reduction, yet more cancers were found in the mammography group, this will be a pure display of length bias. On the other hand, if the same trial shows a mortality reduction with long-term follow-up, then length bias will be a secondary issue, overshadowed by the benefit of screening.

One final word about "interval cancers." While I mentioned the traditional teaching that interval cancers are more aggressive, careful study shows this is not always the case. In fact, only about one-third of cancers occurring in the interval between screenings fit the bill as a "classic" aggressive interval cancer. Most were probably present on the prior mammogram, undiagnosed because the changes were too subtle to prompt a call-back for further evaluation. Or the tumors were large enough to be detected, but were completely lost in a background of dense tissue on the prior mammogram. Or the cancers were flat out missed by the radiologist on the prior mammogram. Still, classic, aggressive interval cancers occur often enough to skew outcomes unfavorably for this group of patients whose cancers emerge between screens.

The allegation that most interval cancers are detectable on the prior screen is supported by the breast MRI screening trials wherein interval cancers nearly disappeared. Furthermore, the MRI screening trials were dedicated to high-risk patients wherein the number of interval cancers with mammography alone is higher than the general population. In contrast to the 20–25% rate of interval cancers with mammography in the general population, the rate can be as high as 50% in women who carry a mutation in one of the BRCA genes. In 6 MRI trials, including one study dedicated entirely to BRCA-gene-positive patients, the range of interval cancer discoveries was only 0 to 9.8%, though there was one sub-group exception (32.3%) in a single trial.[2]

Direct studies of the biology of interval cancers support the notion that only a minority are classic high-grade aggressive tumors that "came out of nowhere" between screenings. Why is it important to study the true character of interval cancers? Because of the direct relationship to *length bias*. If all interval cancers are high-grade aggressive tumors as originally taught, then length bias is a greater force to contend with. If, however, only a minority of the interval cancers are more aggressive than screen-detected cancers, then length bias is not as powerful as originally thought, and the bigger issue is the failure to diagnose cancer on the prior mammogram.

In the last chapter, I introduced the Four Biases with an example of tumors having identical size (1.5cm) and stage, but with prognosis being better if "screen-detected" rather than palpated on self-exam or clinical exam. In this instance, screening gives the illusion of effectiveness when, in fact, it is merely cherry-picking the tumors with lower grade biology. This was an example of length bias and how it can affect outcomes in strange and mysterious ways.

*Overdiagnosis Bias*: In reality, this bias is the same as length bias, with one small difference. Instead of screen-detected cancers possibly being slower-growing tumors that have an inherently better survival (length bias), overdiagnosis takes this concept to the extreme. That is, screen-detected tumors are so slow-growing that they *never* kill the host. In its strictest sense, overdiagnosed tumors (flippantly called pseudo-tumors or fake cancer) reach a certain point where they either stop growing or "regress," such that they never become clinically apparent.

These are the tumors that Dr. Welch and followers claim are diagnosed through screening mammography 70,000 times a year in the U.S. Others, in the hope of appeasement and compromise, arbitrarily pick a number halfway between 0 and 70,000. Those of us who are skeptics about this very high number are still waiting to see our *first case* of an invasive breast cancer that, if diagnosis is delayed or if the patient refuses treatment, disappears—or, simply sits quietly in the breast and does nothing. Discovery of a large reservoir of invasive cancers in preventive mastectomy or autopsy specimens might help bolster claims of rampant over-diagnosis. But clinically, unlike prostate cancer and, to a degree DCIS, for invasive cancer, *we don't see it.* As stated earlier, the disease reservoir hovers around 1%, confirmed from many angles. We will explore overdiagnosis in future chapters where I'll attempt to explain the 70,000.

The discussion in the early days of mammography was all about length bias, not over-diagnosis, even though the two concepts are covering the same base. However, "overdiagnosis" packs a punch far more powerful than the nebulous "length time bias." Overdiagnosis has a major negative impact on the public, as well as physicians, and it has become the word-of-the-day. After all, overdiagnosis implies overtreatment, and now we are clearly in the realm of potential harm.

"Go to a web site you can trust to learn about breast cancer screening" is a recommendation you might hear. Well, on January 11, 2016, I received an e-mail alert to check out the new PDQ® informational web site offered by the National Cancer Institute.[3] There, I read that "of all breast cancers detected by screening mammography, up to 54% are estimated to be results of overdiagnosis." Whenever screwy statements are made, it always helps to check the references. In this case, the solo reference was a 2004 article in the *British Medical Journal*[4] where it was reported that the incidence of breast cancer rose 54% in Norway and 45% in Sweden after the introduction of screening mammography. *This is not overdiagnosis*—this is the expected rise in incidence after screening is introduced as prevalence tumors are discovered, and it must be compared to the rising incidence of the disease in non-screeners. If over-diagnosis exists, it is a subset within this 54%. Indeed, the authors writing in the *British Medical Journal* calculated overdiagnosis to be what they thought to be a very high number—"one-third." Yet the NCI ratchets the number up to 54% instead. This one study is only a fraction of available data on the controversy, and it can be criticized on multiple fronts. As we'll see later, researchers using different methodologies will arrive at overdiagnosis rates between 0–10% for invasive cancer. Even the Task Force offers a wide range of possibilities for overdiagnosis, based on the methodology used, offering values as low as "1 in 8" of screen-detected cancers. So why did the NCI opt to use an article that is already at "one-third" for an overdiagnosis rate, then misinterpret (or misrepresent) the results, rocketing the problem into the stratosphere? Accident? Oversight?

One of the most common criticisms about mammography is that the benefits were over-sold to the public from the get-go. If so, it was well-meaning, and no one died from the sales pitch. But today, what we are witnessing is the *underselling* of mammography in the form of exaggerated claims of harms, sometimes to the point of absurdity. Using the word "overdiagnosis" recklessly to scare women out of screening (under the guise of "proper informed consent") will be a fatal error for some women who opt out of screening. Later, we will explore the different scenarios that can *falsely* place a patient in the overdiagnosis category. Bias creating false-bias, you might say.

## How Do We Throttle the Four Horsemen?

In a nutshell, we throttle the biases through prospective, randomized trials wherein mortality reduction, not "years of survival," is the endpoint. We've already seen how years of survival can be misleading. The only endpoint that deals with the Four Biases is mortality reduction. But what does that mean? What does a 30% mortality reduction imply? Given the inevitable 100% mortality for all of us, the terminology is admittedly short-sighted.

A "33% mortality reduction" is fashioned like this: A prospective clinical trial randomizes women to "mammograms" or "no mammograms" over a defined period of time, then the women are followed for many years. Let's say that 10,000 women are in the no-mammography group and 10,000 are in the yes-mammography group. Ten years down the road, 30 women have died due to breast cancer in the no-mammography group while only 20 died of breast cancer in the mammography group. The 33% mortality reduction is a *relative* term, reflecting the decrease from 30 to 20 (one-third of 30 is 10, then subtract the 10 from 30, leaving 20). A decrease from 3 to 2 would also be a 33% mortality reduction, as would a decrease from 300 to 200.

Although "30 to 20" above is arbitrarily chosen to make a point, the numbers are ballpark figures that reveal concerns that the critics love to point out, even when lives are saved. First of all, 20 women died even though they were in the mammography group. When we talked about this earlier, I pointed out the errant belief that if breast cancer is discovered on mammography, it equates with a cure.

The other point that critics make is this: "33% mortality reduction" is a *relative* term, as opposed to an absolute reduction in risk for an individual. 10,000 mammograms had to be performed yearly for the duration of the study to save 10 lives. For a single person in the study, the chance that she is going to benefit from mammography is tiny.

Let's work with real numbers here. While it is commonly quoted that "1 in 8" women (12%) will develop breast cancer during their lifetime, most will not die of their disease. There is only about a 3% chance that a woman at average risk is going to die from breast cancer. Therefore, if we apply our *relative* 33% risk reduction to this 3%, we see that an individual's *absolute* benefit from screening mammography reduces the chance of dying of breast cancer from 3% to 2%. While I'm going to critique these numbers down the road, maybe it's not so hard now to understand why critics take their position seriously. In spite of the high prevalence of breast cancer, the numbers look different when converted to the *absolute* mortality reduction for an individual.

It is bizarre role reversal, however, for epidemiologists and public health experts to minimize the benefit of screening mammography by calculating numbers that apply to a single person. These experts on public health are traditionally focused on population statistics, and here, the numbers are impressive.

Let's suppose that the annual death rate without mammography in a given country is 60,000 per year. Now let's insist on mandatory mammography for every woman over 40 in our theoretical country. With a one-third mortality reduction, only 40,000 will die from breast cancer. Therefore, we just saved 20,000 lives with screening mammography, even though the individual benefit was negligible. This is usually how epidemiologists think, in terms of the entire population. But if you want to minimize the impact of any intervention, be it a positive impact or negative impact, you publicize numbers that apply to one person, not everyone.

In the U.S., there are 40,000 breast cancer deaths every year, but this already includes those women who are getting mammograms, some regularly and some sporadically. Studies that try to quantify compliance with mammography routinely calculate higher levels than what most of us consider compliance. Compliance may be as high as 75% if you do a telephone survey and ask, "Have you had a mammogram during the last 2 years?" On the other hand, compliance will be shockingly low, 10% or so, if you ask, "Have you had an annual mammogram for the past 10 years straight?" This is the screening behavior that saves lives, not a mammogram every now and then. Critics routinely opt for the high compliance rates in their analyses. Assuming the majority of women are getting regular mammograms makes it so much easier to bash the efficacy, e.g., "Even though mammography compliance in the U.S. is excellent, the incidence of advanced breast cancers has barely been affected."

The breast cancer mortality rate has been declining in the U.S. since 1989, and while some would attribute this to widespread acceptance of mammographic screening in the 1980s, at this same point in time, medical oncologists began aggressive systemic therapy for early stage breast cancer. Both developments share importance in the mortality decline that we witness today. But some argue that mammography should have impacted mortality to a greater extent if the "30% mortality reduction" were truly at work. Again, quoting "75% compliance" puts mammography in the doghouse for not doing a better job of saving lives.

These "number games" will appear again, so for now, let me finish the discussion about the importance of prospective, randomized trials in throttling the Four Biases.

Evidence-based medicine is a relatively new term for an old concept, in brief, relying more on good science, and less on art, when it comes to treatment guidelines. The "new" component of evidence-based medicine is the systematic *ranking* of the *quality* of scientific data, complete with scoring systems. Prospective, randomized controlled trials (RCTs) are near the top of the heap, outdone only by meta-analyses or systematic reviews of multiple prospective RCTs. For many, anything less is "not worthy." More accurately stated, the typical "observational study," where two groups are compared retrospectively, or prospectively without randomization, is ranked well beneath prospective RCTs because this is where the Four Biases do their work most easily.

Although one would think that evidence-based medicine is devoted to examining *all* the available evidence, the reality is sometimes the opposite—ironically, evidence-based medicine often refuses to acknowledge the existence of "lower level" evidence in guideline deliberations, unless there are no RCTs performed to answer the question at hand. Yet it is these same lower level studies that often prompted the higher quality RCTs in the first place. There is something Orwellian about the semantics here, i.e., "evidence-based medicine" that, by definition, excludes much of the evidence.

Editorializing doesn't help clarify our situation here, however. But I do want to comment on the *prospective, randomized controlled trial* since it is the cornerstone of advancements in medical science. *Prospective* = planned in advance, to the point that the number of participants required for the study to show statistical significance can be calculated ahead of time. *Randomized* = "drawing a number out of a hat (or computer)" to determine the group to which a participant will be assigned. *Controlled* = at least one group will receive "standard of care" or no intervention/treatment, while the "study group" receives the intervention/treatment. While we tend to think of these studies as comprised of two groups—e.g., mammograms-yes vs. mammograms-no—prospective RCTs can have 3 or more groups, but always with a control.

One step higher on the stairway to "quality evidence" occurs when the study is "blinded." Single-blinded means either the researcher or the patient is unaware to which group they've been assigned. Better yet, double-blinded means that neither the researcher nor the participant knows which group they are in. Double-blinded trials are common and easily accomplished in pharmaceutical studies where a dummy pill is manufactured that looks like the real thing. We even have triple-blinded studies where the organization responsible for analyzing the data is kept largely in the dark.

However, for trials in surgery and radiology, double-blinding is nearly impossible to accomplish, though some limited efforts at single blinding have been tried, including sham surgeries. More commonly, though, a "blinded" radiology trial would be a study where the clinical outcomes are known, but *not* by the radiologist who examines the X-ray. And, for a radiologist participating in a prospective mammography screening trial, there are no mammograms performed in one of the two groups, so the radiologist automatically knows which group the patient is in. Clinical outcomes are unknown at the time of screening, so the radiologist is effectively blinded. One can easily see how confusing the "blinded" terminology is, and today, researchers sometimes avoid the term entirely and simply describe who knew what and when.

The reason I'm dwelling on this is that prospective RCTs involving radiology or surgery (and other specialties as well) may qualify as "high quality" through their RCT label, but they allow major, unmeasured variables to enter the picture—such as skill of the clinician and the quality of technology. A skilled radiologist will generate different outcomes than one less skilled. Believe it or not, many trials are designed where skill level is intentionally ignored. Why? Because the technology being studied must be "generalizable" to the broad medical community. (Heaven forbid that anyone improve their skill level.) What is particularly vexing about this is when a new technology is handled in a substandard fashion, and results from a prospective RCT, devoid of quality skills, prompt thought-leaders to announce, "*We* can't get this to work, so *you* have to stop doing it."

So do prospective RCTs settle the issue? Often, yes, especially when multiple RCTs performed by different collaborative groups consistently show the same result. Still, there are limitations, and the one most familiar to clinicians is "external validity"—that is, do results apply to the real world experience? There are so many inclusion and exclusion criteria for clinical trials that the final results, in the purest sense, only apply to patients who would have qualified for the clinical trial. These inclusion/exclusion criteria are necessary in order to limit the number of confounding variables in the RCT, but they inherently raise the question of external validity.

Another problem in prospective RCTs is compliance. "Did the patient actually take her pills every day for the full 2-week course?" Some studies compulsively measure indirect evidence for compliance, while in other studies, such as screening mammography, compliance is obvious from the medical record. Remarkably, and not appreciated by all, one of the most rigid guidelines for prospective RCTs is the "intent-to-treat rule," which states that no matter whether the patient was compliant or not, she remains counted as being part of the original group to which she was assigned. If this is not done, then known and unknown confounding variables will come into play.

Many dislike this rule, prompting creative statistical parameters to avoid it. But no matter what gyrations are used to get around the intent-to-treat rule, the purists will dissect a study that violates this premise until there's nothing left but good intentions. The effect is this: patients who did not receive the intervention are counted as if they did, and those who are assigned to no intervention might do it on their own. Now try substituting "screening mammography" for "intervention" in the preceding sentence, and you might be able to guess that I'm going to pounce on this issue later on.

A final word about high-quality evidence (even low quality, for that matter). There is always a statistical analysis between groups. And the result has to be deemed "significant." Many numbers are generated in a clinical trial to assess statistical significance, and the menu of options is getting larger and more complex. But the one number most revered by clinicians (though loathed by many statisticians) is the p-value. In fact, statisticians often mock how we misinterpret p-values in clinical medicine. Hang on for a few pages of math and logic now.

First of all, a p-value (probability value) is not a "score." The definition, or something close to it, states that a p-value is the probability of observing a result assuming the null hypothesis is true. What does that mean? It's the "null hypothesis" part of the definition that makes the human brain incapable of understanding "p-value" the first time at bat.

Let me wade through the oddball terms here. The "null hypothesis" proposes that there will be *no difference* between the groups being studied. Of course, what we're usually trying to prove (except in a non-inferiority study) is the "alternative hypothesis"—that is, a proposed *difference* between two groups. However, the chosen norm today follows a philosophy of science that was cobbled together by Sir Karl Popper (1902–1994) who "solved the problem of induction," at least according to Popper, which carries with it the annoying little caveat that you can never be absolutely certain of a scientific truth, no matter how many observations you make ("All swans are white," or so it was thought). So, rather than buck the system and fight the uncertainty of observations, Popper stated that a scientific question must be *falsifiable* before it is a legitimate query in the first place. We then have adopted a system of double negatives—*falsifying the null (no difference) hypothesis.*

Our p-value is the probability of observing our experimental results assuming the null hypothesis is true. The lower this number, the lower the chances are that the null hypothesis is true, so when we get down to 5% or less ($p \leq 0.05$), by convention, we reject the null hypothesis. That is, we reject the "no difference" concept of the two groups with the implication that there is indeed a legitimate difference. In effect, we are "falsifying no difference" in order to suggest possible truth. (I'm sorry to have to put this stuff in print, by the way.)

Sadly, this is an instance where two negative do *not* equal a positive—a p-value less than 5% does *not* automatically mean that the alternative hypothesis is true. This is where things get confusing, making the p-value ripe for abuse. The p-value may support the alternative hypothesis, but we can't be 100% certain. Stated in p-values, there is no such thing as $p = 0$.

If this concept seems simple and straightforward, then I must have done something wrong. Perhaps now you can better appreciate why we clinicians butcher the terminology and the implications of "statistical significance." And be forewarned—I will slip into misuse of the p-value inadvertently throughout this book. After all, unlike a good statistician, I'm only human.

Believe it or not, I have a point in dragging you through all this. My purpose is to make it perfectly clear that our highly revered p-value of 0.05 (for rejecting the null hypothesis) is completely arbitrary. Nature may abhor a vacuum, but Nature also hates being converted to a dichotomy when it's really a continuum. P-values convert observations of nature and biology into a dichotomy, often referred to as "statistically *significant*" for p-values of 0.05 or less, and "statistically *insignificant*" for p-values higher than 0.05. So, if our experiment ends up with a 4.9% chance the null hypothesis is rejected, we proudly announce that we have performed an experiment with "statistical significance" ($p = 0.049$). But if we come up with a $p = 0.051$, we cannot reject the null hypothesis, so the experiment "fails to reach statistical significance." It's an arbitrary number, and so is the dichotomy it creates.

There's nothing magical about 5%. Karl Popper did not suggest 5%, but another knighted thinker did—Sir Ronald Fisher, an English statistician (among other things) who, in 1925, based his choice on "normal distributions and standard deviations" that you really don't want to hear about. Even though most clinicians know that it's an arbitrary number, it has assumed a rigidity of remarkable strength. Nothing is more disheartening than to hear someone from the podium, or in print, make the statement, "There is no evidence to support such-and-such when, in fact, studies have come painfully close to the 5% threshold, perhaps only having needed more participants in the clinical trial or longer follow-up in order to reach our blurry 5%."

We all prefer study results that are far removed from the watershed 5%, or $p \leq 0.05$. In fact, we like to see p-values with many zeros to the right of the decimal, e.g., 0.0001, as highly supportive of the alternative hypothesis (a "true" difference), while p-values that approach 1.0 are strongly indicative of no difference between groups (I'll let the philosophy of science experts sort out whether or not it's acceptable to have a p-value of 1.0, or if restraint dictates 0.99999...).

Statistical theorists have been pointing out that the *majority* of statements made in the medical literature based on p-values are technically *incorrect*, this in spite of decades of criticism and warnings. We have so misused the meaning of p-values that many statisticians favor moving on to something else. Some have called for an end to p-values entirely. In spite of the overwhelming compulsion for a clinician to claim that a p-value of 0.001 means "there's only a one in 1,000 chance we got this outcome through a statistical fluke," this is a false statement.[5]

Frustrated by the wobbly aspects of the beloved p-value, there is increasing utilization and reliance on "confidence intervals" where, instead of statistical "power," we have "assurance." That is, we have a *range of possible outcomes* associated with a confidence level, usually 95%. Here, the researcher sets the desired level for a range, rather than the data dictating a p-value. While one could pick a 90% or 99% confidence interval (CI), medical research has zeroed in on 95% as a complement to our arbitrary p-value of 0.05. Thus, a 95% CI equals a significance level of 0.05. The CI not only gives you "statistical significance," but also gives you a qualitative "gut feel" about the possible range of "truth," the tighter the better.

Here's an example: a screening study reveals a relative risk (RR) of 0.75 for breast cancer mortality in the screened group (a 25% mortality reduction with mammography), but is this statistically significant? You don't know yet without statistical support. But then you read that the "*95% Confidence Interval is 0.68 to 0.81*," which is a fairly tight range, and the range does *not* cross 1.00 (no effect), so it is statistically significant. Thus, there is a 95% probability that Reality is within our range—maybe as high as 32% (if 0.68) or as low as 19% (if 0.81), but still significant. Had the range, for instance, been from 0.68 to 1.05, the study would have failed to reach statistical significance. This is a different approach than the older p-value, and much preferred.

A tight range with a CI doesn't determine significance, but it helps with one's faith in the outcome. You can have a statistically significant outcome, but if the range is wide (let's say 0.40 to 0.99 in our example above), your confidence is shaken to a degree. The mortality reduction in this instance ranges from 60% to 1%. Likewise you can have an outcome that's barely significant (say 0.93 to 0.99), but the tight range indicates the effect, albeit weak (only a 1% to 7% benefit), could still be legitimate (in fact, a 95% probability).

Going one step further away from p-values, there is swelling support in medical research for Bayesian probability, a complicated approach to statistics distinctive in its inclusion of—get ready—common sense. That's right, this approach allows the statistician to make some assumptions from what "is known" and build from there, generating "degrees of belief." Given the predisposition of statisticians to be rigidly empirical, this deceptively simple concept represents an exciting new development, drawing from a very old theorem by a statistician (and Presbyterian minister) Thomas Bayes (1702–1761), even though it was the French polymath Pierre Simon Laplace (1749–1827) who turned the theory into a mathematical form.[6]

What we're after in science is Reality with a capital R, where truth exists independent of our beliefs, schemes, and observations. This Platonic concept is impossible if we're operating under the social construct of a scientific method that says we cannot prove truth, rather, we can only falsify hypotheses. Even then, we can only do so with a certain degree of probability. If there are 1,000 zeros in front of a number forming a p-value, there is always a tiny chance that the null hypothesis is, in fact, true. The sun may *not* come up tomorrow.

If you enjoy lowbrow movies, you may recall Jim Carrey's response in *Dumb and Dumber* when he searches to define the exact probability of his "not good" chances at "ending up" with the leading lady. After Carrey's suggestion that the odds might be "one out of a hundred," Mary scales down his chances to "I'd say more like one out of a million." Without knowing anything about inductive reasoning, empiricism, or philosopher Karl Popper and falsifiability, Carrey's face brightens as he replies, "So you're telling me there's a chance. Yeah!"

Applied to screening mammography, all clinical trials will have an associated p-value (as well as other stats). It's not enough to say, "This study showed a mortality reduction of 33%." It must be accompanied by an entire host of statistical companions, led by the p-value. And, the more zeros to the right of the decimal point in a p-value, the better we feel even though perhaps we shouldn't. For those of us who see color and continuums, 0.05 is a precarious number to position as the vanguard, and we're better off putting our confidence in Confidence Intervals.

# 6

# The Four Horsemen Are Throttled by Clinical Trials, but O Canada!

The idea of screening a healthy population for breast cancer was controversial from the very beginning. Mammography, from a technical standpoint, was slow and cumbersome, not to mention the concerns about radiation exposure. The earliest versions exposed the breast to radiation levels that, theoretically, could cause cancer if used over many years. Some experts recommended that the idea of screening healthy women be abandoned completely. Others pointed to the remarkable success of the recently introduced Pap smear. From the 1930s to 1950s, the idea of asymptomatic screening with mammography was bandied about, until a landmark publication by Dr. Richard Egan in 1962 reported finding 53 occult cancers in 2,000 consecutive mammograms.[1]

Importantly, Dr. Egan defined "occult cancer" at the very dawn of mammographic screening as *"one which remains totally unsuspected following examination by the usual methods used to diagnose breast cancer, including an examination of the breast by an experienced and competent physician. To qualify for this definition, no symptoms or signs should be present."* The reason I keep stressing this purist definition of "screening" as being limited to patients who are "asymptomatic" is this: we are about to encounter studies that did not comply with this definition, introducing controlled chaos.

In 1963, enthused by Egan's report a year earlier (and a comparable report generated from a private practice group), three individuals in New York City teamed up for a research project that would revolutionize breast medicine with the introduction of screening mammography. At the same time, their initial stumbling steps will leave footprints for the controversies still at work today.

The "engine" of the group was Dr. Philip Strax, a general practitioner[2] in Manhattan whose wife had died of breast cancer at the age of 39. Stunned at the cruelty of this disease, he dedicated his life's work to the eradication of breast cancer deaths. The most obvious way to accomplish that goal in the 1960s was through early detection. Dr. Louis Venet was a surgeon who believed there might be a chance to limit the use of radical mastectomies if small tumors could be identified on mammography, this being a different endpoint, of course, than mortality reduction. This vision of Venet was a sharp departure from the spirit of the times, as radical surgery was deeply embedded in the surgical community, regardless of tumor size, and there was already skepticism about non-palpable cancers being discovered by X-ray: "If I can't feel it, it's not important" was the prevailing mantra. And finally, the official leader of the project was Dr. Sam Shapiro, who served as the director of research and statistics for the Health Insurance Plan (HIP) of Greater New York.

The HIP, within the context of history, is considered a primitive HMO wherein the enrollees were pre-paid and thus somewhat captive, providing an ideal opportunity for a clinical trial. By the standards of the day, Dr. Shapiro's study design was "cutting edge." That is, he was fully aware of the Big Four biases, and therefore, the need to use "mortality reduction" as the endpoint. Yet, while the concept of a control group was well-established, the definition of true randomization to create that control group had not settled upon an acceptable norm. Thus, the HIP was long on "prospective," but short on randomization and controls.

From 1963 through 1966, approximately 62,000 women, ages 40 to 64, were enrolled and "randomized" to one of two groups. More accurately stated, 31,092 women were recruited for the study group, which included 2-view mammography on a yearly basis for 3 years, *plus* clinical exam. The control group, however, was simply drawn from HIP records. The women in the control group never knew they were being studied!

While shocking in today's climate, with strict rules controlled by Institutional Review Boards, this study design was acceptable at the time. Adding strength to the study, however, was the fact that women in the no-mammography control group could be relied upon for their unwitting compliance in that there was *nowhere else to go to have a mammogram.* This "purity" in the no-mammography group would never again be duplicated, in that all other trials will have to contend with non-compliant "control group" patients who seek out mammography on their own.

Given the particularly cumbersome nature of (unproven) mammography, both for the patient and the technologists who developed the film, it is astonishing that this many women in the HIP study were recruited and screened during a 3-year period. Credit here is given primarily to the indomitable and resourceful Dr. Strax who focused heavily on the mechanics of high-volume screening, an assembly line, if you will. In addition to the stationary study sites, Dr. Strax developed the first mobile mammography unit, which he parked on the streets of Manhattan, a sharp contrast to the other vendors.

When the astonishing results from the HIP study were announced in 1971—a 40% reduction in mortality—the world was forever changed. Not only was breast cancer vulnerable to attack, but what about other types of cancer? Maybe early detection could wipe out the cancer scourge entirely. Physician and public enthusiasm ran wild. Dr. Strax proclaimed that the "radiologist has become a potential savior of women—and their breasts."

The National Cancer Act was signed that same year, and Richard Nixon's War on Cancer was underway. Millions of new dollars started flowing to the National Cancer Institute, and fund-raising by the American Cancer Society rose to a new level. The HIP study results were intoxicating, timed perfectly with the passage of the 1971 bill.

The American Cancer Society and the National Cancer Institute teamed up on the back of the HIP results to launch a massive "demonstration" of the feasibility of widespread population screening with mammography. In fact, they used the word "demonstration" in the study's name—the Breast Cancer Detection Demonstration Project (BCDDP). Mortality reduction in the HIP study had occurred with early-stage discoveries—that is, smaller tumors and a greater percentage of node-negativity. Length bias and lead time bias had been accounted for. Proof of mortality reduction was parked in the bank, and it was time now to calculate the interest.

Recall that at the first of this book, I mentioned a sharp divide between *effective* screening and *feasible* screening. The former is deceptively simple—based on X + Y = Z. Or *vulnerable biology + sensitivity of the screening tool = mortality reduction*. But for *feasible* screening, there's a complex host of issues that have to be addressed as to whether or not it is practical to screen the entire population—disease prevalence, acceptance by patients, expertise by radiologists, call-back rates, cancer yields compared to false-positive biopsies, etc. The HIP study had answered the effectiveness question, and now the BCDDP would answer the question of feasibility. As such, the BCDDP was *not* a prospective, randomized trial with a control group wherein a mortality reduction would be measured. *There was no control group.* Every woman recruited was part of the study group. The BCDDP would become, by far, the largest study for screening mammography in history, yet in the end, would play no role in our current controversies.

Meanwhile, back in New York City, Dr. Sam Shapiro was battling the skeptics who didn't buy into the HIP results. Prospective RCTs don't magically make the four screening biases disappear, as these shadowy forces are still at work. Yet the prospective RCT is a *minimum* requirement used to throttle the Four Horsemen.

The critics claimed that Dr. Shapiro had not fully ruled out the effect of lead time bias and length bias. But in this case, time was on Shapiro's side. After long-term follow-up, the 10-year calculations showed a 29% mortality reduction, while the 15-year calculations held onto a 23% mortality reduction. Less than the original 40%, yes, but both calculations reached statistical significance, with the biases effectively held in check.

Perhaps Dr. Shapiro's greatest critic, however, was himself. Forever stewing about the accuracy of his landmark HIP trial, he had the stomach-churning experience of realizing that he and his two associates had forgotten to exclude patients from the study if they had previously been diagnosed with breast cancer. Thus, some of the cancer-specific deaths occurring during follow-up would actually be due to breast cancers that were diagnosed prior to the study's launch.

The consequences would be minimal if prior cancer patients were evenly distributed in the two groups, but therein lies the rub. Women in the mammography group were being seen reliably on an annual basis as part of the study, so it was easy to discover a prior history of breast cancer (not to mention that mammograms would have been unilateral). But remember, the women in the control group *didn't even know they were in the study*. If healthy, they were not being seen by any doctor in the HIP of Greater New York. Contacting the control patients to learn if they had ever been diagnosed with breast cancer was an erratic process, but most observers believe Dr. Shapiro did a fair job.

The thinking at the time went like this: if Shapiro doesn't remove an equal number of prior breast cancer patients from the control group, then more deaths will be recorded in the controls, thus exaggerating the effects of screening mammography. Thus, mammograms aren't saving lives as much as the control group numbers are contaminated. Yet, if anything, students of this history point out that Shapiro might have overcorrected. Regardless, the removal of prior cancer patients from both groups was a relatively small number given the 60,000 participants, but it wreaked havoc on the statistical analysis. All screening trials have large numbers of participants, but the number of cancers discovered is relatively small, and number of deaths smaller still. Thus, a surprisingly small number of deaths can make a huge difference in outcomes, a phenomenon we will encounter again.

The cautious Dr. Shapiro performed the same self-scrutiny when it came to the results for women in their 40s who had participated in the HIP study. His unplanned retrospective analysis of this sub-group, when added to the problems above, showed "no benefit" to screening in the 40s even though the overall study benefit had included the entire range of women, ages 40–64. This is explained by even greater benefits for women over 50, only partially negated by women in their 40s, such that the bottom line is a net benefit for screening overall.

Sub-group analysis, when performed retrospectively, always provokes caution in today's world, but was more acceptable at the time of the HIP trial. Then, in contrast to what one might expect, Shapiro may have overcorrected again, such that many expert epidemiologists today believe that the women aged 40–49 actually did benefit. Others, however, believe the HIP trial is so thoroughly contaminated it should no longer be referenced. What irony that the study that "started it all" with its evidence that mammography saves lives, today, is sometimes relegated to the waste bin of "no useable evidence." But the stage was set. Experts would continue to argue the 40–49 data from all trials for the next half century.

Another issue, not to be taken lightly, is the fact that the HIP study included clinical exam, and many cancers were found in this fashion. Thus, the HIP study does not meet our modern definition of mammographic screening, or even Dr. Egan's definition in 1962, for that matter. Still, data were made available such that researchers for the past 50 years have teased out those cancers that were discovered by mammography alone, and the numbers are still being gnawed upon today.

With the HIP results under fire, skeptics in the U.S. called for another prospective trial, this time with better controls, and with the 40–49 sub-group identified in advance. Too late. The juggernaut of the BCDDP was already underway. This colossal study would vacuum the country so thoroughly, enrolling those women interested in the newfangled X-ray, that there was no interest (that is, no money) left over to prove what the cancer leaders "knew" already to be true. The United States would never again organize a prospective, randomized controlled trial to see if mammography saves lives.

Other countries, however, began tripping over themselves to launch prospective RCTs for screening mammography to see if the HIP results could be more carefully elucidated. With the U.S. out of the picture, given that the leadership solicited patients only for the BCDDP, the banner was carried by Sweden (5 trials, if the 2-county study is split), Scotland (Edinburgh), and Canada (2 trials). These international screening trials were launched in 1976 through 1982.

And now let me present one of the most startling facts in this book—the arguments you hear being played out in the media, or among physicians, revolve around these clinical trials that had their origins in antiquity. In fact, there have been more official meta-analyses (combined studies) of the mammography screening trials than there have been actual trials. It doesn't matter if some expert on TV tells you that "a *new* study from Canada shows no benefit from mammography." If the talking head is reporting on a prospective RCT, then it is not "new," rather, an update or regurgitation of something very old. That is, we are still arguing about the results of trials that used technology, and clinical trial methodology, of the 1970s and 80s, long obsolete.

What about the modern trials, using modern technology? Sorry. The only semi-modern prospective RCT that has a no-mammography control group is the AGE Trial in the United

Kingdom. Launched in 1991 with the final screen in 2004, the AGE Trial included nearly 54,000 women in the mammography group, attempting to answer the question about screening women in their 40s. We will cover the AGE results when we focus on the 40-to-49 controversy. For now, be aware that we have physicians locked in battle over these trials who were not even born when some of the trials were launched.

One of the great ironies today is that, in spite of the controversies about screening effectiveness, there is little interest in a new RCT using modern technology. Why? Reasons include the high cost of long-term follow-up, the technology becoming obsolete again before trial conclusions are reached, the general anti-screening sentiment in progress, and many other reasons. But quietly, no one wants to randomize women to a no-mammography group, given the possibility of sending a woman to her death if randomized to no screening. Sub-groups, such as women over age 75, might be studied with a no-mammography control group, but never again will a general population screening study be performed with a no-imaging control group.

Today, we have clinical trials looking at various screening options—digital mammography vs. tomosynthesis; mammography and ultrasound vs. tomosynthesis; MRI vs. a combination of tomosynthesis plus ultrasound—with some of these trials limited to high risk patients. However, given the difficulty that will be encountered in proving a mortality reduction without a no-screening control group, surrogate endpoints will dominate, most notably "cancer yields," or "cancer detection rates" (CDRs). If a new imaging approach yields significantly more cancers than a standard approach, we will have to act on that information, as was done when the American Cancer Society issued guidelines in 2007 for breast MRI screening in high risk patients. There was no proven mortality reduction, but the vastly superior sensitivity of MRI prompted adoption anyway. And for those who demand prospective RCTs with proven mortality reductions for each new technology, they will never be able to budge from the historical trials of obsolete technology.

One of the basic principles in modern scientific method is "reproducibility." That is, repeat studies should be performed to see if comparable results are achieved. In the case of mammographic screening, the U.S. got lazy, instead deferring to the trials that were introduced in other countries. Cynics claim that self-serving cancer organizations (I won't mention any names, but the initials are ACS and NCI) cut corners and began a massive propaganda campaign in the form of the BCDDP instead of sticking with good science first.

The Breast Cancer Detection Demonstration Project (BCDDP) ran from 1973 to 1980 providing up to 5 annual (free) mammograms to 283,222 women, ages 35 to 74, at 29 centers in 27 cities. Sub-groups that were defined at the formal conclusion of the BCDDP are still being monitored today.

For a while, thermograms were included in this study of screening practicality, but it soon became apparent that there were too many false-positives and too many false-negatives, prompting thermography to be dropped from the BCDDP early on. A knock-out punch for thermography was delivered in 1977 by Stephen A. Feig, M.D., one of the pioneering breast radiologists in the U.S.[3] In a review by Feig and his collaborators addressing 16,000 patients with multi-modality screening, thermograms came in dead last with a 39% sensitivity rate, below old-fashioned clinical exam. This does not mean that this much-maligned modality wasn't grounded in rational thought, as it was apparent early on that some cancers do not show up on mammography. But as it turned out, these hidden cancers show up on ultrasound,

MRI, and molecular imaging, with far superior results to thermography, which, in spite of technologic improvements, has never regained its original hope.

From 1975 through 1980, nearly the entire duration of the BCDDP imaging period, I was a surgery resident at the University of Oklahoma where a pioneering radiologist was a participant in the study. Our role as surgeons was simple. Whenever we scheduled a breast biopsy, we ordered a mammogram and thermogram as part of "some sort of study." We had no idea what the study was or what it meant, nor did we ever see a single X-ray or thermogram (I saw my first mammogram in private practice in 1980). Years later, after establishing a breast-dedicated practice in academia where I was teaching students and residents, I stumbled on the BCDDP data and realized that my co-residents and I had been unwitting contributors, as clueless as the women in the control arm of the HIP trial from the 1960s.

The reason I mention this is to point out, once again, that the BCDDP was not an asymptomatic screening study to determine if mammograms saved lives. In fact, 100% of the patients we surgeons referred for inclusion in the "study of some sort" had palpable lumps. Massive amounts of data poured from BCDDP with regard to feasibility of screening, along with performance characteristics of the test itself. But note that the word "screening" is not part of the study's name, nor is it considered a screening trial. It was, in fact, a demonstration of mass mammography.

Moving then to the prospective RCTs for mammographic screening, one can fill a library with the volumes written on data from these historic trials, and there is no way to do them justice here. In my brief summaries, I've focused on the low points of the 8 trials (after the HIP) in order to highlight the wobbly foundation of all that is revered today (and that doesn't yet count the obsolete technology). In order of launch date, they are:

*Malmö, Sweden (1976)*—pre-existing breast cancers plagued results, as in the HIP; only 70% compliance in study group, while 24% of controls had at least one mammogram.

*Östergötland, Sweden (1977)*—single view mammography every 2 years up to 33 months in women over 50, compliance 89%, with 13% of controls contaminated by mammography.

*Kopparberg, Sweden (1977)*—similar to Östergötland, as part of the "Two-County" study.

*Edinburgh, Scotland (1976)*—randomization seriously flawed on multiple counts, only 61% compliance, sometimes excluded from meta-analyses.

*Canada NBSS-1 for Ages 40–49 (1980)*—randomization came under fire for corruption, with vindication coming from Canadian audits and simultaneous vilification from U.S. audits; compliance good at 100% initially then decreasing to 86% by study's end; 24% contamination in the control group where women underwent screening on their own; strength is in the fact that this was the only trial (until the 1990–1997 AGE trial) that predefined the 40–49 age group.

*Canada NBSS-2 for Ages 50–59 (1980)*—compliance 100% initially, decreasing to 85% by study's end at 5 years; 17% contamination in the control group where mammograms were performed in the no-mammography group.

*Stockholm, Sweden (1981)*—single view mammogram every 28 months X2; compliance 82%, with 25% contamination in the control group, some randomization concerns.

*Gothenberg, Sweden (1982)*—initial 2-view mammography, then single view every 18 months X4, complex randomization complicates interpretation.

So … what were the results?

Well, in spite of the weight from the crushing problems noted above, nearly all of the trials showed a reduction in mortality. Yet these mortality reductions were usually statistically *insignificant*. An exception occurred in the Kopparberg Trial, one half of the oft-referenced Swedish Two-County Study, wherein mortality was lowered by a statistically significant 32%. Recall from our p-value discussion that a lack of statistical evidence can simply occur through the sample size being too small or inadequate follow-up time. Often, the term "maturation" of the data is used to describe the hope that significance will appear over time. This is not an unwarranted hope, as seen in the Gothenberg, Sweden trial where the initial report revealed a 21% insignificant mortality reduction with screening, but when the data matured through long-term follow-up, a 23% reduction finally reached statistical significance.

Now, it may seem that, given all the glitches above, a combined analysis in the form of the statistical technique known as *meta-analysis*, would be a "garbage in—garbage out" phenomenon. Yet statisticians convince us that the garbage is somehow purified in these meta-analyses. And, when the early reports from these trials were combined (pre–Canada), there was a clear-cut, statistically significant 30% consensus mortality reduction for screening mammography in women over 50. Even women in their 40s were found to have a significant mortality reduction, though not to the same degree (15–20%).

The varied deficiencies in the historical screening trials can be loosely grouped into 2 categories: clinical trial methodology and radiologic technology. Flawed randomization would be an example of poor methodology, while single-view mammograms every 2 years is an example of poor use of technology (not to mention that *all* mammograms in these studies were "poor" by today's standards). It is axiomatic that roughly 20% of breast cancers will be missed if only single view mammography is performed. Even a 2-view mammogram doesn't get all the breast tissue on the X-ray plate for evaluation, but the 2-view approach was accepted later on, as a compromise between the proposed 1-view and 3-view strategies.

My point is this: *clinical trial methodologic* problems may be corrected through meta-analyses, but these grouped analyses have more trouble correcting for low quality technology, single views, long intervals between screens, poor compliance, and control groups contaminated by women who sought out mammography on their own. Importantly, all of these uncorrected factors work to the *disadvantage* of demonstrating a benefit through mammography.

Granted, a unique set of numbers are generated and published based on true patient compliance—those who actually showed up for their mammograms—but these are *not the official results of the trial*, and once they appear in fine print, they seem to vanish. Thus, if one has to guess whether or not the benefits of mammography are overstated or understated in these trials, my bet is on *understated*—that, in fact, routine annual mammography using modern technology offers a benefit well in excess of these historic trials.

One other thing might have caught your eye—the duration of active screening in these trials is remarkably short, beginning with the 3-year strategy in the HIP study. The working plan for all studies is to recruit very large numbers and then screen for a short amount of time, sparing costs and getting answers quickly while moving to long-term follow-up. But it is this follow-up that will give us all headaches by the time we're done because it's very difficult to accurately follow 50,000 to 100,000 women for 20 years, not only to monitor breast cancer-specific mortality, but also to measure the impact of mammography habits *after* the study is over, even though long-term outcomes are still being tallied.

What do we really want to know? We want to know the mortality reduction associated with 25 to 35 years of active and compliant screening. It's never been studied, and it never will be. Instead, we have arguments couched like this: "What is the mortality reduction imparted by 3 to 10 years of mammographic screening in this or that group, as viewed long-term even though screening habits vary wildly during that follow-up?"

Do you remember the major weakness of prospective RCTs, even when combined into meta-analyses? The answer is "external validity." The jewel-in-the-crown "prospective RCT" is an artificial construct, which may or may not have application to the real-world experience. Regardless, short-term screening in the prospective RCTs as a substitute for real-world screening is another way in which the power of mammography has been cut off at the knees. What the trials measured is not the same thing as a lifetime of high quality screening performed at regular intervals.

Let's return now to the historical sequence. The year is 1991. Results from the trials above are creeping in, validating what we all believed in the first place—early diagnosis is the key to saving lives, and mammography provides early diagnosis. Thus, screening mammography saves lives. Done deal. Game over.

Then, with all the shock value of Pearl Harbor, the bomb was dropped, this time by our allies to the north. The Canadians announced the results of their NBSS studies in what made headlines worldwide: "MAMMOGRAPHY RELATED TO MORE DEATHS IN YOUNG WOMEN."

# 7

# The Mammography Civil War (1993–1997)

Medical news has a way of breaking the sound barrier, rendering a boom that can catch us off guard, without the means to analyze. Science journalists add their spin, then physicians wait for the publication to appear in print, allowing full scrutiny. Sound bite medicine.

The "killer mammogram" news leaked early in 1991, *prior* to the first scientific presentation that took place at the Second International Cambridge Conference on Breast Cancer Screening. London's *The Sunday Times* was the first to capture the boom, their version headlined "Breast Scans Boost Risk of Cancer Death."

Principal investigator of the Canadian National Breast Screening Study (actually two CNBSS studies) was Dr. Anthony B. Miller, a prominent epidemiologist at the University of Toronto. Fellow epidemiologists had already anointed the CNBSS as the pivotal and premier mammography trial, given the study design that had prospectively defined two age groups, this alone having the omnipotence, as it turned out, to absolve all potential transgressions. As opposed to the retrospective analyses of these age groups in all prior trials, the CNBSS-1 was designed for women in their 40s, while the CNBSS-2 was for women in their 50s.

Radiology experts were not nearly as enthusiastic as were the epidemiologists. Two components to all screening mammography studies have to be considered, and unfortunately, they are prioritized by bickering specialists. On the one hand, epidemiologists and biostatisticians look through their tunnel to scrutinize trial design and methodology. On the other hand, radiologists have the same level of focus directed toward mammographic quality and interpretations. Previously, I referred to these two features as "methodology" and "technology," but to define North from South, make no mistake—this is epidemiology vs. radiology.

"North" will bear no relationship to geography in my treatment here. Canada does not present a united front with regard to mammographic screening. Space precludes the long list of Canadian breast radiologists who were appalled then, and are anguished even today, as to how mammography has been depicted by their country, prompting many commentaries in many journals. No, this is a battle between two disciplines that use different ground rules.

When the tabloid-type results from the CNBSS-1 (ages 40–49) were announced, claiming deaths caused by mammography, the number was shocking, amplified by the use of *relative* terms—"58% higher risk of a breast cancer death than unscreened counterparts!" The alert was widely broadcast, but by the time data made it into print in the *Canadian Medical Association Journal*,[1] with delayed maturation from 7 years in the initial media explosion to 8.5 years

49

of follow-up in the published version, this number "fell" to a still-shocking 36% increase in breast cancer deaths, though statistically *insignificant* (with my pardon to p-value purists). The aftershocks continue to this day.

But wait a minute. How many women actually developed cancer during that short follow-up period? Recall that these screening trials include very large numbers of women. And while the Canadian trial is often described by media pundits as "massive," it's actually quite average, with nearly all trials in the 40,000 to 60,000 range. CNBSS-1 included 50,430 women and CNBSS-2 included 39,405. Even combined, at nearly 90,000 participants, the numbers fall short of the Swedish Two-County trial where participants in East and West combined totaled more than 130,000.

That said, the number of cancers detected during these relatively short studies is quite small, and breast cancer deaths smaller still. Only a handful of cancers in one group or the other can make the difference between statistical significance or not. At only 8.5 years of follow-up in the CNBSS-1, guess how many excess deaths in 50,430 women prompted the Ft. Sumter of mammographic screening?

The answer is 10. Ten deaths out of roughly 25,000 women screened with mammography. Specifically, there were 38 breast cancer deaths in the mammography group and 28 deaths in the "usual care" group. How does this convert to a "36% increase" in deaths? With skills you'll acquire in the next chapter, it's quite simple: 38 divided by 28 = 1.36, which is a 36% increase when expressed in *relative* terms. In *absolute* terms, for an individual woman undergoing 5 years of mammography, at 8.5 years of median follow-up, the excess risk of a breast cancer death was 0.04% (that's 4/100 of a single percentage point, or 4 women out of 10,000). Thirty-eight percent is much more impressive than 0.04%, and though both are technically correct, which would you choose if you wanted to make an impression? But that's not where the story ends when it comes to these wacky numbers. With longer follow-up, even this remote chance of mammograms causing deaths will disappear completely (but I'm getting ahead of myself).

Expert radiologists had been wary about the trial from the beginning, citing very poor quality mammographic technique and interpretations. The trial used second-hand machines, they did not employ grids that control scatter and provide clarity, technologists were not taught proper positioning (cancers must fit onto the X-ray plate to be seen), and community radiologists had little or no training in interpretation. Even one of the CNBSS's own physicists, Martin J. Yaffe, PhD, stated in letter to the editor of the *Journal of the National Cancer Institute*[2] that the quality of mammography in the trial "was far below state of the art, even for that time."

The CNBSS defense rests in the principle of "generalizability"—that is, technology and its interpretation must be studied *as currently practiced* in the real world experience. Centers of excellence sound like a great idea, but are ignored, or even maligned, in studies of "generalizability." But this defense is not supported by Dr. Yaffe in the letter above. The mammograms were "far below state of the art...." Here we are, decades later, still battling data based on untrained radiologists who were reading substandard films derived from substandard equipment, using substandard technique.

In 1984, early in the trial, in an effort to assess mammographic quality, Dr. Anthony Miller, leader of the CNBSS, asked one of the world's authorities on mammography, László Tabár (Central Hospital, Falun, Sweden), to review 50 cases. Although we don't know if anything official was ever recorded, today, in re-living the moment in a video interview on his web site, Dr. Tabár, never one to mince words, said the quality was so terrible that he couldn't get through the 50 mammograms. He flunked the first 15 in a row, and bowed out of having any involvement in the study.

From the epidemiologists' perspective, however, the CNBSS was golden, the best ever, *the* study to end all studies. Enthusiasts today still cling to this notion, unwavering in the belief that study design is the only important half of the equation, conquering all, allowing one to turn a blind eye to mammographic quality issues that comprise the other half. Methodology is half; technology is half. Epidemiologists are fixated on the former, radiologists on the latter.

Dr. Miller did express concern about mammographic quality as the other half of the equation, but neither he nor his right-hand, Dr. Cornelia Baines, have ever acknowledged that it was bad enough to alter outcomes. Quoted in the June 3, 1992, issue of the *Journal of the National Cancer Institute News*, Dr. Miller said, "They [participating radiologists] were all busy people being asked to read large numbers of films. None of them were prepared to make mammography their only occupation." Miller also admitted that some politics were at work, in that the participating radiologists (with little or no training) were resistant to advice from reference radiologists.

But Miller may have been the most resistant person of all. Expert radiologists claimed (and still claim) that he disregarded their advice throughout the study. Linda Warren, M.D., who was the executive director of the Screening Mammography Program of British Columbia, stated that Miller showed the study design to the Canadian Academy of Radiology, and their concern, *even before the study began*, was not trial design or methodology, but misuse of the technology. They told Miller, recorded in the same *JNCI News* article above, that the mammographic technique at the proposed centers was not good enough to support the protocol.

Wende Logan-Young, M.D., director of the Breast Clinic of Rochester, New York, was an early advisor to the program, but quit after 6 months. Not only did her suggestions for improving the technology go unheeded, but also she was eventually restricted from viewing the mammograms. She said, "I even offered to send my technologists to train theirs at my own expense, and they refused." Dr. Miller, of course, cast the blame on Dr. Logan-Young, claiming that she had overstepped her bounds.

Her replacement was Stephen Feig, M.D., then at Thomas Jefferson University Hospital in Philadelphia, today at the University of California, Irvine. He, too, found that his suggestions were ignored. A major concern was the absence of the single most important mammographic view, the mediolateral oblique (MLO). The CNBSS finally caved for the final few years of the study and began using the MLO view that includes the upper outer quadrants where most cancers arise. Still, after 18 months of reviewing grossly substandard mammograms, Dr. Feig resigned, fearing that his name would be forever linked to bad mammography and an inferior study. Still, Dr. Miller later admitted that a "major contribution" was provided through Dr. Feig's insistence that the MLO view be utilized.

In a conciliatory effort, one that American radiologists would probably like to retract, Drs. Miller and Baines of the CNBSS-1 joined with mammography experts Dan Kopans, Myron Moskowitz, Ed Sickles and others to publish an official statement about mammographic quality in the CNBSS, *before* results were announced.[3] All were in agreement that "quality improved" over the course of the study from 1980 to 1987, but the critical point of improvement occurred relatively late, in 1985, when the MLO view replaced the ML (mediolateral) view. This left only 3 years of acceptable mammography toward the end of the study.

But this joint article was not an endorsement by the U.S. radiologists, rather, simple agreement that the tail end of the study was better than the start. For years 1–4, Dr. Kopans stated that *more than 50%* of the mammograms were judged as poor or completely unacceptable. As a result, when the initial bombshell was dropped by the CNBSS, women with the longest follow-up would have come from this early phase of the study.

Daniel B. Kopans, M.D., a Harvard radiologist and pioneer mammographer, had warned colleagues that the CNBSS was going to have results that might be suspect. Certainly, it was a going concern, but after all, mammography quality had not been optimal in the HIP where lives had been saved, nor even in the Swedish Two-County results where only a single view (MLO) was used in the first place, and the screening interval was between 24 and 33 months. In contrast, the screening interval in the Canadian trial was every 12 months. Surely, thought the reviewing radiologists, the power of early detection will overcome all of this, and results will confirm what we've seen in all prior studies.

After the "killer" announcement, there was no more leeway given to the CNBSS. Myron Moskowitz, M.D., a University of Cincinnati mammography expert who had been part of the conciliatory review, summed it up like this: "We're left with a study that can be applicable only to a certain situation—the evaluation of poor quality mammography."

Dr. Miller's enthusiasm for his CNBSS results went unchecked, and while headlines for women ages 40–49 often took care to note the "association" of mammography with increased deaths, as opposed to "causation," Miller regrettably jumped on the causation bandwagon.

In the initial media coverage, he hypothesized that mammograms were squeezing tumor cells into the bloodstreams of younger women and killing them (at least, it apparently did so 10 times), but somehow the squeeze factor did not have the same effect on women in their 50s. The outcry in response to this statement, violating too many principles to list here, prompted Dr. Miller to issue a retraction, a bit late for the millions of women who heard about this deadly potential, but not Miller's retraction.

Not to be dissuaded entirely from causation, as opposed to mere association, Dr. Miller tried his second theory, that perhaps those 10 women had a genetic predisposition (specifically, the A-T gene) toward radiation-induced cancers. At the time, the A-T gene was drawing its first attention in this regard, but there was an overriding problem with Miller's theory— radiation-induced cancers have a long lag time. Any effect in this regard would have been impossible to emerge as a clinical problem with such short-follow-up. A radiation-induced cancer would have had to develop immediately after the first mammogram in order to have time to grow to the point of detection, spread to distant sites, and then result in death, all within this very short follow-up period. His theory was soundly sacked.

It was back to the drawing board for the epidemiologist whose clinical acuity lagged behind his statistical brilliance. One more try—removing cancers in young women took away the anti-angiogenesis factor that primary cancers can produce, keeping their metastatic sites in check. This is a theory still being researched, and while demonstrated in mice and rats as a transitory phenomenon with little difference in outcomes, it has never been a clinical feature described in humans. A considerable portion of the lay population still believes that cancer spreads "only after the air hits it." Believers of the "air" theory are unknowingly invoking principles of anti-angiogenesis. But if you want to see what happens when the air *doesn't* hit cancer, there are century-old medical records for women presenting with palpable lumps indicating near-100% mortality when cancer is left untreated in the breast.

This was Dr. Miller's last theory to explain the bizarre outcome of more breast cancer deaths in the CNBSS-1 for women aged 40–49 undergoing mammography. Of some interest is the fact that this last theory was the first time an explanation was offered where mammograms were not a direct *cause* of more deaths, instead, a mere *association*, with surgery as the actual "cause." Disregarding the basic science of anti-angiogenesis, one still had to wonder why it would adversely affect only those women in their 40s but not their 50s. To my knowledge, no other theories were invoked. By the time that a fourth theory was due, the adverse effect of mammography for women in their 40s had *disappeared* with longer follow-up.

From the mammographer's perspective, the Canadian radiologist Linda Warren, M.D., who had weighed in early about her reservations with the CNBSS, predicted that Miller's study "will have no scientific relevance."

She was wrong. Epidemiologists embraced the CNBSS whole-heartedly. Indeed, the Canadian trials were effectively canonized. Without invoking conspiracy theories, one has to question pre-existing bias, where the "negative" results of screening in the Canadian trial finally validated what some had believed all along. This silent minority dated back to the criticism of the HIP study, especially regarding women in their 40s, and the fact that the U.S. opted to "demonstrate" with the BCDDP, in effect, a military parade, rather than conduct a confirmatory clinical trial that would settle the issue about screening younger women.

After Ft. Sumter, it was a bloodbath—heated letters to editors, blasts from the podium at breast cancer meetings, attacks against the Canadian trial from all angles, with counterattacks by epidemiologists denoting the sloppy methodology of every positive trial that breast radiologists held dear. Note for the military record[4]: *this controversy was 100% confined to CNBSS-1 and women 40–49,* while little mention was made of CNBSS-2.

The Civil War is where I began to take my first steps toward screening epidemiology, through the old-fashioned, often mocked, process of self-education. And the first question I had (for myself) that no one seemed to be asking out loud was this: Why was there *no benefit* to mammographic screening in the CNBSS-2 (ages 50–59)? Granted, a neutral outcome was not nearly as exciting as mammography causing breast cancer deaths, but still…. Women in their 50s more clearly benefitted from screening in the other trials, yet the CNBSS-2 showed no difference in breast cancer deaths between the two groups. With very little in the way of intellectual ammunition, I had one overriding thought: "Something is terribly wrong with both Canadian trials if the 50–59 group did not benefit either."

Emerging from the rubble was a new emphasis on two of the older Swedish studies, Östergötland (County E for East) and Kopparberg (County W for West). From the last chapter, we saw that County W had the most powerful risk reduction of any of the prospective RCTs, a 32% reduction in mortality with strong statistical significance. But County E was not far behind with a 28% reduction that barely missed statistical significance.

These non-contiguous counties in Sweden joined their data into the most powerful of all screening trials when it comes to endorsing mammography, both in sheer number of participants as well as the combined statistical significance. Dr. László Tabár was first author and chief spokesperson for what became known as the Swedish Two-County trial.

Dr. Tabár has a distinctive viewpoint when it comes to Fisher Theory, by the way. Basically, in his opinion, it's bunk. "Yes, lumpectomy and mastectomy have equal outcomes …

equally bad." He points out that the results of the HIP, and its saved lives through early detection, had been announced while the Fisher brothers were busy in the lab, and they should have known they were working on a theory that was being dismantled by screening mammography.

Dr. Tabár's calm, confident, and to-the-point (blunt) style has not particularly endeared him to the world of medical oncology, as he calculates the decline in breast cancer deaths since 1990 as being due almost entirely to early detection through mammographic screening, not systemic therapies. Some medical oncology experts believe the opposite—that is, this decline is entirely due to improvements in systemic therapies. Perhaps this particular issue is best left to a neutral party, such as professor of biostatistics at MD Anderson Cancer Center Donald A. Berry, PhD. With his CISNET collaborators, the group called it a tie, both forces—screening and treatment—having a roughly equal effect.[5]

In spite of his comfort in controversy, Dr. Tabár is the undisputed champion in one arena—worldwide mammography education. One really can't name a contender. After the results of the Swedish Two-County study were available, countries around the world began instituting public health policies to include mammographic screening, and Dr. Tabár saw it as his personal mission to educate the world. His hands-on seminars, with close attention to imaging-histologic correlations, became a staple in the diet of any radiologist planning to read mammograms. If you hadn't done the "Tabár course," you had no business doing breast radiology. As a result of his devotion to this cause, he is probably the most easily recognized household name in mammography. And, due to the success of the Swedish Two-County trial, some refer to him as "the father of screening mammography."[6]

The Swedish Two-County study was a landmark event for several reasons. First, it was already apparent that the HIP trial was hard to interpret because of the fact that it had been a two-pronged (and two-variable) attack—mammograms and exams. Given Dr. Egan's original definition of "screening" being reserved for asymptomatic patients only, the very purpose of a clinical exam at the time of enrollment ought to be the *exclusion* of patients from participation if they have worrisome lumps. If a woman has a breast mass, the mammogram is no longer "screening"; it's a diagnostic study that prompts extra views (and today, ultrasound). So this was the Swedish Two-County Study's first claim to fame—the recognition that we needed to measure what mammography did on its own, independent from clinical exam.

With the two counties considered together, both prospectively randomized, 77,080 women were invited to screen and 55,985 served as controls, for a total participation of 133,065 women aged 40–74. Today, with 29-year follow-up (the longest of all the trials), Dr. Tabár et al. reported a mortality reduction of 31% as calculated by the local endpoint committee data, and a 27% mortality reduction with review by an independent Swedish overview committee, either figure with strong statistical significance.[7] But when women in their 40s are pulled from the study and reviewed retrospectively as a sub-group, the effect is not as strong and the statistical support slips below the key threshold.

Given the need for stronger statistical significance for women in their 40s, the prospective, randomized trials were frequently combined in the process of meta-analysis. Some believed that the Canadian results should not be included at all. Without Canada, there was a clear benefit to screening younger women. And with statistical power sitting on the fence for this controversy, the slightest variable could knock it one way or the other.

Principal investigators of all Swedish trials, for instance, decided that they should combine their data and isolate from the rest of the world (thus, excluding Canada). This was not an overtly biased approach where results were obvious prior to the start, given that the Two-County trial was tops in Sweden. The other 3 trials in that country would actually drag down the Two-County stats on the one hand, while strengthening the modest benefit through larger numbers on the other hand. It was a toss-up when they began. In 1997, the group published their results in the *Journal of the National Cancer Institute Monographs*.[8] For women in their 40s, screening mammography at 18- to 24-month intervals was associated with a 23% reduction in mortality. One problem: statistical significance was missed by a fraction.

One of the chief observations about mammographic screening today, drawing its benefit into question, is that massive data banks don't reveal a corresponding reduction in advanced stage cancers, a strong predictor of screening effectiveness that ought to correspond to a mortality reduction. Anti-screeners love to drag this issue into the open, even though the large data banks don't tell the researchers who had mammograms (and how often) vs. those who didn't. The lack of individual chart reviews prompts multi-layered assumptions as mammography is criticized. But it is interesting to note that in the Swedish Two-County trial, where charts were reviewed and mammography utilization monitored, there was a reduction in advanced stage cancers, to the degree that would be predicted, along with the mortality reduction. This tidbit is rarely mentioned today.

Dr. Tabár's first report on results from the Swedish Two-County study was published in *The Lancet* in 1985,[9] so the resulting enthusiasm for large scale screening mammography had 5 years to gain worldwide momentum before the Canadian bomb was dropped.

With the Two-County trial offering the strongest evidence yet for mammographic screening, it draws frequent criticism from the anti-screening epidemiologists who lash back against the trial's study design with every update, just as the radiologists lash back against every update in the Canadian trial. The Two-County trial was attacked specifically with regard to the process of "cluster randomization" and "end point evaluation," with technicalities that go beyond the scope of this book.

But consider this—the Two-County study was also using primitive mammography by today's standards. However, there's a lot more to the "technology half" of screening trials than the equipment alone. Technologists and interpreters were highly trained, such that they were offering "state of the art" care. Nevertheless, this was a single view study, using the "best" view to get the most critical area of the breast onto the X-ray plate (MLO). Shortly after the trial ended, Dr. Tabár adopted the standard 2-view mammography in use today. One other point—the intervals between screens were remarkably long: every 24 months for women in their 40s, every 33 months for women 50 and older! Yet we still have a strong reduction in mortality for women over 50 and a marginally good reduction for women in their 40s.

In 1993, subsequent to the CNBSS announcement of adverse outcomes, Dr. Tabár would write that, for women in their 40s, "the most likely way to achieve further reduction in mortality is to reduce the interval between screens, possibly to 1 year."[10] He openly stated that, in spite of the stellar results in Sweden, mammography as recommended in the U.S., with modern equipment and short intervals, would likely produce outcomes even stronger than the Two-County trial. Of course, the Canadian trial had used one year as its interval, so many who didn't fully understand the other technologic inadequacies were confused as to why the more frequent screening program didn't work, while less frequent screening in Sweden did.

While I've spoken of the Canadian Ft. Sumter as the initial volley, the Civil War was not formally declared until 1993, with the publication of the Fletcher Report. Now, it was official.

In February 1993, the National Cancer Institute held an International Workshop on Screening for Breast Cancer to review the question of screening women in their 40s. The spokesperson for the group, Dr. Suzanne Fletcher, representing the American College of Physicians, took the brunt of the criticism when the announcement came that, overall, there was no proven benefit for screening women in their 40s. As usual, the announcement came well in advance of the publication that appeared in the *Journal of the National Cancer Institute.*[11]

While Fletcher was vilified by the pro-screening forces, consider that the soap opera of the Canadian trial had not even reached full stride. Without CNBSS-1, the existing evidence was marginally in favor of screening women in their 40s, but the Canadian data was enough to knock the controversy off the fence. How could 10 patients do that? Remember, these large trials have small numbers of actual deaths, especially early on. Small numbers generate weak and friable statistics that chip and peel easily. Even without the 10 excess deaths, the CNBSS-1 would have been a "neutral" outcome, also diluting the data toward the ineffectiveness of screening.

Interestingly, Dr. Sam Shapiro from the old HIP study was part of the 5-person workshop committee that had ruled against routine mammography for women in their 40s, his lingering doubts about the benefits in his own trial still present after 20 years. Others on the committee were accused by radiologists of having long anti-screening track records, raising the question as to who pulled the strings of committee membership. The entire process would haunt us again in 2009 with the déjà vu actions of the U.S. Preventive Services Task Force.

The National Cancer Institute rubber-stamped the workshop's recommendation and announced their new guidelines to begin screening at age 50. They kept their interval option as "every 1-to-2 years," based largely on the Two-County study that showed benefit in spite of longer intervals. For women in their 40s, it was the usual run-around recommendation of "discuss screening with your doctor," a consolation prize for those left out in the cold. The NCI promptly launched an advertising campaign with a positive spin as its cover. "Get Regular Mammograms Starting at Age 50" was the rather lackluster slogan that concealed a more powerful message—"Stop Getting Mammograms in Your 40s!"

The backlash against the NCI was swift, powerful, and devastating. It was a public relations nightmare for a tax-supported institution like the NCI. The American Cancer Society, formerly a colleague-in-arms with the NCI, dating back to their BCDDP, didn't budge in their "start at 40" recommendation. The ACS was the source, by the way, for the "baseline at 35," not only for future comparison, but to offer *something* more than clinical exam to that 5% of eventual breast cancer victims who are diagnosed prior to the age of 40. The ACS recommendation for yearly mammograms starting at age 40 survived the Mammography Civil War and lasted another 20 years before its first major modification in 2015, a subject to be covered as this history progresses.

The lay public was, for the most part, livid about the NCI recommendation to start at 50. Women had been fully indoctrinated about the need for annual mammograms, and simultaneously, new activist groups had recently been established, some for the express purpose of raising money for screening mammography. The Susan G. Komen Foundation was one of those groups that, initially, at least, was focused almost entirely on screening mammograms.

Criticism from the radiologists targeting the NCI was intense. Drs. Kopans and Feig were joined by the American College of Radiology as well as professional organizations in their many points of attack, not the least of which was the fact that the Fletcher Report had looked only at prospective, randomized trials, ignoring the entire body of pro-screening findings in observational studies. This NCI move took place in the era before "evidence-based medicine" had thoroughly permeated guidelines, but was ahead of its time in that the Task Force would adopt the identical approach of hammering this sign on their clubhouse: "Prospective RCTs only—no observational studies allowed."

The mud-slinging was seemingly constant, in journals and commentaries everywhere, back and forth. Pressure from the public and physicians was applied to Congress, and in 1994 the House Committee on Government Operations released this document: "Misused Science: The NCI's Elimination of Mammography for Women in Their Forties."

Then, the world took on a new tilt. Rumors began to swirl about something unthinkable, that the randomization in the Canadian trials had been corrupted. The clinical exam at the time of entry had been performed *before* randomization, and women with advanced palpable cancers had been directly placed in the mammography group, with good intentions, of course, but violating the rules of the game, the very rules that epidemiologists are supposed to cherish.

The Canadian response was swift. In 1994, writing in the *Annals of Internal Medicine*,[12] Cornelia J. Baines, M.D., University of Toronto and right hand to Dr. Miller of the NBSS-1, wrote, "Claims that the randomization process was flawed and more symptomatic women were assigned to screening have been refuted."

Oops. Not exactly.

In his Pulitzer Prize–winning effort *The Emperor of All Maladies: A Biography of Cancer* (New York: Scribner, 2010), Dr. Siddhartha Mukherjee dipped his toes in the water of the Canadian NBSS-1 corruption controversy.

Importantly, the CNBSS protocol distributed to the 15 sites correctly stated that the exam was to take place *after* randomization, not before. Mukherjee writes, "Women with abnormal breast or lymph node examinations were disproportionately assigned to the mammography group (seventeen to the mammography group; five to the control arm, at one site). So were women with prior histories of breast cancer. So, too, were women known to be at 'high risk' based on their past history or prior insurance claims (eight to mammography; one to control)…."

Dr. Mukherjee writes about intended subversion vs. acts of compassion as high-risk women were directed toward mammography. Because randomization was performed "by hand" in a notebook with alternating lines, it was conceivable that women in the room awaiting processing caught onto the scheme and skipped a turn, in order to get in the mammography group, corrupting the process themselves. He notes, "Teams of epidemiologists, statisticians, radiologists, and at least one group of forensic experts have since pored over those scratchy notebooks to try to answer these questions and decipher what went wrong in the trial."

He quotes Dr. Cornelia Baines as a chief investigator in the trial, who said in 1997, "Suspicion, like beauty, lies in the eye of the beholder."

"But there was plenty to raise suspicion," writes Mukherjee. "The notebooks were pockmarked with clerical errors: names changed, identities reversed, lines whited out, names replaced or overwritten. Testimonies by on-site workers reinforced these observations. At one center, a trial coordinator selectively herded her friends to the mammography group (hoping, presumably, to do them a favor and save their lives). At another, a technician reported widespread tampering with randomization with women being 'steered' into groups."

As it turned out, many believe that the CNBSS ended up as a study with more flawed randomization than had occurred in the HIP trial, or the Two-County trial, where some of the women in the control group of those studies didn't even know they were participants.

Yet, remarkably, epidemiologists are willing to forgive this easily identifiable corruption simply because the two age groups had been defined in advance, confirming the virtues of the study's wonderful design. You have to wonder what these same individuals would have said about the study's pure design if the results had been the opposite, strongly supporting mammographic screening.

Dr. Mukherjee, in his *Emperor of All Maladies*, pulled his toes out from the polluted pool in Canada and moved on to one of the Swedish studies rather than describe the wrestling match that continued. In 1995, Robert E. Tarone, PhD, then an epidemiologist at the National Cancer Institute, documented that something went terribly awry in the CNBSS-1 study. From his jarring analysis published in *Cancer*,[13] he concluded that the study was an outlier to every other study of mammographic screening: "an excess of patients with advanced disease diagnosed at initial screenings in the mammography group were not consistent with other randomized trials…. The reason for the excess proportion of advanced disease in the women aged 40-to-49 is still unknown. Because such patients are unlikely to benefit from screening detection, mortality analyses should exclude patients with advanced disease detected by physical examination at the initial screening."

Dr. Tarone had found 47 breast cancer patients with 4 or more positive lymph nodes in the mammography group (14%), while only 23 such patients were in the "usual care" group (8%). This was statistically significant, by the way, and enough to explain the bizarre conclusion that mammograms were causing breast cancer deaths in young women. Surely now, thought critics of the CNBSS, the National Cancer Institute will re-evaluate its position and we will be returning to the "begin at 40" recommendation.

Slam dunk, yes?

No. In 1996, the NCI reconvened in another workshop and hit a brick wall. The battered participants walked out with a different sort of policy, one of considerable confusion … they opted for *no policy* at all. It was a hung jury. You can imagine the forces at play here, but at this point, the science ended. North and South had fought to a stand-off. There was no winner and no loser. It was a tie. In the eyes of the public, our process for government involvement in health care recommendations had demonstrated what it does best—creating impasse shrouded in fog.

In 1997, the National Cancer Advisory Board, one of many appendages of the NCI, having bureaucratic oversight of the stalled process, intervened. Perhaps they had been encouraged by the 98–0 vote in the U.S. Senate calling for a rejection of the new guidelines, or, actually, the lack thereof. In a flash, the National Cancer Advisory Board reinstituted guidelines to resume screening women in their 40s. And just like that, the war was over.

The Civil War had been fought over a single issue—screening women in their 40s. There had been little debate about the *interval* for screening, and no debate concerning screening women over 50.

But while the focus was on the corrupted randomization, with the CNBSS-1 in particular, I was still bothered by CNBSS-2. Why had there not been any benefit for this group either? Did the corrupted randomization cross over to the entire study? Screening in the 50s and 60s had demonstrated benefit in all the other trials, with or without p-values. Maybe the poor technique and poor interpretations affected both the CNBSS-1 and CNBSS-2 equally, but the corrupted randomization, as evidenced by more advanced cancers placed in the mammography group, was seemingly limited to the group in their 40s.

Then, it occurred to me, obvious today, but unspoken then. Forget the intentional placement of women with advanced cancer into the mammography group—women with lumps and/or palpable nodes are not supposed to enter a screening trial at all! Not in either arm—mammography or no mammography. They are to be excluded from the trial at the beginning, as was done in the Two-County study for the first time, well before the start of the Canadian trials. Remember our definition of screening? The HIP study had ignored this definition in its all-out assault on breast cancer. But no more. Screening is defined as "asymptomatic women only."

The Canadian trials, instead of the epidemiologic purity they claimed, actually had more in common with the HIP study. Yet, the HIP study, with its results in favor of screening, has been tossed into the trash can of useless data by the same epidemiologists who have elevated the Canadian trials onto a pedestal made of silly putty. Both Drs. Miller and Baines are planning to defend their study to the death, literally, with both still writing polemics of justification as late as 2015. But the bottom line is this: women with palpable lumps have no business being accepted into an asymptomatic screening trial.

Every time the Canadian NBSS publishes an update, it is whitewashed of its origins and presented as the pristine trial of the century, while those in the know scream silently. Witness its 2014 return when the *New York Times* (G. Kolata, February 11, 2014) called the CNBSS "one of the largest and most meticulous studies of mammography ever done," adding "powerful new doubts about the value of the screening test for women of any age."

Therese Bevers, M.D., is a professor in the Department of Clinical Cancer Prevention at the University of Texas MD Anderson Cancer Center in Houston. Holding many titles and winning many awards, she was asked to respond to the most recent media blitz extolling the virtues of the CNBSS trials. Note that she is not a radiologist and is writing from the position of a neutral judge. On March 13, 2014, in the online newsletter *POST* from the American Society of Clinical Oncology (ASCO), she wrote, "The issues identified, namely concerns regarding randomization and mammographic quality, are considered by most breast cancer experts to have rendered the CNBSS flawed from the beginning, thus eliminating any ability of the trial to accurately discern the benefits and harms of mammographic screening."

She continued, "Screening is, by definition, performed in asymptomatic individuals.... However, women with palpable masses were allowed in the CNBSS. The fact that women with known palpable masses were included in the CNBSS makes the design of this screening trial questionable."

In conclusion, she said, "The strengths of the CNBSS are contrasted by a vast collection of flaws that render any findings, past or present, meaningless. As a result, the study does not provide any data in regard to the benefits of mammography that would influence breast cancer screening recommendations...."

The Civil War ended in 1997, but it was more of a cease-fire than a settlement. It had not been science that had ended the struggle. Instead, it had been politics. The NCI was embarrassing itself, and everyone knew it, or most everyone. With the exception of some last minute gasps for air, the CNBSS had been effectively silenced with its corrupted randomization, or so it seemed. To mix my metaphorical wars, we entered the Pax Romana, and surely we would enjoy 100 years of peace.

Why all this history?

Because it's not history at all. It's the present. It's prologue. I refer to the Canadian trial as the Zombie Trial—you can't kill it. It just keeps coming back. And, as new observers with limited information weigh in and join those who only communicate through numbers, it is very disturbing to hear commentators say, "There was some minimal something that happened with randomization back in the beginning, but it's all been worked out."

As memory fades, ignorance flourishes.

# 8

# The Number Games

*Setting: Medical oncologist's office*
*Year: 1989*
*Characters: Doctor and patient*
*Background: The oncologist is explaining to a newly diagnosed breast cancer patient how chemotherapy is now being given to patients who have node-negative disease, based on new results from clinical trials. This expansion of adjuvant systemic therapies to women who already have a fairly good prognosis is a new concept.*

ONCOLOGIST: From your tumor size and grade, and given your negative lymph nodes, we can say you have an 80% chance of being cancer free 10 years from now. That's if we offer nothing further, now that you're done with surgery.

PATIENT: Is there anything I can do to get that number higher? I suppose that's why I'm seeing you.

ONCOLOGIST: That's correct, and yes, there's something we can do. We have new evidence that suggests that chemotherapy, given up front, before any possible remaining cancer cells have a chance to get a foothold, will improve your survival rate.

PATIENT: I really don't want chemotherapy if I don't have to have it. How much will it help?

ONCOLOGIST: Chemotherapy will improve your survival by 30%.

PATIENT (pausing to perform a quick calculation): But if I'm starting at 80%, and then you're saying that chemotherapy will add 30%, I'll have a 110% survival rate?

¤ ¤ ¤

Though it's hard to believe now, only a few decades ago, physicians made little distinction between relative and absolute risks. It wasn't difficult math. It was a problem *conceptualizing* the numbers, understanding their origins, then translating estimated benefits to patients.

The example above played out in the medical oncology world to the extreme, with surveys showing a wide range of numbers provided to patients faced with the decision of chemotherapy. Our oncologist above, who inadvertently calculated 110%, made the mistake of adding a *relative* risk to an *absolute* risk. In truth, the "30% improvement" should have been applied to the 20% recurrence rate, generating an absolute benefit of 6% ($20 \times 0.30 = 6$). So, without chemotherapy, the patient has an 80% 10-year survival, and with chemotherapy, she has an 86% survival.

The distinction between relative and absolute is critical. Today, the inconsistencies for medical oncology have been corrected through the use of online programs that incorporate patient and tumor characteristics, then generate a range of *absolute* improvements in survival based on different systemic therapies.

Stand-alone relative risks can be perilous. My entrée into this world of remedial math began when I converted to a breast-only surgical practice, and various risk factors were coming off the assembly line of medical journals, and then broadcast daily, it seems, through media outlets. Because relative risks are always higher than absolute risks, often much higher, the percentages were astounding. It was easy to add risks together to find your patient at a 250% probability of developing breast cancer, or higher.

Today, mathematical models calculate risk for breast cancer, and the relative risks are buried deep in the software so that the user only sees absolute risks, a major advance over what patients were told in the past. But relative risks are alive and well on the evening news, and the numbers are used routinely to sensationalize.

For the scientific purists who might be reading, there is a distinction among relative risks (RR), odds ratios (OR) and hazard ratios (HR) that go beyond the scope of this book. My longstanding interest in risks, and how these risks are combined into useable (absolute) numbers, led to an invitation to write my take on risk analysis in the opening chapter of a breast cancer text.[1] As stated in that chapter, after comparing RR, OR, and HR differences (that can sometimes be quite large), from a practical standpoint when converting the numbers to absolute risks for breast cancer, the values are functionally interchangeable. The dry equations I included in that chapter likely sent many readers scrambling on to Chapter 2 where Dr. László Tabár and his team addressed the more popular topic of mammographic screening.

In truth, I am more interested in the *interventions* associated with various risk levels, based on Noah's principle—it does no good to predict rain unless you build the arc. But I inadvertently backed into risk assessment expertise more than 20 years ago when it became apparent that few were paying attention to these numbers and how they could be construed, or manipulated.

And it is "manipulation" that is the reason for this chapter, a short excursion away from the topic at hand.

There are countless ways to churn data to create the desired effect. Importantly, this is not a matter of right or wrong. It's not even a matter of using the sophisticated tools of mystical statisticians. This is simple math. The numbers are valid but at the same time wonderfully pliable by the user. In this chapter, we'll look at two of the most common ways to make the numbers sing the song that you want to hear—(1) absolute risk vs. relative risk and (2) population impact vs. individual impact.

Relative risk (RR) is a fraction, with a numerator and a denominator. In applying RRs to breast cancer risks (either the risk of developing cancer or the risk of death from breast cancer), the numerator is the number of cancers in the "exposed" group, while the denominator is the number of cancers in the "unexposed" group. "Exposure" is the risk factor in question. If the two groups have same number of participants, then simple division generates the relative risk. If the two groups are found to have the same number of cancers, then the RR number will be 1.0. 100 cancers in the "exposed" group divided by 100 in the "unexposed group" is 1.0. Or 3 divided by 3 is 1.0. 647 divided by 647 is 1.0. You can see how "no effect" equals 1.0, *not* 0. There's no such thing as a RR of 0.0. Relative risks *above* 1.0 fall into the category of *risk* factors, but important for our discussion of screening mammography, RRs *below* 1.0 mean the item being studied is a *protective factor*. Our intent is for screening to yield mortality RRs below 1.0.

One trick here is that the denominator is just as important as the numerator. Who made up the control group? For instance, it has become quite common to hear about the RR of mammographic density, placing the risk at RR = 4.0. But compared to what? In fact, the RR of 4.0 is when you compare women with the highest density to women with the lowest level of density, a rather select group and not the "average" woman. If, on the other hand, you compare breast cancer risk in the highest group to the average woman, you get RR = 2.0. For the patient with 50% density on her mammograms, however, the RR = 1.0, or no risk at all, when the average woman is considered as the "referent." Choosing the referent for the denominator is every bit as important as the numerator. As I said earlier, relative risks can be perilous.

But the most important thing to remember is that the equation for RR does *not* include the number of participants in a study. You can have 50,000 women in your study (as with mammographic screening), but the only thing that matters for the RR is the relatively small number of women who developed cancer, and then if they were "exposed" to mammography or not. If only 45 women in the mammography group die of breast cancer, and 60 in the no-mammogram group die of breast cancer (and the groups had an equal number of participants), the RR = 45/60 or 0.75. Because the RR is below 1.0, screening mammograms are a "protective factor," or beneficial (assuming statistical significance). This is stated as "mammography resulted in a relative risk reduction in mortality of 25% (the converse of RR = 0.75)."

Returning to our medical oncologist at the start who ended up with 110% survival, critics of mammography today are pointing out that the word "relative" has been left out of the discussion for mammography benefit when interacting with the public. And on that point, the critics would be correct. Women have been told to get mammograms because of the "25–30% reduction in mortality" without any mention that this is a relative number. It's not an incorrect number by any means, but the accusers claim that it's misleading, and that we should be following in the footsteps of the medical oncology computer programs that calculate individual *absolute* benefit.

The point is well-taken, but it ignores the vast difference between treatment of a disease and prevention or early detection. By definition, screening is going to include large numbers of people who do not benefit, a vastly higher number than treatment of established disease. If one converts the relative benefit to the individual in any screening program, the result is minimized to the point of "dilutional nihilism," the phrase used by Dr. Dan Kopans, whom we've already introduced and will be circling back time and again. Dr. Kopans is a pioneering breast radiologist at Massachusetts General Hospital and a 5-star general of the Mammography Civil War.

Yet critics charge that we should doing just that—offering informed consent to patients based on their absolute individual benefit. In our example above, in a trial of 50,000 women where 25,000 were assigned to the mammography group, only 15 lives were saved, so the benefit for an individual is a tiny fraction of a single percentage point. This small benefit is unlikely to prompt a mad rush to the local mammography center, but that's exactly what critics want to point out. (As mentioned earlier, it is most peculiar that epidemiologists and public health experts have suddenly become so interested in individuals and the statistics that go with them.) Population screening is more akin to vaccination programs in public health than it is to cancer treatment benefits, so it depends on your analogy as to whether or not relative risks have been out of line in promoting mammography.

These mathematical tools work to the convenience of the user. If you want to amplify a benefit or a risk, then use *relative* risk. If you want to minimize a benefit or a risk, use *absolute* risk. Both are legitimate, and in many articles published today, authors who foresee the allegations of bias will use both.

Many years ago, I came across the masterful use of relative vs. absolute risks in a commentary endorsing the use of tamoxifen to prevent breast cancer, a legitimate option still today. The challenge with tamoxifen risk reduction is establishing a risk:benefit ratio, given that this drug can cause uterine cancer while preventing breast cancer, albeit the latter far more likely. In the editorial, the author pointed out that tamoxifen causes uterine cancer in "only 1%, while cutting the risk of breast cancer by half." Marvelous rhetoric. In a single sentence, the author minimized risk by using the *absolute* 1%, then maximized benefit by using a *relative* 50%.

The second potential for manipulation is applying risks or benefits to an entire population vs. risks and benefits at the individual level. This can work however you want it to work, and we will be going through many examples in the remainder of this book. The recommendations of the U.S. Preventive Services Task Force, for instance, will have minimal impact at the individual level, based on the comfortable position that the vast majority of women are never going to deal with breast cancer in the first place. On the other hand, when the same numbers generated by the Task Force are applied to the entire population, we'll be doing a body count.

Relative risks/benefits vs. absolute risk/benefits, population impact vs. individual impact, all combine to allow skewed rhetoric. All approaches are technically correct, but effectively chosen for a purpose—to make a bigger or smaller impact, depending on the user's intent. That's why balanced presentations will reveal both "relative" and "absolute" risks, as well as "population impact" vs. "individual impact."

Another calculation that has gained wide popularity among the public health planners is the NNT, number needed to treat—that is, the NNT to prevent disease. In preventive medicine, this sounds like a population statistic, but it's not—it's a hybrid that combines both the population and the individual. Many of the preventive measures used in medicine today are cast in a new light through the use of NNTs. For example, a recent Cochrane (one of the independent "think tanks") report calculated that when low risk patients take statins to prevent a coronary death, it requires treating 1,000 patients for one year, or NNT = 1,000/year to prevent one death. Clearly, it is a stat that provides perspective, and with it, a touch of "dilutional nihilism."

For the mammography debate, NNT is converted to NNS—number needed to *screen*—where, in fact, there is more room for manipulation, as much of the data is based on women *invited* to screen, whether they actually screen or not. NNI (or NNIS) is what epidemiologists prefer to use, as this follows the intent-to-treat rule. Actual compliance with screening is no major concern when using NNI, while the radiologists' camp prefers NNS, the actual number of screenings performed to save one life.

As you can imagine, these NNS and NNI numbers cover a wide range, and to no one's surprise, the better numbers come from the pro-screeners, while the worse numbers come from the anti-screeners. A critical and obvious component of calculating NNS or NNI is the mortality reduction that one uses in the formula. So, if you use the lower end of the range, say, a "15% mortality reduction," the NNS is going to be much higher.

To use one example, in the 2011 update on the Swedish Two-County trial, with 29-year follow-up,[2] there was one life saved for every 1,334 mammograms performed (1,677 using a different approach), or NNS = 1,334. A variation that Tabár used was this: if you screen 1,000 women from age 40 to 69, between 8 and 11 lives will be saved. These NNS calculations will rattle all over the place when we get to the Task Force.

At the beginning of this book, I made a crude stab at calculating the *absolute* benefit of screening for a lifetime in an *individual*. If 12% of women who live to age 90 are going to develop breast cancer, but only 3% are going to die from breast cancer, then the entire world of breast cancer screening is trying to lower the 3%. Not much room for improvement (unless you're going to be one of the 40,000 women who die each year of breast cancer—a population focus rather than an individual). If we then apply a 33% *relative* reduction in mortality through a lifetime of screening, we are trying to lower the 3% to 2%, or a 1% benefit of a "saved life" to an individual who agrees to be screened over the course of her life.

This may be a bit pessimistic, as this 1% absolute benefit has actually been demonstrated in the Swedish data, for a shorter duration than "lifetime." And we'll explore ways to get a 2% reduction instead of 1%, again minuscule for the individual, huge for the population. Nevertheless, this 1% mortality reduction happens to be roughly the same benefit that an individual gains over the course of a *lifetime* of seat belt use, lowering the risk of dying in an auto accident from 2% to 1%.

Seat belts have long been a point of reference for academic radiologists performing cost-effective studies of mammography, concluding that seat belts, now with air bags, are *less* cost-effective than mammographic screening. The recent recall of 34 million air bags (responsible for 8 deaths and more than 100 injuries) probably tips the scale even more in favor of mammography's benefit. Dr. Stephen Feig,[3] whom we met earlier when he resigned in protest as advisor to the Canadian NBSS, has been a leader in cost-effective analyses, publishing a number of comparative studies, relating mammography to other accepted health and safety measures. Cost-effectiveness, by the way, does not mean that mammography saves the health care system money in raw dollar amounts. Through various approaches, it means that the benefit is worth the cost, with conventional and acceptable levels in the cost containment literature.

A recent article in the *Journal of the American Medical Association* (*JAMA*),[4] however, prompted me to pull out the old seat belt analogy, not with regard to cost-effectiveness, but with regard to the 1% mortality reduction. In brief, this article on mammographic screening described harms-to-benefit ratios, with a heavy emphasis on the harms, coupled with the negligible benefit of mammography at the *individual* level. In my view, harms were inflated, while benefit minimized (although an absolute 1% at the individual level is already minimized). Still, the authors admitted to possible underestimation of benefit as they had to draw from antiquity when it came to the mortality reductions seen the original prospective screening trials. Their reasoning, of course, was the usual: "It's all we have."

Had this article been just another hatchet job on mammography, I would have let it pass. But the endpoint to be measured in the study, after what was considered a balanced informed consent, was how many women opted for *less* screening. In short, the study was a success. Women, now fully informed, opted to screen less often, and it even reached a significant p-value!

Perhaps the endpoint should have been mortality rates after this informed consent, as less screening should translate to more deaths. Mathematical modeling is wonderfully deductive, and in later chapters we will be computing body counts directly correlated to screening intervals.

Nevertheless, the satisfaction that the authors displayed in de-programming women out of annual screening prompted me to write a letter to the editor of the *JAMA*, drawing on the old seat belt analogy. I've included the letter in its entirety here.

To The Editor:

Re: Pace LE, Keating NL. A systematic assessment of benefits and risks to guide breast cancer screening decisions. *JAMA* 2014;311:1327–1335.

Inspired by the approach of Drs. Pace and Keating with regard to mammographic screening, keeping in mind that lifetime mortality risk for breast cancer approximates the lifetime risk of dying in an auto accident, I propose the same rationale be used to limit mandated seatbelt utilization. Admittedly, there has been a mortality reduction associated with the introduction of seatbelts, but the campaign to diminish drunk driving coincides chronologically with seat belt adoption and could be the primary beneficial factor at work. And, while seat belts are widely promoted as reducing mortality by 50%, this is using the deceptive "relative risk reduction," rather than more realistic absolute risks. Indeed, when this 50% risk reduction is applied to the 2% lifetime risk of dying in an auto accident, seat belts provide only a 1% survival benefit, in spite of buckling up more than 50,000 times during a 60-year span of driving.

Furthermore, seat belts can cause considerable harm by transferring what used to be catastrophic head injuries into catastrophic abdominal injuries, only partially obviated through the use of shoulder straps and air bags. Even worse, seat belts can, in and of themselves, result in death that would not have occurred if unbuckled.

Perhaps we can resolve the overutilization of seat belts through selective use. For instance, one could opt to wear seat belts on even days of the calendar, thereby cutting harms in half. Given the fact that odds are overwhelming that one is not going to be in a wreck anyway, little will be lost and harms will be cut by one-half. And, of course, why wear them at all after the age of 75? Only minimal lifetime risk remains at this age, and co-morbidities are much more likely to cause death than an automobile accident. At the other extreme, we have new, young drivers where accidents are a serious problem, so a personalized approach is warranted— teen-agers should wear seat belts even when stationary, whether in a car or not.

Lastly, no one should be forced to wear seat belts given the tiny benefit unless first being informed of the harms. A brochure should be developed to explain these harms, and post-test behavior should be monitored, with the only measure of success being if the reader uses seat belts *less* frequently, indicating a true grasp of the meager 1% benefit.

In recent years, the complexity of human bias has been distilled into dollars and cents, so for my two cents' worth, I should mention I have nothing to disclose financially with regard to the seat belt industry.

Alan B. Hollingsworth, MD

Medical Director, Mercy Breast Center, Mercy Hospital—Oklahoma City

In this era of online submissions, the response from journals can be lightning-quick, and that was certainly the case here. In a blink of the electronic eye, the editors issued a swift rejection. Apparently, they did not find the letter nearly as amusing as did I.

# 9

# The (Over)Selling of Mammography

It's been stated many ways, and for different reasons.

"America has a love affair with screening."

"Mammograms have been oversold to the American public."

"If people only understood the small benefit of mammography, they'd think twice."

But no matter who says it or why, people are talking about different things and coming from different angles.

Often, it's the new initiate to the controversy who is startled to discover the numbers we've known for decades, unaware that these elastic numbers often apply to preventive health and screening, in general. Yes, the odds of a call-back after a screening mammogram vastly exceed the chance that a life will be saved. The numbers haven't changed much at all. What has changed is the societal shift to *do less*, a trend so powerful that even the use of military metaphors in writing about breast cancer (as I've done liberally) is frowned upon. It's a kinder, gentler approach toward cancer where we focus more on physician-induced harms than on benefits. And with focus comes inadvertent magnification.

A prime example of "over-selling" was the use of relative benefit rather than absolute benefit. As we learned in the last chapter, this is where master manipulation can take place. If you want to inflate a risk or benefit, go with relative numbers. If you want to minimize risk or benefit, go with absolute numbers. And if you want to annihilate either risk or benefit, go with absolute numbers as pertaining to mass screening (as opposed to treatment) where dilutional nihilism erases reality, if not the very meaning of life.

"After all, our medical oncology colleagues were forced into a corner on this issue, and now they use absolute benefits exclusively," say many physicians who are beginning to question screening. This claim is not so misplaced as to invoke apples and oranges, but it is Granny Smith compared to Red Delicious. Chemotherapy used for treatment of a known life-threatening condition is not exactly comparable to screening an asymptomatic population with mammography.

Why not use both "absolute" and "relative" risks in patient counseling? It's not that hard. We do it in our high-risk program where we give absolute risks for breast cancer, then cut those risks by a relative "one-third" to "one-half" with various interventions. Then, we do the math in front of the patient, taking a relative bite off calculated risk, and giving the patient her new *absolute* risk.

Otis W. Brawley, M.D., F.A.C.P., is the chief medical and scientific officer for the American

Cancer Society, known for his blunt honesty. He has broken ranks with mainstream medicine on many occasions, most recently in a book that covers a wide variety of controversies.[1] Dr. Brawley has stated on several occasions that mammography was oversold to the American public, a remarkable confession coming from one of the most pro-mammography organizations in America. In an October 21, 2012, article in the *New York Times*, Dr. Brawley said, "I'm admitting that American medicine has overpromised when it comes to screening. The advantages to screening have been exaggerated." That does not mean he is *opposed* to screening, only that the benefits have been overstated, while harms understated. He continued in that article with "Mammography is effective—mammograms work and women should continue to get them."

In fact, Dr. Brawley had previously pointed out the arbitrary dividing line between women in their 40s and women in their 50s (*OncologySTAT* online from Elsevier Global Medicine News, November 16, 2009) when, in response to the 2009 Task Force, he said: "The USPSTF [Task Force] says that screening 1,339 women in their 50s to save one life makes screening worthwhile in that age group. Yet [the] USPSTF also says screening 1,904 women aged 40–49 in order to save one life is not worthwhile.... The America Cancer Society's medical staff and volunteer experts overwhelmingly believe the benefits of screening women aged 40–49 outweigh its limitations." By 2015, Dr. Brawley will be munching on those words, when new guidelines were announced by the ACS.

Of course, it had been the American Cancer Society of 40 years prior, in league with the National Cancer Institute, that had launched the massive Breast Cancer Detection Demonstration Project (BCDDP) in lieu of confirmatory clinical trials in the U.S. Conspiracy theorists have no trouble accusing the ACS (and NCI) of self-interest in sponsorship of this effort, yet consider the times. Breast cancer incidence was on the rise (prior to screening), while mortality rates went unchecked. Adjuvant systemic therapy had not yet found a place in the armamentarium, so the *only* apparent method available at the time to lower breast cancer mortality was early detection through mammography as evidenced in the HIP study. Admittedly, the HIP was inconclusive without "validation by others," and the minority who objected to the BCDDP felt that their cautionary notes were squashed. Contemplative caution doesn't appreciate being steamrolled, and some of these thoughtful individuals are at work today as activist anti-screeners, their caution fully converted now to a cause.

Although captured by a less pervasive media at the time, public controversies swirled about the BCDDP every bit as much as the Canadian NBSS to follow. The greatest objection to the BCDDP in principle and practice came from epidemiologist John C. Bailar, III, Deputy Associate Director for Cancer Control at the NCI. Out on a lonely limb, employed by one of the sponsoring organizations of the BCDDP, Dr. Bailar raised the specters of lead time bias and length bias as possible distortions that had colored the HIP study, calling for confirmatory studies rather than demonstrations. Washington, D.C., journalist Jack Anderson took up the cause and printed excerpts from some of Bailar's writings in 1976.[2] The objections were virtually identical to what we hear today from critics of mammographic screening, a sad testimony that these things were not worked out back in the day when it still would have been acceptable to randomize women to "no mammography."

Of the myriad controversies that arose from the BCDDP (including some mammography equipment that had delivered radiation far above acceptable limits), a premier issue that persists to this day is "overdiagnosis." As we will see, this issue is far more complex than what many observers sprinkle into their rhetoric. In fact, the most common scenario to explain "overdiagnosis" probably doesn't occur at all, i.e., invasive cancers that allegedly "fester" in the breast and do nothing until discovered by mammography. We saw the refutation of this concept in an earlier chapter wherein multiple autopsy series, when combined, showed that only 1% of women are undiagnosed with occult invasive cancer at the time of death, the identical number as one would predict with zero overdiagnosis.

Instead, a very real problem of overdiagnosis was made evident in 1977, during the BCDDP, when a prominent breast pathology expert, Dr. Robert W. McDivitt (co-author of a favorite reference book of breast pathology at the time—the "AFIP breast fascicle"[3]) was asked to review 506 "minimal breast cancers." This minimalistic term was coined while I was a surgery resident in the 1970s, with the inexplicable grouping of 3 different entities—LCIS (lobular carcinoma in situ), DCIS (ductal carcinoma in situ), and invasive cancers under 0.5cm (some chose 1.0cm as the cut-off)—that made absolutely no clinical sense at the time for 3 separate entities to be shoved together under one moniker.

Other than a 95–99% survival when lymph nodes were negative, what did these entities have in common? Surgical care at the time made little distinction. If it was cancer we were dealing with, the breast was nearly always removed, unless one was a participant in the NSABP B-06 trial. But some experts were thinking well beyond the larval stage of us surgery residents. Indeed, it had already been identified that the common denominator for these 3 entities was mammographic discovery, and that these "minimal cancers" might not be acting like cancer at all.

In his microscopic review of the 506 "minimal cancers," however, Dr. McDivitt found that 66 of the lesions, 53 of which had prompted mastectomy, contained no cancer at all, not even carcinoma in situ. The 506 lesions were controversial enough, but what Dr. McDivitt claimed was incomprehensible—minimal cancer was not the root problem, it was the total *absence of cancer*. A firestorm was launched, with back-and-forth claims and counterclaims, but the majority of the 66 lesions in question stood the test of additional review. Dr. McDivitt correctly pointed out that mammography was not to blame. Instead, the problem was coming from the pathology department. His words of wisdom apparently went unnoticed, and blame has been placed squarely on the back of mammography for the past 40 years. Journalists of the day picked up the story within the context of "unproven mammography," and some of these writers are still at work on the same theme, with the same misconception as to the valid issues surrounding overdiagnosis.

After that extraordinary mess, did we learn anything practical from the BCDDP? As you might imagine, a mountain of data was generated, with all sorts of indirect evidence for both the benefit and feasibility of widespread population screening with mammography. Remember, the BCDDP was as much about Demonstration as it was Detection, so the mere practicality of general population screening was the major focus. Without a control group, the study would never be able to address the bottom line: Do mammograms save lives? Furthermore, this was not even a screening trial, given the large number of women who entered with palpable lumps. Five years of annual mammography in a quarter of a million women thus created a data windfall, but without definitive answers regarding asymptomatic screening.

However, the BCDDP did suggest that the technology was improving over time when compared to the earlier HIP study. More than 90% of the cancers detected were visible on mammography, and 50 percent had been detected by mammography alone. Interestingly, the BCDDP revealed that mammography could detect cancer in women under age 50, with a greater percentage of patients being found to have cancer in their 40s than had been seen in the HIP. But don't jump to conclusions. The leadership from what would emerge as the Canadian NBSS had an alternative explanation for this better detection in younger women— rather than a benefit of mammography, this finding "may have been due to less efficient physical examinations."[4]

In a way, the BCDDP was similar to the Canadian NBSS in that both studies included women with palpable masses, and the respective contribution of exam or mammography, or both together, is thus part of the evaluated data. Both were prospectively designed, but with the major distinction being no control group in the BCDDP.

Still, it is important to note that the BCDDP, while intended to affirm screening mammography, identified cancers most commonly as Stage II, the stage usually associated with palpable cancers. Mammographically discovered cancers are usually Stage I (or even Stage 0). In fact, in the BCDDP, there were more Stage II cancers (1,375) discovered than Stage 0 and I combined (1,306). This is *not* early detection. And when we get to the details of the Canadian NBSS, and its "statistically significant" smaller cancers discovered by mammography that did *not* save lives, we will find tumor sizes more in line with the BCDDP tumors than what modern mammography can accomplish.

In spite of the bitter scientific controversies surrounding the BCDDP, the fact remains that we are a celebrity-driven society, especially when it comes to breast cancer. In 1974, one year after the BCDDP launch, Betty Ford and Happy Rockefeller were both diagnosed with breast cancer, and their impact was felt at the BCDDP where enrollment in the study jumped abruptly as did the incidence of breast cancer diagnosis nationwide. The momentum would continue with Nancy Reagan's mammographically discovered cancer (7mm DCIS) in 1987, for which she underwent a modified radical mastectomy (prompting the observation of overtreatment, even at the time).

There was less debate about the outcomes of the BCDDP at the American Cancer Society where routine mammographic screening was advised in 1980, with a baseline to be done at age 35 to 39. In 1983, the baseline was de-emphasized, but screening was recommended every 1–2 years starting at age 40, then annually after 50. Later, this would become "annually starting at 40, for life" until the 2015 revision.

The American College of Radiology and other organizations joined with similar recommendations and, collectively, began public awareness campaigns, initially for enrollment in the BCDDP, then for the general population. The data for "earlier stage disease" in the BCDDP was all that was needed for many, adding indirectly to the notion of a mortality reduction as seen in the HIP study (keeping in mind that "length bias" can be responsible for lower stage disease that does *not* necessarily translate into saved lives).

Once upon a time, there were no pink ribbons. Mammography found its home prior to pink ribbons and the organizations that went with them. Yet they emerged hand-in-hand with aggressive campaigns to get women to comply with yearly mammograms. Some prominent breast surgeons and medical oncologists actually shied away from this movement, believing that mammograms were being oversold at the outset. Some breast cancer specialists defected completely, talking about the "post-mammography era" as if that era were right around the corner.

In fact, one organization has been so bold as to call for complete eradication of breast cancer through systemic therapies by 2020, a deadline rapidly approaching and doomed to fail. I'm in total agreement with the research goals of this organization, but there is no reason to denigrate screening mammography in the process. This is the same error made by those who were talking about the "post-mammography era" 30 years ago. It's nowhere close to happening. Once the disease is eradicated, *then* there will be no need for screening. It is a grievous mistake to get this order of events backwards, made worse by honoring studies that irrationally malign screening. We can do both. We can improve screening in the decades to come, while working on "the cure" at the same time.

A more ominous version of mammographic screening is that it is a dark plot, organized by the military-industrial-oncology complex that rules the United States, keeping the cure for cancer top secret. The picture here is radiologists rubbing their hands together in scrumptious glee, salivating at the loads of money being raked in. While "vast conspiracies" might occur, this is not one of them. Breast radiologists believe in their heart of hearts that they are routinely saving lives. But if one chooses to turn this controversy into strict dollars and cents, how big is the piece of pie that goes toward mammographic screening? Figures vary widely from source to source (no surprise), but a fair estimate for the industry of breast cancer screening ranges from $6 to $8 billion.

How does this compare? Well, it's always interesting to see where our priorities lie. The entire industry of mammographic screening, including all the "unnecessary biopsies," would represent less than 1% of Apple's market capitalization. Hurray for our smart phones! But to keep it real, how does it compare to our spending in other areas of medicine? Surprisingly, it's comparable, or perhaps a little higher, than the National Cancer Institute's entire budget devoted to cancer research. In this light, it makes us fidget a little, and one can better understand the "cure it, don't take photos of it" activists who believe the money "wasted" on screening could be used to get rid of the disease instead. Yet this $6–8 billion is government-sponsored research only. The private sector is able to raise untold billions for medical research, and many of the gains made in biotherapies are developed through that industry.

Also, diagnostic and treatment costs are always much larger when compared to research funding, with $35 billion going to the drug rehab industry, $175 billion for diabetes treatment, and $290 billion for cardiovascular disease. In the end, mammographic screening amounts to 0.2 cents of the health care dollar. The problem is that everyone wants their piece of the pie to be larger, and if that means coveting 0.2 cents, so be it.

From the standpoint of a general surgeon practicing in the 1980s, the acceptance of mammography was swift and intense. I recall magazine ads with a series of black dots, starting dime-sized on the left, progressing to a pinpoint on the right. The implications were obvious. Enthusiasm for early detection ran wild.

Yes, mammography was able to find pinpoint cancers, but with a big "if." *If* the cancer presented as a small calcium cluster. Or *if* the cancer had developed in a zone of fatty replacement so that it stood out as a bright point. But no one included these 'ifs" in the promotional efforts. In fact, no one bothered to ask what percentage of cancers were showing up at all. If you could see 2–3mm cancers, this must be one powerful tool. However, what was *not* discussed is the fact that, sometimes, cancers are invisible to mammography and can get so large that you feel them before you see them on a mammogram. This scenario was not considered by the average practicing surgeon. We heard one number loud and clear—Mammograms detect "90%" of cancers. In fact, the false belief in mammographic Sensitivity launched its own malpractice crisis with doctors telling patients not to worry about palpable lumps if the mammograms were negative.

The definition of "overselling" mammography varies from person to person. To draw from the phrase we heard earlier with regard to corruption in the CNBSS ("suspicion is in the eye of the beholder"), perhaps we should say, "Overselling mammography is in the eye of the beholder."

Certain examples are tossed into this ring where they don't belong. These are the public misconceptions that were never sold by anyone, to anyone—examples include the belief that mammograms detect 100% of cancers and always result in a cure, or, more shocking, that mammograms actually prevent cancer. While surveys document how prevalent these erroneous beliefs are, often to fortify the "crisis of overselling," it is not appropriate to lay blame on the medical community any more than it makes sense to lay blame on NASA for the 7% of the population that believes the moon landing was a hoax.

I have my own definition, and it marks a departure from the majority. In fact, it's the crux of my entire platform, and a primary reason for writing this book. It's a deceptively simple question I've already proposed: "What percentage of detectable breast cancers are picked up by mammography?"

Although I agree with Dr. Brawley that mammograms have been oversold, we are not talking about the same thing. He is referring to the lay public, where expected benefits have been exaggerated, and harms minimized. Many authors of many articles have re-characterized the mammography experience through a reversal of the historical approach—inflating the harms and minimizing the benefits. This seems to say, "You were oversold the benefits of mammography for years, so in order to keep the karma cool, we are now going to undersell it by focusing on harms. In a few decades, we'll be back to a zero balance, and all will be fair."

No, my version of "overselling" is not so much to the lay public where interest in our mathematical calculations of harms and benefits is not nearly as interesting as we think. Instead, my contention is that we have oversold mammography to ourselves. We physicians, even experts, believe mammograms are finding a greater percentage of detectable cancers than we're willing to admit. Dr. Brawley of the ACS has stated this Sensitivity number as 80%, a slight adjustment from the original 90%, but still far in excess of evidence that is both easily available and readily ignored. For many years, the American Cancer Society has published its *Breast Cancer Facts and Figures*, loaded with references, but no reference was offered when it came to defending the statement in that publication that mammograms detect "80–90%" of cancers. In the current version, a specific percentage is no longer offered.

The American Cancer Society is not alone here, with many expert breast radiologists quoting the same, though acknowledging the number may be as low as 50% in young women or in those with extremely dense tissue. The full revelation will not occur until a later chapter, and I mention it now, not only as a teaser to keep you reading, but also due to the fact that our topic in this chapter is selling and overselling. It's my contention that no one has acted maliciously or deceptively in putting mammography on the map. It has been a good faith effort to save lives. That said, we have oversold the detection rate of mammography to ourselves. And while the "mortality reduction" controversy is the endpoint that deserves the most attention, we are stuck in the past by a pothole of ancient data in that regard. Improvements will come only when we acknowledge true detection rates.

**Biology (interval) + Sensitivity (detection rate) =
Screening Benefit (mortality reduction)**

$$X + Y = Z$$

As Richard Feynman, PhD, Nobel laureate in physics, 1965, said, "The first principle is that you must not fool yourself—and you are the easiest person to fool."

# 10

# The Evidence for Evidence-Based Medicine (or, How to Raise the Bar of Bias: An Editorial)

For in much wisdom is much grief: and he that increaseth knowledge increaseth sorrow.—Ecclesiastes 1:18, *King James Version*

Lovers of wisdom (philosophers) have toyed with this Biblical notion of inverse relationships, including the paradoxical twist: As wisdom increases, knowledge decreases. The knowledge question—that is, how do we know what we know (labeled *epistemology* by philosophers to make sure we don't know what they are talking about)—was one of the earliest questions asked, dating back several thousand years at least. In fact, one could argue that modern philosophy is engaged in the drab exercise of re-stating the ancients.

Unbeknownst to nearly all clinicians and most medical scientists, at the same time that the mammography Civil War was underway in the 1990s, the philosophers of science were locked in their own battle, today called the "Science Wars."

The controversies, as with mammography, had been brewing for years in academic philosophical circles. What is true scientific knowledge? What is the best process for arriving at Reality with a capital R? Or do we ignore Reality altogether, and simply confirm that if something works, that's good enough (or is that the definition of "technology")?

We noted earlier that Ptolemy's Earth-centered model worked beautifully as a predictor of movement in the solar system, so why move on? If it works, it works. Copernicus and Galileo didn't buy into the functionality standard, instead favoring Reality. And, though closer to the truth in terms of 3-dimensional Reality with circular orbits, they were in turn trumped by Kepler who reasoned elliptically (a theory dismissed by Galileo). But the Reality vs. Functionality argument marches on.

The academic debates of philosophers in the Science Wars centered on post-modernism and its impact on scientific method. Modernism, of course, had "reason" at its core, or rational thought. Reason had been the foundation of the Enlightenment of the 17th and 18th centuries. On the other hand, post-modernists, in brief, claimed that there were no objective truths. Taken to its extreme, the traditional scientific method is nothing more than a social construct, and it became the post-modernists' task to deconstruct that construction.

Most working scientists had no interest in this sort of debate whatsoever. But in 1996, concurrent with our Mammography Civil War, a physicist named Alan Sokal[1] perpetrated a hoax to expose what he felt was post-modern gibberish. Sokal submitted an article to an academic post-modernist journal, proposing that quantum gravity was nothing more than a social construct. The article was published, whereupon Sokal immediately announced the hoax, along with the fact that he had used "a pastiche of left-wing cant, fawning references, grandiose quotations, and outright nonsense."

Those who had been humiliated struck back with claims of unethical and immoral behavior by Sokal, and the War was on. Notably, the line in the sand was not drawn between scientists and post-modernist philosophers. There were scientists on both sides of the issue, and there were philosophers on both sides.

The point here is that the much revered "scientific method" is not universally agreed upon. The Science Wars set many to thinking about the definition of Scientific Truth, with the intent to separate science from pseudo-science. But no matter where the arrow is placed along the ruler, a strict definition of scientific truth will exclude many of the greatest scientific discoveries of all time. And if the arrow is adjusted to include those great discoveries, then countless examples of pseudo-science must be welcomed to the family of scientific truth. It's an unsolvable problem.

So the "scientific method" that most have learned at least once must get some degree of scrutiny. Where did it come from? Who came up with the following (one version of many):

1. Ask a question based on your observations.
2. Gather what is already known or believed.
3. Form a hypothesis.
4. Test the hypothesis through experimentation and collect data.
5. Analyze the data and draw conclusions.
6. Publish results.
7. Repeat the study (best done by others).

While Francis Bacon (1561–1626) is given credit as the "father of the scientific method," that moniker sometimes spills over as the "father of empiricism," which is not exactly the case. And he certainly was not the "father of evidence-based medicine." First of all, Bacon was a lawyer, serving as attorney general and lord chancellor in England, first in a precarious dance to save his head from Queen Elizabeth's inclinations, then knighted when King James came to power.

In brief summary, Bacon was very much interested in the scientific revolution underway, and he formulated basic principles that are still valid today. Bacon believed that the primary blockade that could prevent scientific truth was the human mind itself. *We* are the problem, due to our inherent biases that prevent us from critical thinking. Bacon's "4 Idols of the Mind" (idols = "false images," not pagan worship) represent history's tagline, but without some explanation, a rote listing of the 4 Idols strike us today as peculiar—Idols of the Tribe, Cave, Marketplace, and Theater.

Suffice it for our purposes to summarize the 4 Idols as *The mind is the problem, experience is the answer*. Rather than call Bacon the "father of empiricism," it is more accurate to say that he first articulated the process of *inductive reasoning*—that is, observing particular events and drawing generalized conclusions from that experience, independent of the powerful biases of the mind.

There is some baggage with this approach. No matter how many times you observe something and draw generalizations, there is always the possibility that there's an exception to any rule you make. "All swans are white" was used in teaching rhetoric until black swans were discovered in Australia. This uncertainty with inductive reasoning is only a hop and a skip from skepticism, and before you know it, you've jumped into post-modernistic nihilism. Given that lawyers and the judicial system are predicated on the *deductive* method of reasoning, as opposed to *inductive*, it is most peculiar that an inductive philosophical approach to science was formulated by an attorney.

While Bacon has been immortalized for his contributions, his intellectual opposite has been reduced to a multiple-choice question on college exams: Question: Who said, "I think, therefore I am." Answer: René Descartes, a French philosopher who held the converse position—*Experience is the problem, the mind is the solution.* Witness the false impressions one gets by watching the sun and stars move across the sky—*they* seem to be moving, not us. Furthermore, if you a throw a ball in the air, why does it fall in the same spot if Earth is rotating? Why is there no wind if Earth is spinning so fast? Observation can be very deceiving. The answer for Descartes was *not* in observation, but in the mind. After all, where did mathematics come from? Math came from the mind as rational thought, not through inductive reasoning.

No greater example of deductive reasoning can be found than in Euclid's geometry, where absolute truths (Reality, until non–Euclidean geometry emerged) are proven in sequence. You begin with an absolute truth, and deduce reality from that point on. In fact, Euclid's geometry would seduce many philosophers who believed the same rational deductive process could be applied to all science, including the social sciences.

Today, in medicine, we think of mathematics and probability as the talons brandished by the biostatistician who then feeds the prey to the epidemiologists. But the irony is that this is not Baconian at all; in fact, historians note that Bacon was uncomfortable with the mathematical explanations of nature, and some claim he would have been horrified by probability statistics (which had not yet been "invented"). In contrast, mathematics was at the very core of the deductive reasoning of Descartes.

The reason for this detouring loop from our main road is to point out that scientific method is not pure empiricism, a point of some importance, given that "evidence-based medicine" is heavily weighted toward empiricism, *if not synonymous.* In the 7-point list above for "scientific method," several of the steps are purely rational thought. Indeed, good science is a combination of both rationalism and empiricism. As a matter of fact, Bacon proposed this very combination. In his parable of the spider (pure rationalism, spinning a web from within), the ant (pure empiricism, collecting and organizing dirt particles), and the honeybee (the ideal blend of collecting pollen, then producing honey), Bacon chose the honeybee as the ideal symbol for the scientific method.

Well, hang on, because in this era of "evidence-based medicine," we have killed the spider, glorified the ant, and the honeybee numbers are in rapid decline.

What is evidence-based medicine? Haven't we been doing this all along? Haven't we been trying to base good medicine on some sort of science?

Growing up in a family with a physician-father and medical technologist-mother (who was later a writer), I heard the phrase, "Medicine is both a science and an art," and somehow got the impression that "art" meant bedside manner. I now subscribe to a different definition of art—it's the chewing gum used to plug the holes left by good science. Alternatively stated, it is the rational thought used to back up and organize empiric data. Ground rule: it is going to be impossible to prove everything done in medicine through prospective, randomized trials. Therefore, there will always be holes, there will always be art. We will always need chewing gum.

Much has been written (by science writers) about doctors as poor scientists, and it's easy to draw from examples, such as annual Pap smears after complete hysterectomies that once were the norm. Nonetheless, a doctor who is a pure scientist and nothing else is going to be useless, unable to complete diagnosis and treatment on a single patient, paralyzed by the uncertainties left by the lack of randomized trials.

But the stage was set for "evidence-based medicine" through several simultaneous forces at work. First, rising health care costs in the face of limited resources mandated a system of priorities and, thus, quantification. Physician-led groups decided to police themselves rather than wait for bureaucrats to make medical decisions. Then, the computer revolution added its part by revealing the massive amount of information in the published medical literature, making it very difficult for an individual physician, even when highly specialized, to keep up on all developments. Most notably, sophisticated mathematics in the form of biostatistics began a relentless creep into the medical literature, validating the epidemiologist and public health expert in many instances, but sometimes pushing aside rational thought.

Although Robert L. Egan, M.D., is often considered the "father of mammography," Gerald D. Dodd, Jr., M.D.,[2] must be listed as an accessory, perhaps the "uncle of mammography." While still a radiologic faculty member at Thomas Jefferson Memorial Hospital in Philadelphia, Dr. Dodd is credited with participating in the first needle-directed surgical excision of a non-palpable mammographic mass. In 1955, he was recruited to MD Anderson Cancer Hospital in Houston where he eventually became chairman of the Department of Diagnostic Radiology. But as he left Thomas Jefferson, he dragged with him a promising radiology resident who had yet to complete his training—Dr. Robert L. Egan would go on to finish his radiology residency at MD Anderson and, while at that location, emerged as the "father of mammography."

Dr. Gerald Dodd, in his role as editor of *Breast Diseases: A Year Book® Quarterly*, responded in 1994 (Volume 5, no. 3, page 47) to the Canadian NBSS brouhaha with these words: "It is vital, however, that personal clinical experience be included in the appraisal. Over the centuries, the majority of advances in medicine have been made through clinical investigation. The recent importance given to epidemiologic and statistical data is appropriate but cannot totally replace clinical experience."

In a word, medicine is both an art and a science. It is rational thought combined with empiric evidence.

What Dr. Dodd was witnessing was the infiltration into clinical medicine of epidemiologists ("medicine without the blood") who do not have clinical experience. Epidemiology and public health had originally addressed, well, epidemics. But the expansion of these disciplines into the clinic was heralding a new phenomenon in the 1990s, which would extend to the present day where the balance of power is now placing the clinician in a subservient role. Dr. Dodd had been prophetic in his warnings, but alas, his words have been lost.

The shift of influence from the clinician to the epidemiologist is part of a larger picture. It is a change in focus from the importance of the individual to society at large. The Hippocratic Oath has been experiencing a death rattle for years when it comes to the individual patient as top priority,[3] though few will acknowledge it. Paradoxically, researchers tout the worthy goal of "personalized medicine," while epidemiologic think tanks outline recommendations for the population as an amorphous blob. While not mutually exclusive, the two trendy banners waving in the breeze of "evidence-based medicine" and "personalized medicine" do not easily blend. Evidence-based guidelines are not created for individuals; they are designed for populations. What may be best for an individual is not necessarily what is best for all, and vice versa.

This societal change is inbred in medical training today. Whereas cost containment was rarely discussed during my years of residency (thus our current problems), new doctors are groomed to be the custodians of the pot of gold designated for health care delivery. They cut their teeth now on medical care based on what's good for the whole population given limited resources. There are political words used to describe a society where the masses are always more important than individuals, but let me stray no closer to politics, returning to the origins and definition of "evidence-based medicine."

Related to information overload introduced by the personal computer and internet, public health guardians began to publish studies of practicing physicians as to how well they understood the results and limitations of clinical trials. In essence, they were evaluating the epidemiologic and statistical skills of the average doctor. The results were rather alarming, in that many physicians could not transfer the basic information to be gleaned from a clinical trial and apply the correct numbers to the individual patient sitting before them. (We know from Chapter 8—The Number Games—how tricky those numbers can be.)

Bottom line: academically-inclined physicians, interested in helping their mathematically naive colleagues, joined forces with epidemiologists and biostatisticians to formalize the process of judging evidence according to its "quality," drawing from the insurmountable pile of published data. What's "new" about evidence-based medicine is this: (1) the *ranking* of evidence into a hierarchy of quality, and (2) the establishment of "neutral" *think tanks* that will review the evidence not only to generate this hierarchy, but also to create guidelines for clinical management.

Okay, sounds good so far. And, when those "think tanks" are composed of expert physicians who actually practice what they preach, things work fairly well. In the world of cancer management, one of the most commonly referenced set of guidelines comes from the NCCN, the physician-led National Cancer Comprehensive Network. Guidelines work quite well here for the practicing medical oncologist who can be overwhelmed by countless prospective trials for multiple types of cancer, all while the market is being flooded with new biotherapies, perhaps the most exciting time in the history of oncology.

But what if each hospital had to manufacture its own chemotherapeutic agents and biotherapies? Then, you would introduce staggering bias into the system, given that one hospital might be making a "better" version of the same drug. That's what happens, to a degree, when guidelines are created for surgeons and radiologists, where major differences can exist from one location to another. This is why the Canadian NBSS was comfortable with substandard mammography, drawing on the principle of "generalizability" that endorses mediocrity out of practical necessity. Excellence falls by the wayside in this system, and we see the "tall poppy syndrome," where the head is lopped from the strongest plant to keep all flowers at the same low level.

Witness the tribulations of Dr. Mel Silverstein, one of the nation's top authorities on ductal carcinoma in situ (DCIS) of the breast. While the prospective, randomized trials found benefit to adding radiation therapy to lumpectomy, Dr. Silverstein pointed out many years ago that a subset of patients could be identified where radiation had little to add. Indeed, the recurrence rate was lower in this subset than the general population of irradiated women in the NSABP trials. His system was highly methodical and regimented, and it made perfect rational sense. Many surgeons, skeptical already about radiating everyone with DCIS, adopted his approach immediately after his first publication that introduced the "Van Nuys Prognostic Index."

Yet there were no prospective, randomized trials to provide "high quality" data. For many, it was heresy to delete radiation therapy for DCIS. It took Dr. Silverstein 12 years of active campaigning through presentations and publications before his approach was effectively adopted by the NCCN. Even then, it is listed as Category 2b (lower level evidence). Many champions have arisen today, leading the charge to limit breast radiation in selected women with DCIS. Such an effort to *do less* is fashionable now, but when Dr. Silverstein and his pathology collaborator, Dr. Lagios, began the crusade, they were in direct conflict with the most powerful organization in the history of breast cancer—the NSABP. It was David vs. Goliath, but it was also rational thought vs. strict empiricism.

Even physician-led groups can stumble and falter when you move away from pharmaceutical agents, in that "drug studies" have standardized manufacturing and pristine clinical trials where compliance is high, contamination low, and the design is double or triple-blinded. In contrast, for radiology and surgery, the clinical trials may be anointed with "prospective, randomized trial" winning the hearts of many, but the scientific purity falls short of a blinded drug trial.

Another scenario occurs when a clinical trial is performed to perfection, but experts differ on the interpretation. Witness the ACRIN 6666 trial for using ultrasound and/or breast MRI to improve mammographic screening in high-risk women with dense mammograms. Both ultrasound and MRI improved outcomes substantially, but there was sharp disagreement as to the winner—some believe the trial supported adjunct whole breast ultrasound, while others consider it a clear victory for breast MRI. The evidence from this excellent trial design is questioned by no one, but the results are open to wide interpretation by top experts. The problem is not a lack of evidence. The problem is that pure empiricism has its limits, that is, it must be engineered by human beings.

From a practical standpoint, the expert physicians who serve on the NCCN committees have been a blessing for oncologists treating cancer. *Preventive medicine and cancer screening,* however, have largely fallen into the hands of non-experts working through organizations other than the NCCN. In fact, one of the working principles in preventive health and screening has been the exclusion of experts from these "think tanks" to avoid bias. In the minds of the bean-counters, one only needs beans. The bean farmer can squawk all day about size and quality, but the person who grew the beans plays no role when it comes to counting. This is where evidence-based medicine can be unsettling. Imagine stripping the judgment about systemic therapy options from the medical oncologist and instead, establishing panels of non-oncologists to decide how and when chemotherapy should be administered. Well, that's exactly what has already happened when it comes to screening.

Making decisions about proper clinical care, as defined by M.D.s and PhDs who don't have anything to do with that specialty, is a stretch for rational thought, yet has already found its comfort level in medicine today. At a more subtle level, these "neutral" think tanks harbor a self-perception of intellectual superiority ("we only look at good science") casting their knowledge over a sea of minions.

Practicing experts are excluded from membership in these "think tanks," with some going so far in the name of banishing bias that they don't even allow *testimony* by experts. Thus, we have in place a glorified system that, in the name of banishing bias, actually elevates reverse bias. It is a system of trial without a judge or witnesses. The lay jury decides it all. It should be easy to see why physician groups have organized their own sets of guidelines, often in direct opposition to the "neutral" think tanks.

As with many social movements, there is an inherent *in*ability to restrain the momentum. The ranking of evidence by think tanks, or even expert-led physician groups, graded by numbers and/or letters, creates the potential to simply ignore "lower level evidence" if "higher level" is available. This is where the nebulous word "judgement" can do so much damage. The ranking itself can be controversial, knowing that a certain level of quality will translate to specific guidelines.

This exclusion of lower level evidence, to continue with the legal analogy, is akin to disallowing all circumstantial evidence at trial. Given that eyewitnesses, even with videotapes (direct empiric evidence), can be unreliable, our judicial system relies heavily on supportive evidence that can surround an alleged crime. Not so with evidence-based medicine when used by the "neutral" think tanks. Circumstantial evidence is to be condemned wherever it rears its ugly head. Only top quality evidence is admissible to the jury that needs neither witnesses nor a judge.

What data are at the top of the rankings? Prospective randomized trials, at a minimum. Preferably, studies that have combined these trials into overviews or meta-analyses. Lower level evidence provides the bulk of published data, by far, when it comes to mammographic screening, but these observational studies are very much prone to the 4 Horsemen of Potential Bias we talked about earlier. But rather than keep the limitations of these studies in mind, the evidence-based think tanks often toss the evidence out the window.

At this point in the controversy about screening, I've focused almost entirely on the historical prospective, randomized trials for mammography, but does anything so far that we've talked about seem like high quality evidence in those trials? By today's standards, absolutely not. There are *no high quality* studies for mortality reduction with screening mammography, including the Swedish Two-County, and certainly not the Canadian NBSS. So, for the remainder of this book, keep in mind that without the empirical evidence we need to make a decision, we need to be honeybees—collecting as much pollen as possible, but then using rational thought to create something like honey.

If evidence-based medicine simply ended with helpful guidelines, all would be right with the world. But that is not the case. Guidelines have a way of becoming rules. As you might imagine, third party payors use the guideline-turned-rules to decide when and where they are going to pay. When a physician goes "off-guideline" with a clinical decision and recommendation, then insurers use an offensive word, like "experimental" or "investigational," to cast the doctor as the enemy, a mad scientist indeed. And if the government is the third-party payor, you can imagine a circular system wherein guidelines from government-supported think tanks are skewed in favor of those approaches that allow less reimbursement. This is not conspiracy theory; it's simple human nature performing on the political stage.

There is an underlying reason why axioms and truisms and clichés emerge, usually because there is some truth hidden in there somewhere. So do the following phrases sound familiar? "You can prove anything with statistics." Or a favorite among statisticians themselves, "If you don't like your statistical results, then torture the numbers until they talk." Or my favorite, "80% of statistics are made up."[4] Medicine is not either/or when it comes to science. The human body is not a bundle of numbers that can be sorted into dichotomies. Clinical experience is important.

Don't interpret my editorializing to mean that I am opposed to evidence-based medicine. In contrast, I embrace it as a helpful tool. What I'm opposed to is this—the total preoccupation with evidence-based medicine *to the exclusion of rational thought.*

Perhaps *Calvin and Hobbes* sum up the wisdom vs. knowledge issue the best. The syndicated cartoon took its title from theologian John Calvin and philosopher Thomas Hobbes, the latter being one of those thinkers drawn to Euclid's geometry and how deductive reasoning could be applied to political and social science.

This particular *Calvin and Hobbes* was published September 21, 1993, at the start of both the Science Wars and the Mammography Civil War: In the first scene, the tiger Hobbes is watching Calvin studying a book, and the young boy comments, "The more you know, the harder it is to take decisive action. Once you become informed, you start seeing complexities and shades of gray. You realize that nothing is as clear and simple as it first appears." And then, perhaps the most memorable line from the career of cartoonist Bill Watterson, Calvin says, "Ultimately, knowledge is paralyzing." And, in an act of defiance in the final panel, Calvin throws the book over his shoulder and concludes with "Being a man of action, I can't afford to take that risk." By this time, the tiger Hobbes is resting with paw against jowl as he says, "You're ignorant, but at least you act on it."

Dogma does not have a good track record in the history of science. Richard Feynman, PhD, the 1965 Nobel Prize winner in physics, is perhaps best remembered for his wisdom on the philosophy of science. One of his most consistent themes revolves around one word: uncertainty.[5] The moment you get an experimental result, he would say, try to think of every possible explanation *other than* your hypothesis. Dr. Sam Hellman said the same thing in his Karnofsky Memorial Lecture in 1994 where he introduced the concept of "Spectrum Theory" as applied to breast cancer biology. In fact, his words were blunter: "Dogma is the enemy of science."

So, if *uncertainty* is the most revered quality of the wise physician-scientist, why are we turning over the control of medicine to those who worship certainty, believing that all biologic continuums can be converted to dichotomies with confidence intervals, and that our colorful world can be made black and white with p-values?

# 11

# Blame It on Canada (and Something's Rotten in Denmark, Too)

Breast radiologists and pro-screeners were lulled into complacency by the exposed corruption in the Canadian NBSS randomization process (albeit with intended benevolence). It didn't last long. The CNBSS initiated a border skirmish that threatened the Pax Romana on September 20, 2000, when the 13-year follow-up results of Study-2 (screening in ages 50–59) appeared in the *Journal of the National Cancer Institute*, indicating no benefit to screening mammography above and beyond what is provided by physical exam alone.

Two tidbits should be remembered at this point: (1) there has never been a screening trial demonstrating a reduced mortality through exam alone, so the desired endpoint by the CNBSS (clinical exam alone) has been wobbly from the onset, and (2) all other trials besides the CNBSS-2 have shown a mortality reduction in this age group, even if not always statistically significant. In fact, the over-50 benefits of mammography are widely accepted. Why was the CNBSS unable to demonstrate a mortality reduction even in the 50–59 age group?

Although most of the focus throughout the years has been on Study-1 (where, initially, mammograms were alleged to be *causing* breast cancer deaths in women 40–49), the key to appreciating why this trial is an outlier lies in Study-2, not Study-1, where the former, addressing women in their 50s, has an outcome that shouts: "Something is wrong with this trial!"

The CNBSS routinely presents their data to confirm that mammographic detection finds smaller tumors. This is a critical point. If mammographic tumors were the same size and stage as tumors that were palpated, this would completely validate the claims that mammographic quality in the CNBSS was nothing short of terrible. It is thus critical for the CNBSS to reveal "earlier stage" disease through mammography, but *without a concomitant reduction in mortality*, in order to call upon "length bias" as the explanation not only for their trial but also playing an important role in other trials as well.

The CNBSS-2 update was followed by the Study-1 update, appearing September 3, 2002, in the *Annals of Internal Medicine*. Magically, the "mammography kills" effect had disappeared, leaving only the ashes of neutrality. No one was hurt by mammography allegedly squeezing tumor cells into the bloodstream, but no one was helped either. CNBSS-1 was a neutral study this time around, just like Study-2. For women in their 40s, there were 105 breast cancer deaths in the mammography group and 108 breast cancer deaths in the "usual care" group (remembering that "usual care" patients are free to get mammograms on their own—26% had mammograms outside the clinical trial).

82

With the uncanny resilience worthy of the zombie title, the CNBSS was reanimated and on a lumbering roll. The CNBSS wasn't about to sit idly by while their life mission was being torn to shreds. Notably, this was not, and is not, a xenophobic battle on the part of the United States and its leading radiologists against our neighbors to the north. Canada is not a monolithic force opposed to screening mammography. Screening mammography is widely utilized in Canada, and some of the harshest critics against the CNBSS come from Canadian radiologists.

Nonetheless, the CNBSS fought back on many fronts, one example being the hiring of security firms to analyze the documents used in the randomization process, claiming victory. Not surprisingly, security experts on the CNBSS payroll confirmed the CNBSS position, while critics dismissed these findings and pointed out that the proof was in their uniquely neutral mortality outcomes, given that the rest of the world had witnessed a benefit to mammographic screening.

The original claims of overt malfeasance in randomization, primarily in Study-1, were trivialized by many observers, a phenomenon that continues to this day. Dr. Tarone's study from the National Cancer Institute had confirmed a statistically significant number of patients with advanced cancer who were directly placed into the mammography group. Furthermore, he stated that unless these patients were excluded from all future analyses, the CNBSS would not be able to draw conclusions from their mortality data. Today, those patients have been lost in the melee, with the CNBSS claiming that if you exclude those who were inappropriately placed in the mammography group, the results are the same. But we're still left with the 50–59 age group where, unique to the CNBSS, there was no benefit seen with mammographic screening.

The real culprit in the CNBSS, all along, has been substandard mammography, even for the day. Remember: X + Y = Z.

**Biology + Sensitivity = Screening effectiveness (mortality reduction)**

Notice that "study design" is not part of that equation. Sensitivity (Y) is all-important since you can't control biology (other than to change the screening interval). If your screening tool misses too many cancers, you will not be able to generate a mortality reduction. Study design is a methodologic *tool* used to prove X + Y = Z, yet in the case of the CNBSS, for many, the tool has become an authority unto itself. And, since the *intent* of the CNBSS was to have the best study design ever, many supporters have enthusiastically embraced the "negative" results in spite of all evidence indicating massive compromise in the quality of the mammograms.

Study design and study execution are two different things, however. And while the *design* of the CNBSS might have been the best yet up to that point, randomization of advanced cancers into the mammography group was merely the most dramatic finding. There were other issues as well, touched on earlier, bringing the entire study into question.[1]

In 2002, the World Health Organization *excluded* the CNBSS (both studies), from their analysis of screening mammography and its impact on mortality from breast cancer. But you wouldn't know it, would you? American journalists and editors of both traditional and online periodicals keep the door wide open and greet the CNBSS with welcome arms.

Enter Peter Gøtzsche, M.D., from Denmark.

Dr. Gøtzsche is professor of clinical research design and analysis at the University of

Copenhagen. Without passing judgment good or bad, it's fair to say that he is a screening nihilist, not only for breast cancer, but medical screening and much of therapeutics as well. To his credit, he is consistent. As I mentioned early in this book, it may be more intellectually honest to claim that harms outweigh benefits in screening (thus, stop it) than it is to say that screening saves lives but we should do *less* of it.

While his books are euphemistically called "ground-breaking," it may be more revealing to point out that Dr. Gøtzsche makes our American near-nihilist, H. Gilbert Welch, M.D., look like a gentle lamb. *Mammography Screening: Truth, Lies and Controversy* (London: Radcliffe, 2012) has helped anti-mammography forces in North America and Europe rally around the flag, as his version of "truth" appeals to wider and wider audiences who have become disenchanted with the promise of mammographic screening. Standing ovations are not uncommon when this charismatic speaker charms an audience, even though he may be delivering a sentence of doom to some whose clapping hands eagerly embrace his words.

In 2000,[2] and again in a 2001 update,[3] both in *The Lancet*, Dr. Gøtzsche and Ole Olsen, the latter a statistician at the University of Copenhagen, reported their "meta-analysis" of the prospective mammography screening trials, announcing to the world—no benefit to mammographic screening whatsoever. For many, the report was instantaneously comical—the duo had excluded the trials that showed a strong benefit with mammography, while including the CNBSS as the anchor study, adding only one other study in the so-called "meta-analysis." To justify exclusion of the Swedish overview, the two authors felt that there were features in those trials that "raised the possibility of bias" (no problems with the CNBSS, of course). This type of speculative language permeates the article. As expected, worldwide media captured the story and magnified its impact beyond anyone's imagination.

A new battle was launched. In the *International Journal of Epidemiology*,[4] investigators from the University of California, Berkeley (David A. Freedman), Kaiser Permanente of Southern California (Diana B. Petitti) and Harvard School of Public Health (James M. Robins) analyzed the "meta-analysis" from Gøtzsche-Olsen, the Nordic branch of the Cochrane collaboration (a think tank). Their results? "The basis for the Gøtzsche-Olsen critique turns out to be simple. Studies that found a benefit from mammography were discounted as being of poor quality; remaining negative studies were combined by meta-analysis. The critique therefore rests on judgments of study quality, but these judgments are based on misreading of the data and the literature."

Even prior to this put-down, some players in the screening world, including screening minimalists, began to distance themselves from the Gøtzsche version of the truth. In a 2003 review article on "Mammographic Screening for Breast Cancer" in the *New England Journal of Medicine*,[5] the authors expressed satisfaction that Dr. Gøtzsche's "criticisms of all but one of the trials excluded from the meta-analysis have been answered. In-depth independent reviews of the criticisms concluded that they do not negate the effectiveness of mammography, especially for women older than 50 years of age." The lead author of this review? Dr. Suzanne W. Fletcher of the famed "Fletcher Report" that had launched the Mammography Civil War. Although still not ready to give up on the 40–49 controversy, Dr. Fletcher's report remains a strong statement in direct opposition to the study by Gøtzsche-Olsen.

If these statements were not strong enough, we can always turn to Dr. László Tabár who claims that Dr. Gøtzsche did not inform the Cochrane Breast Cancer Review Group of his planned 2000 article in *The Lancet*, even though drawing upon the good reputation of that group as the "Nordic branch," of which Dr. Gøtzsche was director. Furthermore, the review group refused to approve the 2001 Gøtzsche article to *The Lancet*. Dr. N. Day, professor of public health at the University of Cambridge, said, "The *Lancet* paper by Gøtzsche and Olsen ... is not simply controversial, it contains a number of serious statistical mistakes. It is a worthless piece of work which if it had been produced by one of our masters students, would have been sent back with demands for a complete rewrite." And finally, from the article "Gøtzsche's Quixotic Antiscreening Campaign: Nonscientific and Contrary to Cochrane Principles" written by Peter B. Dean, M.D., of Turku University Central Hospital in Finland, in the *Journal of the American College of Radiology*,[6] we read, "Evaluations of evidence-based medicine should be performed by individuals who have personal competence in the subjects they choose to evaluate."

From Dr. Tabár's web site, we have this final blow to indicate something is rotten— Denmark has one of the highest breast cancer death rates in Europe, similar to that of Serbia. In contrast, Finland and Sweden are among the lowest mortality groups, even though all Nordic countries use identical breast cancer treatment guidelines. The health care delivery systems among these countries are similar, too, but with the specific difference that Finland and Sweden introduced nationwide screening more than two decades ago. As Dr. Mukherjee says in his book, *The Emperor of All Maladies*, in quoting a Swedish resident, mammography is "somewhat of a religion here."

Yet, even if you actively search medical news releases, you heard none of this. The nearly universal condemnation of the Gøtzsche-Olsen "meta-analysis" was never introduced to the public sphere, only the initial proclamation that reverberated worldwide—"mammography at any age does not save lives."

Although the Gøtzsche-Olsen "meta-analysis" was laid to rest, something changed. That something, I believe, was tolerance for the opposing viewpoint. Breast radiologists had survived the Mammography Civil War, but they were still licking their wounds when the Canadian NBSS rose from the grave with renewed vitality, prepared for a duel to the death. These pro-screening radiologists were not fighting for an unpopular position. They were fighting for the majority position. They were fighting for the default position, in that breast cancer staging, unlike many other cancers, is highly predictable for outcomes based on anatomic extent of disease. Early diagnosis = earlier stage disease = improved survival, so the rational position, without empiric evidence of any kind, would favor mammographic screening. Yet their position was being ignored with increasing frequency, by journal editors and journalists alike, while clumsy papers like the Gøtzsche-Olsen "meta-analysis" were being canonized by the ill-informed and/or strongly biased.

Frustration rose to new levels. A group of 41 screening experts, perturbed by the nonstop flow of non-scientific criticism, published a letter—"Effect of Population-Based Screening on Breast Cancer Mortality"—in the November 19, 2011, issue of *The Lancet*: "Although the wider scientific community has long embraced the benefits of population-based breast screening, there seems to be an active anti-screening campaign orchestrated in part by members of the Nordic Cochrane Centre."

And where a pioneering radiologist like Dan Kopans, M.D., might have once used the term "randomization flaws" to describe the CNBSS, new words like "fraud" replaced the old, and emotions took center stage. No longer were "challenges" placed before screening mammography, instead, "attacks against mammography" were tossed into the fray then countered as ridiculous hyperbole. Clearly, though, radiologists were fed up. Editorials with titles like "Enough Is Enough" and "It's Just Wrong" began to appear. Tolerance began to disappear.

At the same time, those without vested interest could afford to remain calm, inventing new ways to get beneath the skin of breast radiologists. We all learned this technique in the sandbox. If someone's a hot head, either avoid them or needle them, whatever your pleasure. In the mammography debates, it became a new sport for the cooler heads, no matter how empty, to bait breast radiologists into an argument. Often, to the unwitting observer, the cooler heads prevailed.

In 1988, I made the decision to leave the private practice of general surgery and morph into a dedicated breast surgeon when I was hired to return to my alma mater. My assigned task was to convert the mammography screening unit (born as one of the original BCDDP sites) into a multi-disciplinary breast cancer program fashioned after the model that had been established by Dr. Jay Harness at the University of Michigan. My position at the University of Oklahoma, however, was not open for another six months after my decision to accept the new role. Given that I had trained in an era where "surgical technique" was the only thing one had to know about breast cancer, I decided that I should get some didactic information under my belt before returning to Oklahoma from Los Angeles.

Back then, there were precious few textbooks devoted to breast cancer, but I picked one that was hot off the press, and read it cover to cover. Quite the eye-opener, I should mention, as virtually everything in the book was news to me.

Anyway, *Breast Diseases* (edited by Jay R. Harris, Samuel Hellman, I. Craig Henderson, David W. Kinne [Philadelphia: J. B. Lippincott, 1987]) has stayed in my library for the past three decades, and I still refer to the book when I'm curious about historical data that may not appear easily with online searches. In refreshing my memory about details from the BCDDP for this current book, I opened the text to the screening chapter where I found my answers. However, I noticed something else.

Everywhere, there was an undercurrent that was skeptical of mammographic screening. Not only the beneficial skepticism of good science, but also an odd preoccupation with the role of physical exam. Old observational studies of screening, long since dismissed due to small sample size, were reviewed as evidence of no benefit to mammography. In contrast, the newly reported Swedish Two-County results were included (31% reduction in mortality, statistically significant), but with clear disbelief: *"they leave unanswered the question of the amount that mammography adds to the benefit of physical examination, and there has to be concern that the relatively high interval cancer rates noticed are at least in part due to the absence of physical examination."*

What? Again, the very definition of mammographic screening minimizes the role of the unreliable and unproven clinical exam. This is a *strength* of the Two-County study as being the first to evaluate mammography as the sole screening tool, not a weakness. As for the high *interval* rates in the Two-County trial, this is far more likely due to the exceedingly long *intervals*—33 months for women over 50—the longest interval in any of the historic trials.

The author of the chapter then stated that all these problems would disappear once the results were available from the upcoming Canadian NBSS trials, elegant in design like no other study.

Who wrote this stuff, I wondered?

I flipped back pages to find the name of the sole author of the chapter, entitled "Early

Detection of Breast Cancer." It was Dr. Anthony B. Miller, chief architect of the Canadian NBSS, revealing his personal bias long before any results from the CNBSS were available.

No one is immune. We bring our bias to the table. Evidence-based medicine brings great sophistication in raising the bar of bias; it does not eradicate it. Sharpening the sword of rhetoric does not necessarily give us Reality. The problem is in our minds, said Francis Bacon more than 400 years ago. Bacon's answer, of course, was not strict empiricism, rather a fusion of rational thought and empiricism.

Why do the two studies of the Canadian NBSS—the only two prospective studies of mammography with no measurable benefit at all—become the bedrock of belief for so many? Eight other prospective RCTs show measurable benefit, some significant and some not, but altogether, a statistically significant mortality reduction with screening mammography. Why cling to Canada?

As we're about to see, the zero impact on mortality as described in the CNBSS is the perfect springboard from which to dive back into the Four Horsemen of Bias. Specifically, without the messy problem of saved lives obscuring the statistics, length bias and overdiagnosis bias resume their positions front and center, ready to tarnish results from all trials. One bad apple, or in this case, two bad apples (Study-1 and Study-2) are setting the stage to prove that something rotten goes way beyond Denmark.

# 12

# Overdiagnosis: Embracing Your Inner Malignancy

Nothing yanks the chain of the breast radiologist like "overdiagnosis," one of the "Four Horsemen That Inflate the Power of Mammography" from Chapter 5. Unfortunately, debate has stalled in crossfire where the combatants are talking past each other. Most have not come to grips with the fact that our language does not currently allow for shades of gray in this area, clumping a variety of scenarios into one rancid bouquet.

So let me draw upon that great philosopher, Calvin (the one with the tiger friend), who proclaimed, "Ultimately, knowledge is paralyzing." When it comes to overdiagnosis, we are paralyzed. Some experts place the figure at 0–5%, others are convinced that it's 20–30%, while extremists ratchet the toll up to 50%. How could the range be so wide, a tip-off that something's amiss? These are all smart people coming up with wildly different numbers. The greater the discrepancy, the more we distrust the process. Yet true believers quote this or that number with total conviction. What's going on?

The concept of overdiagnosis is not new. Epidemiologists were concerned about it from the earliest days of medical screening, especially cancer screening. Quite simply, overdiagnosis is the detection of disease that will never cause symptoms or death during a patient's lifetime. And while the definition might sound simple, the reality is not. What do these fake cancers do if there is no screening? Sit there quietly for a lifetime? What if the patient is young with decades of remaining life? Do they disappear? They certainly look like "real" cancers under the microscope—that is, screen-detected invasive cancers look exactly like palpable cancers.

One cannot detect which cancers are "harmless," so to speak, when addressing individual patients. Overdiagnosis is a phenomenon that can only be evaluated through the study of large populations, which is a mine field of caveats. This is a perfect time to re-work the forest vs. trees cliché—clinicians are dealing with individual trees, while epidemiologists, in claiming overdiagnosis, are looking at the forest. The problem is that they are viewing that forest indirectly through fun-house mirrors. Even at the population level, you can only conclude a rate of overdiagnosis *indirectly*. You can't see it, and you can't prove it.

Because overdiagnosis is so closely related to length bias (a.k.a. length time bias), it helps to review the latter. Length bias is the tendency of screening, by virtue of long intervals between screens, to detect slower-growing tumors (the aggressive ones pop up between screens), thus rendering an apparent advantage to screening that is an illusion. As an aside, when recommendations for screening use longer intervals, this bias will *increase*, as will the opportunity for more aggressive cancers to arise in between screens, a.k.a. "interval cancers."

Length bias can have a powerful effect, and for anti-screeners, it's a wonderland for mammography bashing. When there is a proven mortality reduction in a prospective randomized trial, such as the Swedish Two-County, then length bias has minimal impact on the interpretation. Right or wrong, through circular reasoning, it adds legitimacy to using "downstaging" (earlier stages) through screening as a surrogate endpoint for lives saved.

But when there is no overall mortality reduction, as in the Canadian NBSS, "downstaging" and "better survival" for those women with cancer detected by mammography can be attributed 100% to length time bias and overdiagnosis. It is these spin-off conclusions from the CNBSS that make it so popular for anti-screeners. Thus, the fingers of the CNBSS are far more penetrating than a simple outlier where, uniquely, there was no mortality reduction. No, the CNBSS serves as a playground for the study of these biases, which are revealed in all their might. Supporters of the CNBSS, as we watch the data mature in upcoming chapters, will extract data for mammographically-detected cancers to bolster claims of length bias and overdiagnosis bias, while at the same time, attempting to dispel "myths" about poor mammographic quality.

In order to make a distinction between length bias and overdiagnosis, it helps to divide the cancers into "slowly progressing" for length bias, and "never progressing" for overdiagnosis. Thus, it takes much longer follow-up to demonstrate overdiagnosis, perhaps explaining, in part, why it has leap-frogged over length bias when it comes to "popularity" in recent years as we now have long-term follow-up on the original RCTs performed in the 1970s and 1980s. As to the distinction between the two, the implications are vastly different. Length bias "simply" distorts the benefit of screening. Much more concerning, overdiagnosis has treatment implications, specifically, *overtreatment* for a cancer that was never going to hurt the patient. As stated earlier, of the 4 biases, only overdiagnosis is a potential harm.

With all that said, is it real? Do we really have overdiagnosis in breast cancer? Nearly all experts would agree that this occurs in ductal carcinoma in situ (DCIS), which is best described as a "non-obligated precursor" for invasive breast cancer. That said, there are strong disagreements as to the likelihood of future invasion by DCIS and its panoply of biologies. But I'm going to focus on *invasive* breast cancer and overdiagnosis because this is what is "new," making tempers fly.

First, be aware that epidemiologists consider overdiagnosis a "given" in screening for medical diseases in general, not limited to cancer screening. Consider it a side effect. A necessary evil, if you will. And consider it guilty until proven innocent. It's always going to be there for the epidemiologist, so the key questions are "How big is the problem?" and "Does it lead to overtreatment?"

H. Gilbert Welch, M.D., whom we've met already from his study of autopsies in 1997 that suggested overdiagnosis of DCIS (but *not* invasive disease), is a gifted communicator. And when he begins his sermon, he starts with an idealized "picture" of the astronomic entity we know as a black hole. Of course, we cannot confirm black holes through direct visualization since the power of gravity is so great that light cannot escape. Yet black holes are accepted as scientific reality through multiple indirect measurements, confirming their existence from many angles. And this is how it works for overdiagnosis in invasive breast cancer. You can't actually see "overdiagnosis" in an individual; you can only theorize its presence through indirect measurements in populations.

One of these approaches is to monitor the number of "excessive" cancers in the screening limbs of the prospective RCTs over the long haul. For instance, in the Malmö trial (one of the Swedish studies), there was a persistent excess of 115 cancers in the screened group 15 years after the trial was completed, translating to a 10% rate of overdiagnosis.[1] Dr. Welch, however, looked at the same data and managed to wrestle a 25% rate of overdiagnosis,[2] demonstrating the pliable nature of the overdiagnosis label. Critics of Welch dismantle his high numbers based on a variety of false assumptions and methodologic errors, but we won't need to travel that far to challenge the staggering rate of overdiagnosis as calculated by Dr. Welch.

Estimates of overdiagnosis began pouring out for the various trials, with numbers all over the map, ranging from "0 to 54%" (we saw in an earlier chapter how that 54% was misquoted, but it adopted "truthiness" long before that). Rather than sort through the morass with intended discernment, some public health experts have chosen an "average" of 30% as a recommended value to include in educational materials when warning patients of the harms of screening. Women don't seem to be buying into this "information." In fact, the studies have already been done to better understand why women fail to appreciate the ogre of overdiagnosis. Editorials in major journals have worked hard to treat the rampant overdiagnosis problem as a crisis in comprehension. But rather than join the fashion trend, let's dig deeper.

There is a clear reason why we have such a wide range of calculated overdiagnosis. A helpful resource comes from an article by Dr. Stephen Feig, breast radiologist at University of California, Irvine, who, as we previously noted, has extended his expertise to cost-effective analyses as well as the epidemiology of screening (and who resigned in protest from the Canadian NBSS).[3] Due to some breast cancer biologies that are slowly progressive, at least 25 years of follow-up are needed to calculate overdiagnosis rates, and ideally, the last 10 years should be without screening in both groups—those originally screened vs. not screened.

This "no screening period" allows women in the unscreened group to "catch up" with those who underwent prior screening. This is the "natural" way to adjust for lead time. (Yes, *lead* time works at the end of studies, just like it works as a bias at the front end of screening studies.) If this "natural" method is not used (and it's nearly impossible to do so), then epidemiologists have ways to correct for the lead time that would otherwise cause excessive cancers in the screened group. Even this correction is not straightforward because mean lead times (1–4 years) used in these adjustments do not always account for the very broad range of biology. Some breast cancers can recur up to 20–25 years after diagnosis.

Additionally, corrections in trials that are not randomized must include risk status of the patients, as the "screened" group may include a disproportionate number of women who are motivated to get mammograms due to their heightened personal risk. More cancers will be discovered in this group as a result. In an overlooked article from 2009,[4] Dr. Puliti and colleagues from the Cancer Prevention and Research Institute in Florence, Italy, reviewed 16 studies that had calculated overdiagnosis rates. In the 10 studies that had not made the proper adjustments for lead time and patient risk status, the overdiagnosis rates ranged from 30% to 54%. However, among the 6 studies that made appropriate adjustments, overdiagnosis ranged from 1% to 10%.

While all this was brewing behind the scenes, so to speak, with the public privy to very little of the debate, the controversy went viral on November 22, 2012, with publication in the *New England Journal of Medicine* of an article by Archie Bleyer, M.D., of the St. Charles Health System in Oregon, and H. Gilbert Welch, M.D., of Dartmouth.[5] From a massive

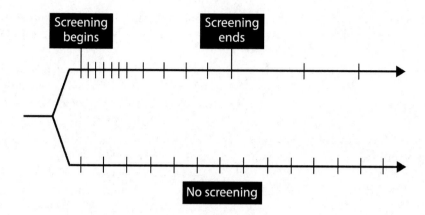

**Correction for lead time. Hash marks represent newly diagnosed cancers in a screening trial where the top limb is screened and bottom limb is not screened (both limbs have 14 marks). The institution of screening always generates more diagnoses up front until a "steady state" is reached. At the end of a screening trial, there will always be more cancers in the screened group, prematurely implicating overdiagnosis. If no one in either limb is screened subsequently (for 10 years or so), then the "no screening" limb should catch up to the screened limb. Rarely can this be observed, given that patient screening habits after the study period cross over between the two limbs, with non-screeners opting for mammography while those in the screening limb may opt out of mammography. Therefore, epidemiologists have tools to adjust for the lead time problem, and the more attention paid to this adjustment, the lower the overdiagnosis rate.**

database called SEER (Surveillance, Epidemiology, and End Results), examining trends from 1976 to 2008, a comparison was made between the increased incidence of early-stage breast cancers and the decrease in late-stage breast cancers.

The premise was this—if every cancer detected by mammography was clinically significant, then there should be a concomitant decrease in late-stage disease matching early detection. Instead, Bleyer and Welch found a large excess of early stage cancers, and from this, came the staggering conclusion that, in 2008, 70,000 women (or 31%) with a new diagnosis of breast cancer had been overdiagnosed. Applying this over the long term, 1.3 million women in the U.S. over the past 30 years had been overdiagnosed. Soon, Dr. Welch was giving his "black hole" pitch to breast cancer specialists everywhere. For many, it was the first time they had considered the concept of overdiagnosis for invasive disease. And the *New England Journal of Medicine* article served as a complement to Dr. Welch's book, *Overdiagnosed: Making People Sick in the Pursuit of Health* (Boston: Beacon Press, 2012).

As often occurs in complex biologic problems, a charge can be levied that sounds simple and plausible, yet it takes a high degree of sophistication to answer. Stated alternatively (and repeatedly in this book), slinging mud is easy, cleaning it off is hard. Big Data sometimes leads to Big Mistakes due to Big Caveats and Bigger Holes of Missing Information.

One question tossed into the ring immediately after the Bleyer-Welch article was "What were the screening habits of those women? Was each chart reviewed to document long-term screening compliance?" Of course not, and SEER does not distinguish women who were screened and who were not screened. The authors had no clue as to which tumors were screen-detected and which were palpated. It was an indirect look at indirect evidence, whereupon a black hole appeared. There were so many "assumptions" and "best-guess estimates" that Dr. László Tabár publicized that the authors had used 71 terms of imprecision in the article (nonetheless, the *New England Journal* would not print Dr. Tabár's response that criticized the Bleyer-Welch article, demonstrating once again how hard it is to buck the fashionable trend.)

The true endpoint we're after is mortality reduction. Advanced cancer, as used in the Bleyer-Welch study is only a surrogate. But the reasoning of the authors goes like this—when you look only at mortality, you can't tease out the effect of adjuvant systemic therapy (which, by the way, was not routine in the early years of their study). But if you focus only on the Stage at the time of diagnosis, you should see a direct effect—for every early diagnosis, there should be one less advanced cancer. In fact, cases of advanced cancer did decline over the years in the Bleyer-Welch study, but "only" 8%, less than expected based on the increase in "early detection." Thus, massive overdiagnosis.

Cleaning off the mud is a task best left to other epidemiologists, but for some reason, their voice is rarely heard. At the 2014 American Society of Breast Surgeons meeting, where I previously mentioned participating in an ad hoc committee on screening, I had the opportunity to interact with the luminaries in this debate. Representatives from each camp had delivered formal presentations to the Society earlier in the day. One of those luminaries was H. Gilbert Welch, M.D. Measuring overdiagnosis had sounded so simple when described by Dr. Welch, but when other epidemiologists and biostatisticians in the room began countering with complexities, it became clear why the calculated overdiagnosis rate ranges from 0 to 54%.

For example, Robert A. Smith, PhD, lead epidemiologist for the American Cancer Society sat on the committee as well, and he pointed out that the Bleyer-Welch study had assumed the underlying breast cancer incidence was flat. In fact, considerable evidence was available to indicate that breast cancer incidence was on the rise even without the introduction of screening mammography. This would skew results toward higher rates of overdiagnosis. Even more importantly, he pointed out the failure to correct for lead time, something he later published,[6] where Dr. Smith's estimate of overdiagnosis from the same data used by Dr. Welch was only 5%.

One of the major problems in this overdiagnosis mayhem is the inability to monitor mammography habits of women after a trial has concluded its (relatively short) active screening period. Controlled chaos is already underway *during* a prospective, randomized trial with women crossing over against study design. But afterwards, the problem is worse. Do the women who were randomized to the mammography group continue more reliably with lifetime mammograms than the women who were assigned to no mammography during the trial? If so, then there will always be an excess of cancers in the screening limb, until one of two things happen—(1) the aforementioned 25-year follow-up with the final 10 years of "no screening," or (2) one must correct for lead time. Only #2 can be performed from a practical standpoint.

One more point of interest about the Bleyer-Welch article—their 31% calculation for overdiagnosis applies to *all* women diagnosed with breast cancer, but only half of these cancers were mammographically-detected (50% being an assumption from population statistics). Thus, to apply their findings to the mammography-detected group alone, the overdiagnosis rate would be double their published conclusion, or 62%. Why was this not their final overdiagnosis rate? Was it because it would convert an intriguing, semi-believable 31% and turn it into a preposterous 62%?

Overdiagnosis would be more acceptable if it were not so potentially harmful through its implicated tie to *overtreatment*. If women are undergoing mastectomy for a cancer that doesn't kill, it's a big deal. Breast conservation lessens the impact only a little, as there are still complications of lymph node assessment and radiation therapy, not to mention endocrine therapy, chemotherapy, and biotherapy.

Let's come clean, though. Overtreatment is a mainstay of cancer therapy, and it forces breast radiologists to draw upon this fact in their written defense statements, incidentally stepping on the toes of radiation oncologists and medical oncologists. After cancer has been removed, patients are given a baseline survival rate if they do nothing else. Then, they are told the benefit of adding radiation and/or systemic therapies, but we really don't know who has residual cancer and who does not. Therefore, the longstanding principle has been to treat with adjuvant therapy ("blindly," after tumor removal) and, as it turns out, we have better outcomes … for the population as a whole. For the individual, however, most don't benefit in early stage disease.

Unthinkable? Not at all. We've simply done it for so long, we don't give it much thought. If a calculated survival rate after lumpectomy is 80% already, then it follows that the greatest possible benefit of additional therapy is only 20% in absolute terms. If adjuvant therapies get you to 90%, that's a 10% absolute improvement. However, cancer recurrence is all-or-nothing—if you're in that 10%, you have greatly benefitted, perhaps you've been cured. But if you don't respond to the additional therapies, you're in a different 10%, that is, the tumor will recur in spite of the adjuvant therapy. So 80% didn't require the adjuvant therapy in the first place, then for another 10% it didn't help, while 10% benefit greatly—that's 90% "overtreatment." This has not gone unnoticed, of course, and huge efforts are being made to precisely determine who needs what therapy and when.

All aspects of cancer diagnosis and treatment have, in the past, congregated under one large tent. And while outposts are under construction to group patients with specific needs, we are still in the early stages. If an invasive cancer is diagnosed by mammography, there is no possible way to be certain as to whether it's deadly or not. So the rhetorical questions are "Why slap numbers onto the possibility of overdiagnosis during the informed consent process, as is being recommended today?" "With numbers from '0 to 54%,' with very little understanding as to how this unreliable range is derived, who benefits?" "Why is overdiagnosis of '30%,' let's say, being treated as a certain Reality when it's anything but?" "How can providers deliver informed consent for screening mammography when they are being misinformed?"

Dr. Dan Kopans, the outspoken Harvard breast radiologist, will turn red-faced and steam will pour out of his ears when inflated numbers for overdiagnosis are publicized. He's never seen a single cancer that festers in the breast without progressing, nor have I. But what if the epidemiologists are talking about something else? What if they are describing a different phenomenon than what we see in prostate cancer, where "festering" is common?

In the next chapter, I'll propose 3 different scenarios for "overdiagnosis," and for lack of a better name for each type, I'll default to Type I, Type II and Type III.

Proposed in the 17th century, one of Francis Bacon's "Four Idols" was the "Idols of the Marketplace," his term for the problematic nature of language—that is, words used as currency in the exchange of ideas. Bacon expressed doubts that science, then called "natural philosophy," could ever achieve consensus due to the fact that words would not be understood in the same way by warring parties. So, with a nod to Francis, I'm going to be painfully precise in my attempt to classify overdiagnosis.

Epidemiologists might object to my proposed system, but I can rest in the comfort that the words they use in their objections will be so obtuse as to defy understanding by regular people.

# 13

# Overdiagnosis Part 2:
# A Way Out of the Wet Paper Bag

## Type I Overdiagnosis (a.k.a. "Festering Cancers")

This is the commonly conceived portrait of overdiagnosis—that screening will find invasive cancers that, if left alone, would "fester" and never kill the host (patient). These lesions meet the definition of cancer under the microscope, in fact, they look the same as cancers discovered by palpation, but looks are deceiving—they're allegedly harmless. Drs. Welch and Bleyer have offered up the bizarre claim that this happens 70,000 times a year, prompting outcries from every breast radiologist in the country. Note the pure definition of overdiagnosis does not allow for a slow-growing tumor (length bias); it mandates that the cancer *never* become clinically apparent—thus, my use of the term "fester" to describe a tumor that sits in place and does nothing, as we have already seen as a rather common occurrence with low grade prostate cancers. The only other scenario to explain this pure definition would be if invasive breast cancers spontaneously regress, something very real to certain epidemiologists who practice numerology, but a near impossibility for those who actually see untreated breast cancers.

Speaking for Dr. Welch, he might say, "How would you know if cancers were festering or regressing? You take them all out after the diagnosis."

The answer: "Oh, no, we don't."

All breast radiologists, and other specialties as well, have encountered two scenarios where we get to witness the natural history of untreated breast cancer. Neither scenario is pretty, but facts are facts. The first is the delayed diagnosis, where cancer is missed on the first mammogram, then picked up a year or two later when the tumor is more obvious. And the second situation is when patients consent to biopsy, whereupon the invasive cancer is diagnosed, but then all treatment is refused (collectively, a fair number nationwide). In these instances, we get to watch the natural history of breast cancer unfold.

Breast cancer can sometimes grow quite slowly. So-called "doubling times" are based on tumor volume ($V=4/3\pi r^3$), not diameter. Diameter can change very little over time, increasing only slightly while volume doubles. But over this protracted course, be it a diagnostic delay or a treatment delay, we don't see invasive cancers regress[1] and we don't see them stay the same size when missed earlier. They get larger. And, as they get larger, they are eventually felt. Now, they may not have the potential to spread and kill, but they will become clinically

95

evident if the patient lives long enough, prompting diagnosis and treatment without mammography having been performed.

This clinical emergence of a "harmless cancer" violates the basic definition of overdiagnosis, which states that these pseudocancers *never* become clinically apparent. That is, not only are they harmless to the host, but also they remain hidden clinically. *This definition mandates that, if cancers don't regress, a high reservoir of invasive cancers must be found at autopsy or in preventive mastectomy specimens.* If not, then we're dealing with length bias, not overdiagnosis.

Remember, too, the data from Dr. Sam Hellman and his Spectrum Theory, where tumors "de-differentiate" as they get larger. That is, they become "more malignant" over time, with new mutations occurring in the tumor cells *after* cancer has already developed. This was recognized long before genetic analyses became available, simply by looking at tumor grade with an old-fashioned light microscope. As tumors get bigger, a greater proportion will be higher grade.

If we quit screening for breast cancer, are we really going to entertain the notion that 70,000 cancers a year would regress, or not grow to the point of palpation, if we had simply not screened? This is exceedingly improbable. Where is the footprint of this stance? There should be an enormous reservoir of undiagnosed cancers in autopsy series, as seen with prostate cancer.

Instead, as introduced earlier in this book, the primary autopsy review was performed, ironically, by Dr. H. Gilbert Welch in his early anti-screening days, in an effort to discredit the detection of DCIS. While some DCIS may fit the bill of "festering," only 1.3% of women at autopsy were found to have undiagnosed *invasive* breast cancer, the exact prevalence of undiagnosed breast cancer in the living. Invasive breast cancer does not fester! And the proof came from Dr. Welch. We don't know the screening habits in these autopsy series, but the earliest were prior to the mammographic era. Even assuming good screening compliance later on, a large reservoir of invasive cancers should have been present, in line with the DCIS data.

Indeed, Dr. Welch did find a reservoir of DCIS (9%; range 0 to 14.7%), though even this was nothing in comparison to the prostate cancer data. We are unlikely to see more autopsy data emerge, given that this practice has been dwindling away for many years. So it is most remarkable that the strongest argument against classic overdiagnosis comes from a long-forgotten study by the chief architect of overdiagnosis in invasive cancer, rendering a big black hole in the deductive rhetoric.

Today, when trying to inflate the evidence for overdiagnosis, some authors will reference the Welch autopsy study and make the claim that "up to 15% of women die with undiagnosed breast cancer." What these sophists are doing, of course, is quoting the DCIS study with the highest number and calling it "breast cancer" with the unwritten implication that this is invasive disease, or that it consists of the usual ratio of invasion:DCIS. It makes you want to cry.

In this era of evidence-based medicine, it is remarkable that there is no direct evidence to support allegations of massive overdiagnosis through screening for invasive cancer. Indeed, the only semi-direct evidence indicates quite the opposite—a mere 1.3% autopsy incidence for invasive cancer, the exact number one would expect with little or no overdiagnosis. While it may take a PhD in epidemiology to identify the methodologic flaws in calculating 70,000, even a lowly M.D. can understand that a 1.3% autopsy incidence of invasive cancer should put an end to the incredulous rates of overdiagnosis being perpetrated today as scientific fact.

Type I overdiagnosis is clearly at work in low grade prostate cancer, and this is why I devoted an entire chapter earlier to the cautionary note to keep prostate and breast separate.

Recall that autopsy series show occult cancer present in men roughly equivalent to their age, such that an 80-year-old man has an 80% chance of harboring occult cancer, "festering" at the time of death. Urologists even offer "observation alone" for low grade prostate cancer, but you'll never hear this option from an oncologist after needle biopsy confirms the presence of invasive breast cancer—the biology is different and so is the screening.

As for DCIS and its modest reservoir in the same autopsy study, the argument can be made that mammographically-detected DCIS is a different animal—by laying down calcifications, or by presenting as a mass due to reactive inflammation and fibrosis, the DCIS found by radiologists could be more committed to becoming invasive than the incidental findings at autopsy. DCIS found by MRI might be even more biologically significant, as it is associated with angiogenesis that surrounds the ducts even at the pre-invasive stage.[2] The natural history of various forms of DCIS is an active area of research, and we should all be mindful of the extremely long natural history of this entity,[3] making sure to include extended follow-up in the planned studies of observation alone for DCIS.

## Type II(A) Overdiagnosis (Pseudo-Pseudocancers)

Since, *unlike* prostate cancer, invasive breast cancer doesn't regress or fester, how could we explain the 70,000 from the Welch analysis, if we accept that number as a possibility? Well, how many options are there? In other words, let's pick a single invasive cancer and figure out how it behaves such that it gets counted as overdiagnosis, especially given the fact we know it doesn't fester or regress (Type I). The options are pretty limited.

Let's go back to Chapter 2 where I discussed Dr. Hellman's Spectrum Theory. In that diagram, which is a merger of two older competing theories (Halsted and Fisher), there was a Biologic A (local, spreading only late), a Goldilocks biology where A converts to B during the clinical window, and Biologic B (spreads early in its course, prior to early detection).

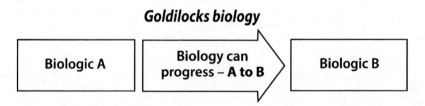

Spectrum Theory. Biologic A tumors are unlikely to progress to systemic disease, until very late in their course. They will not be affected by early detection through screening because they will still be cured after becoming palpable. Biologic B tumors have already become systemic early in their course, so they too are unaffected by early detection. The Goldilocks tumors in the center demonstrate progression from A to B during the clinical window. Enlarging that window to include early detection through mammography is where mortality can be impacted.

Now let's suppose that the Biologic A tumors are responsible for overdiagnosis. The numbers match up fairly well, though they are so speculative as to be illustrative only. Still, I propose, while dangling from a mathematical limb, based on mortality reductions through screening mammography (30% for compliant patients) that 1 in 3 patients have a Goldilocks biology that makes their tumor vulnerable to early detection. Women in this group, however, must be compliant with mammography as the tumors will eventually convert to systemic disease. If we place roughly one-third into each of the 3 groups, and an estimated 240,000 women will be diagnosed with invasive cancer each year, then we have 80,000 women in each group. Could it be that Bleyer and Welch are measuring the number of women who have Biologic A tumors? That is, cancers that do not kill even when discovered relatively late?

Now let's imagine what would be the natural course if we take the 70,000 excised pseudo-cancers hypothesized by Bleyer and Welch, and now re-insert those tumors that were discovered by mammography back into the black hole left by the lumpectomy (or mastectomy). They don't fester, so what do they do? What would be their natural history? *They grow.* But they grow without metastasizing. These Biologic A patients are still cured after the cancers become palpable.

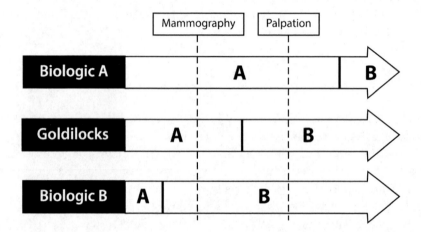

Another way to conceptualize Spectrum Theory as it relates to the impact of mammography and over-diagnosis. In this schematic, all tumors progress from A (local) to B (systemic), but the point at which that occurs varies widely depending on the inherent biology of the tumor. In Biologic A tumors, it does not matter whether the cancer is found by mammography or later on by palpation, the patient will likely be cured of her disease. For Goldilocks tumors, if mammography is performed in the A phase, this is where lives are saved. For Biologic B tumors, metastatic disease has already established itself prior to the mammogram, so there will be no benefit from screening.

With regard to *overdiagnosis*, Biologic A tumors might be regarded as overdiagnosis in statistical analyses of large populations, but technically, these tumors are progressing very slowly, and if the patient lives long enough, most will become palpable (and still curable) years later. This is length time bias at work more than true overdiagnosis. Some will convert to systemic disease very late in their course. By strict definition, overdiagnosis means tumors do not progress at all (or regress), and thus, they are always *overtreated.* The near total absence (99%) of "reservoir" cancers in autopsy studies, however, makes this scenario very unlikely for invasive breast cancer (nor do invasive cancers regress). But in this Type II scenario, where overdiagnosis might appear in large population studies, the fear of overtreatment is mostly unfounded, as the patient will eventually receive the same treatment once the tumor becomes palpable.

Recall the distinction between length time bias and overdiagnosis—the former occurs with tumors that progress very slowly, while the latter occurs with tumors that don't progress at all. Thus, 70,000 seems less bizarre if one considers these as the "slowly progressing tumors" we've acknowledged for many years. But these are not "pseudocancers" as alleged by Dr. Welch and others. I'm proposing that they're nothing more than the same Biologic A tumors that are described by Spectrum or Fisher theories, something we've accepted for decades. Type II is thus more accurately characterized as "length time bias," occurring in those breast cancers with a very long natural history.

Now, if you're still with me, the question arises—what does it matter? After all, if these Biologic A tumors were never going to harm the patient, then mammography is still dredging them up and forcing unnecessary treatment. It's not overdiagnosis alone that's the problem, it's the overtreatment that goes with it.

And here's the most important statement in this chapter, and the reason I've spent so much time on the relentless "growth" of invasive breast cancer (as opposed to festering)—without mammography, these indolent Biologic A tumors *still grow* to the point that they become palpable, thus they will be treated eventually anyway, *if the patient lives long enough.* We don't have the means to confirm Biologic A tumors face-to-face, so to speak, so the treatment will be the same whether it's through mammographic discovery or by palpation later on. Thus, mammography is not forcing overtreatment, rather, it is simply moving treatment up earlier than what would have been.

Tumor growth and systemic metastases are only loosely linked in breast cancer. Dr. Bernie Fisher was working only with clinically palpable tumors in his formative research days. It was apparent that very small tumors could kill early, while other large tumors did not. The critical issue at play for Fisher was the host-tumor relationship. It wasn't the tumor alone. Great enthusiasm exists today for defining biologic sub-types based on genetic profiles within the tumor, but that's only half the story. The other half is the host and her immune surveillance system. How is her body going to respond to a particular biology? Different people will react to the same biologic tumor in different ways. Yes, tumor size is a prognosticator of outcome, but it's only one of many variables. A woman with a *large* Biologic A (local until late) tumor is going to do much better than if she has a *small* Biologic B (systemic early).

So, for the Biologic A tumors, if they are found at 1.0cm on mammography or 3.0cm by palpation, it doesn't matter because the patient is cured regardless. The danger of overdiagnosis is overtreatment, but all Biologic A tumors are "overtreated" if you want to get technical, regardless of whether they were found on mammography or palpated. That said, Biologic A tumors, very late in their course, untreated, will eventually grow and metastasize, causing death if the patient lives long enough, something known from historical data generated at Middlesex Hospital in London.[4]

Yet these 70,000 women with Biologic A tumors appear on the books through Big Data as overdiagnosis. Without mammography, though, the tumors would have eventually appeared clinically by palpation, though perhaps many years later. Thus, there is a fine and shaky line in the distinction between length bias (slowly progressing) and overdiagnosis bias (never progressing), the latter far more anxiety-provoking and thus, more popular as a focus for anti-screeners with its overtreatment implications. Yet, in summary, what we're probably observing is length bias with Biologic A tumors where the natural history can be quite protracted.

And that brings us back to the requirement that if you don't have 25-year follow-up, with 10 years of "no screening" at the end, then you'd better correct for lead time. If you don't, you're going to generate high numbers for overdiagnosis. Even if you correct for lead time, you will still register some overdiagnosis due to a little problem I'm going to call Type IIB (a.k.a. death).

## Type IIB Overdiagnosis (Death)

Suppose you are diagnosed with breast cancer through mammography, and it so happens you had a Goldilocks biology and your life will thus be saved through screening. Upon discharge from the hospital after your lumpectomy, though, you are hit by a bus and do not survive your injuries. Guess where you end up when it comes to the epidemiologist's ledger? Overdiagnosis. That's how the epidemiology of screening works, and that's how overdiagnosis works. Hard to believe? I had not thought this through until I read an interview with Anthony B. Miller, M.D., of the Canadian NBSS who was asked the question point blank, admitting that if this scenario were to occur, yes, it would be counted as overdiagnosis.

The bus accident is extreme, so how often does this really happen? How often does unrelated death intervene and skew the data toward overdiagnosis? Not so often in younger women, but death due to competing mortality *from any cause* is a big deal when you get older (thus, the efforts to define the optimal age to stop screening). So how about the 70-year-old who is diagnosed with a Goldilocks tumor and her life saved by mammography, who then dies of a heart attack 5 years later? Same thing. Overdiagnosis. How long does this problem exist after mammographic detection? Since low grade tumors can take 20–25 years to run their course, it's not an uncommon event at all. It very likely accounts for a big part of the Big Data.

So, in this age of exhaustive informed consents, are we are to dwell on Type IIB overdiagnosis so that our patients think twice before mammograms? Is this the message? "You must consider the fact that if we save your life with mammography, but you die from something else in the meantime, then we've overdiagnosed and overtreated you, so let us apologize for that in advance." Technically, it may be true, but what purpose does it serve? You can apply co-morbidity and unrelated mortality to many things in medicine, an unsolvable problem given the eventual mortality rate of 100%.

Distinguishing Type IIA from Type IIB is not really possible, given overlap due to very slow progression of some breast cancers. Let me give you a commonly encountered example, though, using a tumor that is likely Biologic A—tubular cancer—and see how this "very slow progression" plays out in Big Data.

A 75-year-old patient is found to have a 0.8cm tubular cancer on screening mammography and is treated with lumpectomy. What would have happened if there had been no mammograms? Odds are that she would die of unrelated causes before the tumor became life-threatening (Type IIB overdiagnosis).

Tubular carcinoma is a very well-differentiated invasive ductal cancer, a slow-grower. Growth from one year to the next on a mammogram might be nearly imperceptible. Furthermore, a thorough literature review would come up empty-handed in trying to document a single death from a "pure" tubular cancer under 1.0cm in size. Wait a minute! That fits the definition of a Welch pseudocancer, Type I overdiagnosis, a tumor that never progresses.

Not so fast. Back in the day when pathology cancer research was pretty well limited to the light microscope, someone noticed that there were precious few large tubular cancers. Screening mammography really brought tubulars to the forefront, much as had been done with DCIS. In fact, the "minimal cancer" concept included many tubulars, always small. Well, the natural history was worked out by correlating tubular cancer size to "purity," i.e., how much of the surface area on the microscope slide fits the definition of "tubular" and how much is ordinary invasive ductal cancer?

Routine (usually Grade 1 or 2) invasive ductal features on the same slide as the tubular features represented "de-differentiation" of the tumor—that is, a cancer that becomes "more malignant" over time (a critical feature of Spectrum Theory, minimized in Fisher Theory). Malignant cells have many genetic mutations, but time allows many more. In de-differentiation, or worsening Grade, the pathologist sees the cells as more and more abnormal. So, in this correlative exercise, the larger that tubulars grew, the less pure they became, representing progression, or de-differentiation. Tubulars under 1.0cm were "pure tubular," those between 1.0cm and 2.0cm were part tubular and part "garden variety" invasive ductal, and tumors larger than 2.0cm had only partial remnants of the original tubular cancer. How many tubulars are there larger than 3.0cm? Very few. Breast cancer can de-differentiate over time.

Back to our patient with a 0.8cm pure tubular cancer. If this had not been removed, it would have taken a number of years before it de-differentiated and picked up growth speed to the point of palpation, maybe as long as 5–10 years. For our patient, then, we are looking at palpation by age 80 to 85, now perhaps a surgical risk from co-morbid conditions that developed since age 75. But that aside, she would still be treated if she lives long enough. If she doesn't live to the point of palpation, this scenario is then tallied by Big Data as Type II overdiagnosis due to mammography. In fact, it was length time bias, but death allowed overdiagnosis to win on a technicality.

You might be one step ahead of me already at this point. Overdiagnosis is a greater issue in the elderly by virtue of fewer years to allow the natural history of these low-grade lesions to evolve. Take our 0.8cm tubular cancer, or DCIS, and put it in a 40-year-old, whereupon competing mortality is not going to have much of an impact at all. The natural history will evolve. This *lower* rate of overdiagnosis in younger women has been well-documented and serves as a tremendous thorn in the side to anti-screeners who work hard to tally the "greater harms of screening mammography in younger women."

More rhetorical questioning: Why are public health aficionados insisting we give women in their 40s informed consent about mammography that includes the higher rates of overdiagnosis based on Type IIA and Type IIB overdiagnosis that is largely drawn from the elderly? Why, too, are we using the term "overdiagnosis" so liberally when we're really observing length bias played out in older patients?

Finally, there's a third type of overdiagnosis, but it's a misnomer. It would be more accurate to call it a "false positive" or "misdiagnosis," but I include it here because it's another reason why there are "excessive cancers" in screened populations, so the epidemiologists count them and lay blame on the breast radiologists. Indeed, this is the most serious issue of all, yet the problem is not with mammography, the culprit is pathology.

## Type III—Misdiagnosis as Overdiagnosis

Type I overdiagnosis is what many physicians picture when they hear the term "overdiagnosis" ("just like prostate cancer," only it's not); Type II is where epidemiologists can generate massive numbers, which may simply be exaggerated length time bias through uncorrected lead time or patient death; but Type III—benign disease misdiagnosed as cancer—is what many lay people fear. And, for a small number, they're correct. But just how often does this occur? How often is cancer diagnosed when there is no cancer?

In the BCDDP study, recall that breast pathology expert Dr. Robert McDivitt was asked to review 506 cases of "minimal breast cancer" (a term used during that era for LCIS, DCIS, and small invasive cancers, all three entities largely a function of screening mammography). Controversy was already brewing as to how to manage these "minimal cancers." However, exposing an entirely new problem, Dr. McDivitt claimed that 66 of the lesions in question were not cancer at all—not LCIS, not DCIS, and not invasive cancer. 53 of the 66 women had already undergone mastectomy. Was this an aberration of the 1970s, long since corrected?

After a surgical pathology fellowship at UCLA in the academic year 1977–78, I returned to Oklahoma to complete my surgical residency with an entirely new perspective. And if I had to reduce that year in pathology to one word, it would be "subjective." Clinicians who have never rotated to that planet do not appreciate how much subjectivity enters into the diagnosis of disease, in what is generally considered the "most scientific" of the medical specialties. This is especially true in breast pathology where the distinction between precursors and cancer can be subjective, with disagreements even among the experts.

The difference between atypical hyperplasia and carcinoma in situ is not nearly so subjective to a patient, where nothing might be recommended for the former and mastectomy for the latter. Yet there is one step more treacherous than putting labels on the continuums found in breast "premalignancy," and that is a group of lesions that can mimic invasive cancer yet are completely benign. These mimics can trick any pathologist who does not happen to be considering them at the moment of diagnosis. Microglandular adenosis, sclerosing lesions with distorted proliferative epithelium, yes, an entire family of tricksters can appear to be cancer on X-ray with confirmation coming, incorrectly, in the pathology lab.

Many, if not most, of these errors go undiscovered. The patient undergoes surgery with pathology revealing "no residual tumor," then radiation, maybe even chemotherapy or endocrine therapy. Then, she is "cured," forever grateful to the breast radiologist who saved her life. When the problem is discovered through second opinions or cross-checking within the department (most pathologists today double-check routinely), the error is sometimes discovered not with the needle biopsy but, unfortunately, after the entire lesion has been removed as part of the cancer surgery. Juries have little sympathy for the great difficulty we have with some of these mimics, holding pathologists to a standard of human perfection.

Over the years, there have been efforts to address these problems—both the difficult continuum between atypia and carcinoma in situ, as well as the mimics of invasive cancer. White papers have been written, discussions have taken place, but very little makes it into print in major journals to see how we are doing with this problem, a challenge known to exist long before the McDivitt controversy (by the way, the involved surgeons fought McDivitt bitterly to defend their pathologists). But that was nearly 40 years ago! "Certainly, pathology training has taken us beyond that," you might think.

Sorry, it's not so much the science. It's the humanity. And it's the inexact nature of disease. When it comes to the mimics, unless a pathologist thinks, "The first thing I'm going to do is rule out a benign mimic," when looking at a suspected cancer, then it slips to the deeper parts of the brain. Oddly, these mimics are best diagnosed, not at high power (greater magnification), but at low power, where one steps back to look at the big picture for an overall "Gestalt" before zeroing down on the details.

Rarely put into print, this topic was addressed recently in the March 15, 2015, issue of the *JAMA*[5] where interestingly, the lead author, Joann G. Elmore, M.D., MPH, has published cautionary articles on screening mammography, turning here to breast pathology, with the mammography implications being indirect. This labor-intensive study was an attempt to quantify disagreement among pathologists in the interpretation of breast biopsies (4 categories—benign, atypia, DCIS, invasion).

The "official" diagnosis for 240 cases (1 slide per case) was generated by 3 internationally recognized breast pathology experts where, interestingly, they did not agree unanimously in 25% of the cases at first glance, though this number was reduced to 10% disagreement after open discussion. It should be unsettling when I tell you that one of the disagreements surrounded a mimic lesion where 1 of the 3 experts believed an area of invasion was present, the other 2 disagreeing, calling the lesion completely benign.

Then, 115 pathologists got a crack at the same slides, demonstrating a 75.3% concordance with the expert panel. The best concordance occurred in those slides with invasive cancer, but 1% of the invasive calls by the pathologists being studied were considered completely benign by the 3 experts. If one then includes DCIS, then 3.2% of the "cancers" were completely benign according to the experts.

Perhaps more concerning was the nature of some of the completely benign mimics. For Case #60, it appears from the graph in the article that 20% of the pathologists considered a benign lesion as "invasive cancer," while in Case #69, *40% of the 115 pathologists* called a completely benign lesion "invasive cancer." When I use the word "mimic," I hope you can see how difficult this can be. Certainly, as occurs in malpractice trials, juries simply do not believe this can happen. Yet even the experts used in this study did not agree among themselves.

This was a fascinating and pristine effort by Elmore et al., with many more conclusions and inferences. While the findings are certainly applicable to the historic screening trials where these misdiagnosed cases are tallied by today's epidemiologists as "overdiagnosis," the problem persists.

To offer a measure of comfort today, the pathologists in the study were limited to the slides that were offered. In their home court, they could have ordered deeper cuts and special stains that can help make distinctions. For instance, p63 immunohistochemistry allows the pathologist to distinguish normal myoepithelial cells, which surround normal ductal structures. These myoepithelial cells might be partially absent around the ducts in the intermediate stages of DCIS, but are clearly absent in invasive carcinoma. Furthermore, in the real world, pathologists readily send their difficult cases to experts for second opinions.

In summation on this difficult issue of overdiagnosis, *Type I* does not exist, in any practical sense, when it comes to invasive breast cancer, in that it does not "fester" and it does not "regress." The now infamous "70,000" is impossible to explain using this definition, a phenomenon that might be applicable to low grade prostate cancer, but not invasive breast cancer. *Type II(A)* is routinely overstated due to failure to correct for patient risk and lead times, but even if the "70,000" is valid based on Fisher or Spectrum theory, or partially so, the tumors are not truly overdiagnosed (non-progressive) since they would eventually grow and become palpable (slowly progressive), being treated anyway, even if not lethal. Thus, overtreatment of Type II is not the hazard as would be the case with Type I. Moreover, a good proportion of these cases evident in Big Data likely come from Type IIB overdiagnosis in older patients where mortality cuts short the natural history of slow-growing cancers. *Type III*, or "misdiagnosis" of mammographically-generated lesions, is the most troublesome scenario, with valid overtreatment criticisms. This scenario is becoming increasingly rare through the use of special studies by pathologists, along with increasing awareness of the problem. In spite of a few confused journalists who believe this is what is meant for all instances of "over-diagnosis," Type III is responsible for only a small fraction of the total, but having the greatest of consequences.

We will return to our historical sequence covering the evolution of screening recommendations in the next chapter. But to recap, after the bizarre Gøtzsche-Olsen "meta-analysis," where the prospective RCTs that showed mammography benefit were excluded, the temporary flare of tempers and tantrums subsided. Even those cautionary experts who favor less screening had to admit that the Gøtzsche-Olsen paper, and its conclusion that mammography had no benefits whatsoever, wasn't going to fly.

Peace settled over the world of mammographic screening once again, lasting roughly five years. I even began working on a different book about breast cancer screening, tentatively titled *A Bridge Half-Built*, with the intent to explore ways to improve our detection rates while, at the same time, improving cost-effectiveness. My premise was simple: now that we're reasonably settled on current mammography guidelines, what can we do to make things better?

It was not to be. My writings became obsolete overnight. As it turned out, we weren't "settled" on current guidelines for screening mammography at all, so there was no point in building the other half of the bridge when the first half was being bombarded. In November 2009, the U.S. Preventive Services Task Force announced their recommendations, similar to what the National Cancer Institute had done in 1993 to start the Mammography Civil War, that is, start mammographic screening at 50, then screen every 2 years. Here we go again.

# 14

# The Task Force Opens Fire

The U.S. Preventive Services Task Force stunned the world of breast cancer screening with their November 2009 announcement to (1) stop routine mammographic screening for women in their 40s, and (2) switch from screening every year to every 2 years, starting at age 50.

The volleys were swift and intense. Dr. Dan Kopans couldn't believe it—not again, not after all these years, they're starting the same argument that was settled in the 1990s? For breast radiologists, the announcement was nothing short of being told that the United States, upon second thought, had decided to return to Vietnam and finish what we started decades ago. In an unbridled act of total frustration, Dr. Kopans referred to the Task Force as "idiots." And at that point, it can be argued that the 5-star general of the Civil War lost any vestigial remnant of a soap box. Journal editors, with the exception of those dedicated to radiology, refused to publish counter-position editorials by Dr. Kopans (and other pro-screeners), effectively cutting the dialogue in half.

For the vast majority of breast radiologists, and perhaps breast cancer specialists in general, this was the first that they had ever heard of the U.S. Preventive Services Task Force, making the hoopla all that much more surreal. How could this merry band of unknowns get so much publicity, so quickly, out of nowhere, after this controversy had been beaten to death for more than 40 years, and with recommendations already in place by all major medical organizations dealing with oncology? To draw from Paul Newman as Butch Cassidy, the question was "Who are those guys?" And when the noise didn't die down, the question would be raised again and again, "Who are those guys?" Everyone wanted to know, it seemed. Few sought the truth.

"They're a bunch of government bean-counters who reviewed the clinical trials over a weekend of beer and pizza. Weekend warriors, if you must. Dilettantes."

And so it began, with one bizarre statement after another. All in all, I think there have been more mistakes made about the Task Force and their recommendations than any area in breast medicine. It was as though emotions, unshackled, ran free and frenzied, blocking simple assessment of the facts. Here's my take.

First of all, "Who are those guys?"

I became aware of the Task Force through their 2002 publication in the *Annals of Internal Medicine*[1] where, in a very well-researched study of the prospective RCTs, they proposed no major shake-ups in screening recommendations. This will be a curious point to remember when we get to 2009, where a negligible change in raw data prompts a radical change in recommendations.

I had stumbled on the article for a reason not directly related to "screening recommendations." Years ago, I began the practice of looking up references whenever a value for mammographic Sensitivity was quoted. This Task Force article contained important references in this regard that will play a major role later in the book. For now, however, I mention it only to point out that by the time I first learned of the Task Force, comparatively early, they had already been a working group for 18 years! And, by the time that the general public heard about them, they'd already been around for 25 years. Who are those guys?

In 1953, President Eisenhower added the Department of Health, Education, and Welfare to his cabinet, later re-organized as the Department of Health and Human Services (HHS). The HHS includes such well-known operating divisions as the FDA, the CDC, and the NIH. By far, the largest division is the Centers for Medicare and Medicaid Services (CMS), funded at nearly $1 trillion, while the smallest division is the little-known Agency for Healthcare Research and Quality (AHRQ), appropriated for a measly $400 million per year. The U.S. Preventive Services Task Force was created to serve as a group of *independent, non-binding advisors* to this "small" government agency and the HHS in general.

Within hours of the 2009 Task Force announcement, its members were defending themselves against the accusations that they were government stoolies. They pointed out, "We are not government employees!" True, as the 16 members are, in fact, volunteers who are experts in preventive health and evidence-based medicine, most of whom are in private practice (internal medicine, family medicine, pediatric medicine, behavioral health, obstetrics/gynecology, and nursing, according to the AHRQ web site). Yet the group is 100% government-funded and government-appointed (by the director of AHRQ).

From a practical standpoint, the Task Force is an autonomous unit that offers its recommendations directly and openly, *without* the burden of AHRQ or HHS approval. The Task Force addresses evidence for and against preventive health measures and screenings. By their organization's charter, they are not allowed to perform studies of cost-effectiveness. Instead, they are restricted to evaluating evidence for and against various public health measures, whereupon they provide a Grade for each service:

A = a recommended service, with high certainty the net benefit is substantial
B = also recommended, but either the certainty *or* the benefit is only moderate
C = in 2009, it meant a position "against *routine* screening," but the definition changes
D = a recommendation against the service (without qualifiers)
I = insufficient evidence

Over the years, the Task Force has amassed recommendations dealing with nearly 100 preventive health measures. Oh yes, one other thing—according to the rules of evidence-based medicine, *no experts are allowed on the Task Force* when it comes to the specific service being studied (the premise is this: You cannot have service providers evaluating the data!).

This exclusion principle is a sociologic trend playing itself out in many venues, prompting reactions that range from horror to enthusiastic complicity. In essence, many proponents of evidence-based medicine are saying, "We do not want bias, therefore, we are willing to exclude insight, nuance and wisdom in order to make our own judgments." The problem is that it's impossible to exclude bias, no matter who you are, as the very act of judgment is an exercise in human bias.

In the case of breast cancer screening, the "neutral" Task Force sits in judgment about a technology about which they know very little, toying with numbers pertaining to mammography as performed generations ago—indeed, they are a judge and jury that needs no witnesses. Statistics suffice for the think tanks, as is true for evidence-based medicine in general, under the improbable notion that numbers can neither be manipulated nor interpreted differently by different observers. This brings up the theme I've introduced already—empiricism to the exclusion of rational thought.

It is also important to realize that membership on the Task Force rotates, such that when the 2016 update was provided for breast cancer screening, only one member of the 2009 Task Force—the immediate past chair—served as liaison to the new 16-member committee (17 names are credited on the 2016 update, 12 males and 5 females for those who are curious). With nearly 100 topics covered by the Task Force over the years (some inactive or being updated), where members serve only four years before rotating off, I have to wonder about the depth of understanding for each of the volunteers on each of the preventive measures (I can barely keep up with the evidence surrounding one policy, and I do it full-time).

The Task Force serves as the guiding light on such screening controversies as screening for vitamin D deficiency, screening for chlamydia and gonorrhea, screening for asymptomatic carotid artery stenosis, screening for suicide risk, screening for cognitive impairment in older adults, screening for thyroid dysfunction, and so forth. I encourage you to visit their web site to fully appreciate the enormous spectrum of their expertise. How do they do it? Remember, they don't have to be experts in the actual disease process, only the numbers that accompany the clinical trials and the methodology of those studies. Even so, what is the depth of knowledge of each and every committee member on each and every guideline? Or are there only a few key individuals who drive the consensus with quiet approval or dissent among others?

Perhaps this ongoing rotation of members explains the Task Force's flip-flopping of recommendations for screening women in their 40s, beginning with their first opinion in 1989. Then, it was yes, followed by "no policy" in 1996, yes in 2002, no in 2009, no in 2016. And while we had two "no's" back to back in 2009 and 2016, the definition of "no" changed. That is, the definition of a C recommendation changed from "against *routine* screening" (the operative word being "routine") to a kinder, gentler "selectively offering this service to individual patients based on professional judgment and patient preferences." Semantics aside, kinder and gentler is not going to matter other than to trick critics into quiescence, given that the Affordable Care Act is not required to cover C-recommendations. This legislation is where the power of the Task Force was launched. However, when accusations were made that the 2009 move was motivated by "Obamacare," committee members at that time defended themselves by noting that their work began on the mammography data during the prior Administration.

The 2009 Task Force announced that "new data" had prompted their two major changes in screening recommendations: (1) start at 50 rather than 40, and (2) every 2 years instead of annually. So let's examine that new data.

## Begin Screening at 50 Rather Than 40

We've already covered the basic debate here, dating back more than 50 years to that odd moment in screening history when Philip Strax, M.D., parked his mobile mammography unit on the streets of Manhattan. 40 to 49 screening has *always* been controversial. At the time of the 2009 Task Force and their C-recommendation (against routine screening), there were at least 8 meta-analyses of the 40–49 question, including the one by the Task Force. Recall that none of the individual screening studies have shown a statistically significant mortality reduction in and of themselves for this age group. It's only when the studies are combined into a meta-analysis that we see a benefit. And while 7 of 8 of these meta-analyses indicated benefit, only 3 of 8 reached statistical significance. Here's the peculiar part—*the Task Force is one of the three that shows a statistically significant benefit to screening women in their 40s!*

Furthermore, their calculated 15% statistically significant (relative) reduction in mortality in 2009 was *identical* to the 15% reduction calculated by their predecessors serving on the Task Force in 2002. Yet they opted for a reversal in policy. If this seems fishy to you, it should.

The Task Force stated that "new data" had emerged from the AGE trial, and this played a role in their decision. Yet the AGE trial, a U.K. study designed to settle the 40–49 question, at the time of the 2009 Task Force, had reported a non-significant mortality reduction of 17%, similar to the other trials with the exception of the Canadian NBSS-1. It does not take any training in statistics to know that if your baseline benefit is a 15% mortality reduction drawn from hundreds of thousands of women in multiple trials, then if you blend in one more trial with a 17% benefit, it's not going to alter your calculations one bit. In other words, the so-called "new data" didn't change a thing! The 2009 Task Force calculated an *identical* number to the 2002 Task Force, yet reversed their opinion and their recommendations.

This 15% relative risk reduction, by the way, is the same relative benefit the Task Force calculated for women ages 50–59, begging the question as to why draw the line at 50 if the benefits are the same below and above. The answer is that the incidence of breast cancer is higher during the 50s. Remember, this 15% is a *relative* number, so when you apply it to the actual number of breast cancer deaths in order to calculate the absolute benefit, more women in the 50–59 age group will benefit than those in their 40s.

But how big is this difference? As we learned in Chapter 8, The Number Games, we can express data as lives saved in the general population (a large number) or as the potential benefit for a single person (a tiny number). However, the other method previously introduced, easy to envision, is the use of "number needed to screen" (NNS) to save one life, a hybrid that considers both the population and the individual. In general, values for "number needed to screen" are inherently large in screening and preventive health (a surprise to many) and can vary widely from study to study. But they do seem to help conceptualize the controversies.

The 2002 Task Force calculated the NNS for women in their 40s to be 1,792, while for women in their 50s, the NNS was 1,224. That is, you must screen 1,792 women in their 40s to save one life, but "only" 1,224 women in their 50s to save one life. Obviously, a lot of mammography has to be performed *at any age* to save one life, so one can see why screening is under such fire when resources are limited.

One also must be aware that there is a difference between NNS and NNI, the latter being the "number needed to *invite* for screening." NNI is always higher (worse) as some women invited to screen in the prospective trials did not comply, yet were still counted in the screening group to maintain randomization, according to the intent-to-treat rule of RCTs. This opens the door to considerable trickery as articles and commentaries often do not bother to make the distinction between NNS and NNI. The 2002 Task Force used both NNS and

NNI in their review. In *2009*, the Task Force focused on NNI (invited to screen) rather than NNS (actually screened). Media outlets failed to appreciate this distinction.

Now, instead of 1,792 actual mammograms performed to save one life, we were given the number that 1,904 women in their 40s had to be *invited* to screen to save one life (realizing that some never had mammography performed), and the NNI for women in their 50s was now 1,339, instead of the NNS of 1,224 reported in 2002. The difference may seem relatively small, but the claim was made that this was based on a new review of the literature, whereas one can also question the use of NNI instead of NNS, and how this was translated to the public.

Are we really to deny screening for women in their 40s based on this? The Task Force is saying, "It's proper to invite 1,339 women to have mammograms to save the life of one woman in her 50s, but it's not worth it to invite 1,904 to save the life of one woman in her 40s." This is a chilling conclusion, but it's exactly what the Task Force is telling us.

The Task Force acknowledged that the incidence of breast cancer rises sharply during the decade of the 40s, but then uses this truth to explain why screening in the 40s is more inefficient. Yet, if one looks at incidence curves over the decades of life, and if there was *no data available* about screening benefit, one would not draw the line *after* the steep curve upward between 40 and 50. An untutored person looking at the curve would say, "We should start screening at 40, before that sharp rise in incidence." This is why women in their 40s were included in prospective clinical trials to begin with.

As stated previously, there's a big difference between 40 and 50. Draw the line at 40, excluding women in their 20s and 30s as we do today, and you're already disenfranchising 5% of women destined for breast cancer. But draw it at 50, and now you're disenfranchising another 20%, or 25% total. One out of 4 eventual breast cancer victims are denied screening mammography when access is limited to age 50 and older.

While NNS and NNI numbers are intriguing and easily pictured, don't be fooled by any semblance of strict accuracy. The Confidence Intervals (more accurately called "credible intervals" in this situation) in the 2009 NNI data from the Task Force for women in their 40s ranges from 929 mammograms to 6,378. For women in their 50s, the credible range is from 322 to 7,455. Recall that the wider the range, the less reliable the numbers. And, with less reliability, the more these numbers allow themselves to be massaged and manipulated. Pro-screening advocates can easily calculate the NNS at the low end of the range, while anti-screeners draw from the same data to calculate numbers at the high end of the range. So the numbers are best used for making comparisons, rather than stand-alone accuracy.

Moving on. No matter how repugnant it might be for the epidemiologist and statistician, many believe the Canadian NBSS should be excluded from these analyses due to the afore-mentioned issues of "benevolent corruption," but more to the point, the trial is technically not about mammographic screening as an independent tool, having enrolled women with palpable lumps. As of this writing, Drs. Miller and Baines are still locked in open battle (e.g., letter to the editor, *The Breast Journal,* June 2015) with Dr. Tabár et al. as to the significance of the advanced cancer cases that inexplicably appeared in the mammography limb of the CNBSS.

"You can't exclude the CNBSS when it is the only trial to have defined an age group prospectively," say the epidemiologists in a chorus of adulation for the Canadian trials.

Interestingly, that claim is no longer true. That is, the CNBSS is not the only trial with

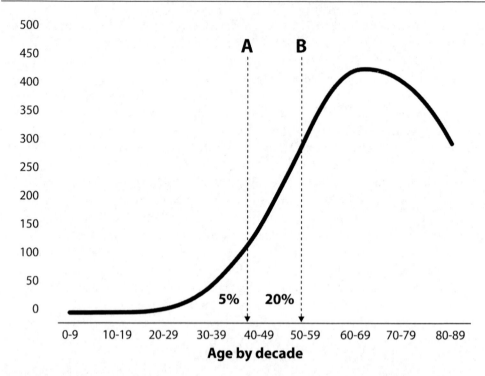

Age-specific SEER incidence rates for breast cancer, 2003–2007. This is a schematic representation of data from the Surveillance, Epidemiology and End Results program sponsored by the National Cancer Institute. The incidence rate (new cancers per 100,000 women) are listed on the Y-axis, while age by decades forms the X-axis. Arrow A depicts the point when screening begins at age 40, whereas B applies to age 50. 5% of eventual breast cancer patients are excluded from screening when we start at 40, and 25% are excluded when we start at 50. The sharp rise in incidence during the 40s is what prompted inclusion of women in this age group into the screening trials in the first place. In fact, the *relative* risk reduction in mortality with mammographic screening is essentially the same for women in their 40s as it is for women in their 50s. The difference is that the baseline incidence is lower in the 40s, so the absolute benefit is less. Stated alternatively, it takes screening more women in their 40s than the 50s in order to save a life.

predefined age groups. Appropriately named, the AGE trial in the U.K. is designed entirely for women in their 40s, and while still using obsolete mammography, the trial is the "newest" of the old studies. While an official rendering at this point in our story said "no benefit" (17% mortality reduction, but not statistically significant), the final tally will come later as a punchline. For now, however, this was the "new data" that didn't alter one thing in the final analysis by the 2009 Task Force.

The *2002* Task Force publication is an excellent read, as it provides a detailed analysis of the 8 prospective RCTs (although no data yet from the ninth RCT—U.K.'s AGE trial). Keep in mind that even the 2002 Task Force did not analyze the overwhelming bulk of published data on mammography, as this group opts to focus almost entirely on prospective RCTs, if available. The only way some think tanks will stoop to an observational study (non-randomized) is if there are no available RCTs.

In this 2002 Task Force article, Table 1 notes that the Canadian NBSS had an enrollment methodology that "made subversion possible," and that "17 women in the mammography group vs. 5 in the control group had tumors with 4 (or more) nodes on initial screening." Under "external validity," it is further noted that the CNBSS used "poor mammography technique; only a third of cancer cases were found by mammography alone." Criticisms are not limited to the CNBSS, of course, but I mention the 2002 effort as remarkably thorough and accurate.

When it comes to the 2002 discussion on the 40–49 problem, admitting it has always been controversial, here's a quote of interest (p. 356): "In the early years, it (the 40–49 controversy) centered on the lack of evidence that observed risk reductions were statistically significant. That argument has dissipated over time as more evidence has shown a significant separation in survival curves with longer follow-up." Critics have charged that this benefit does not appear for more than 10 years post-screening, so why not wait until age 50 to begin? To that, the 2002 Task Force replied, "We found little evidence to convincingly address this concern and some evidence that some benefit from screening women 40 to 49 years of age would be sacrificed if screening began at age 50 years."

So what happened between 2002 and 2009? (Disregard the fact that volunteers rotate off the Task Force committee.) What prompted the reversal? Could it be that a general anti-screening sentiment has been at work, permeating our belief systems? Is this a sociologic phenomenon rather than scientific? While "new data" was the defense that the 2009 Task Force promoted, we have already seen that the only new data when it came to the *benefit* of screening was the AGE Trial that didn't alter benefit one way or the other!

In fact, the "new data" that prompted the reversal in position came from a new way to calculate the *harms* of screening. Thus, the *benefits* of screening are chained numerically to primitive trials, with archaic mammography, including the bizarre CNBSS story and its powerful dilution of data that otherwise would have shown a stronger benefit. At the same time, the 2009 Task Force opted to use new and sophisticated tools of mathematical modeling to calculate the "modern" harms of screening, rather than the actual harms encountered in the very same trials used to calculate benefit.

It's a ratio—benefit-to-harms—and it doesn't take altering the benefits one bit in order to reverse a stance. Simply change the harms. The 2009 Task Force kept the benefits intact from 2002, but then elevated the harms to a new level. How did they do that? Through utilizing CISNET, the Cancer Intervention and Surveillance Modeling Network, a consortium of NCI-sponsored biostatisticians that use mathematical modeling to help assess the impact of cancer control strategies. The Task Force "sub-contracted" the responsibility of calculating harms to this group, the details of which go beyond the scope of this book. For the record, I am a strong advocate of mathematical modeling (which involves, heaven forbid, deductive reasoning), and I have no objections to any of the CISNET numbers generated for the Task Force.

Here's where I depart from the Task Force—not in their calculations, but in their final step of announcing that harms exceed benefits for women in their 40s. That's a judgment call, not science. When the 2009 announcement was made to begin screening at 50 instead of 40, there was an extraordinary backlash, and Task Force members were put on the defensive. Some acted "surprised," apparently believing that most women would welcome the news about less mammography. *USA Today* called the response an "unprecedented furor." One spokesperson from the Task Force, in his own defense, stated, "We only look at science," followed by the remarkably patronizing comment that if women choose to ignore the recommendations and get mammograms based on emotions, it was certainly their right.

In those immortal Nixon words, "Let me make this perfectly clear"—this is not about science, it's about the subjective interpretation of statistics. They are not the same thing, no matter how sophisticated the stats might be. And it's about using those statistics to address politics, limited resources, and a rising anti-screening sentiment. Yes, you can use good science to calculate a benefit (although analyzing mammography as performed in the Dark Ages is remarkably prone to error). Then, you can use science to calculate harms. But the moment you put benefits and harms on each end of the teeter-totter, "science" and "statistics" exit the process.

How many "unnecessary biopsies" (a pejorative term in its own right) does it take to equal a saved life? What is the anxiety of a breast biopsy when compared to the anxiety of a delayed diagnosis of breast cancer and resulting death? How many points do you assign to a mammographic call-back in order for the total to equal the identification of a lumpectomy candidate rather than mastectomy? The final step is 100% judgment, in spite of the attempt by the Task Force to hide behind the skirts of science. And given this new era of policy-generating committees that insist on a "no experts allowed" membership policy, it's all rather creepy.

In 2002, the U.S. Preventive Services Task Force, in an admirable study and thoughtful discussion of the prospective RCTs addressed the 40–49 question in detail, noting it was a close call, but the benefits outweighed the harms. The 2009 Task Force looked at the identical benefit, calculated the harms differently, then as a matter of pure opinion, stated the opposite. Under attack, 2009 members then backpedaled with softer wording, which many radiologists misconstrued as a retraction. There was no retraction—screening women in their 40s stayed put as a C-recommendation.

Nearly everyone agrees the benefit of screening women in their 40s is more difficult to demonstrate than older age groups, but the difference is marginal. In fact, you don't see a strong jump in screening benefit as women age until the decade of the 60s where the number needed to screen (NNS) to save one life is at its lowest (best).

The artificial division at age 50 seems to be a compulsion based on the average age of menopause, with the attendant belief that premenopausal breast cancer is a different biology than postmenopausal. And that mammograms are denser (thus, missing more cancers) in the premenopausal years. Dr. Kopans has expended a great deal of effort studying these two allegations, publishing evidence that the biologic aggressiveness of breast cancer in the decade of the 40s is not significantly different from the decade of the 50s, nor is there a measurable difference in density between those two decades either.

That said, if one were to compare a large group of 40-year-olds vs. a large group of 60-year-olds, there would be some differences at these extremes. The point is that 50, while compelling in its surrogate role as the definition of menopause, does not appear to be a natural cut-off when it comes to the reality of screening (indeed, some minimalists have suggested screening only for a 10-year time period—the decade of the 60s). Too, we have not yet addressed any of the observational evidence (non-randomized studies), which favors screening women in their 40s. And while this evidence is ranked lower on the scale of "quality," to the point that rarified "think tanks" won't even acknowledge its existence, how can one claim to be devoted to "evidence-based medicine" while, at the same time, refusing to acknowledge the bulk of the evidence—and in this case, all the evidence when assessing modern technology?

In 2002, it was a B-recommendation from the Task Force. In 2009, the same organization but with different members made it a C-recommendation. In spite of their attempt at kinder, gentler wording, it might as well have been a D-recommendation (a flat-out "don't do it") which is where PSA screening for prostate cancer has landed per the Task Force. After all, the only difference between C and D was the word "routine," as in "against *routine* screening." In the publicity that followed the 2009 Task Force, "routine" was lost in translation.

In their 2016 update, the (new) Task Force didn't meddle with the 2009 analysis of women in their 40s. However, the C-grade was made softer still, tossing out the negative wording, and replacing it with this fluffier version: "selectively offering or providing this service to individual patients based on professional judgment and patient preferences. There is at least moderate certainty that the net benefit is small." Hmmm ... sure sounds better. In fact, some evidence-based radicals felt betrayed—that the Task Force had gone soft, calling for older wording, more rigid recommendations, and most disturbingly, calling on the Task Force to be given greater power and broader scope to perform cost-effective analyses (since this is the real issue at hand anyway). In the end, the wording doesn't matter, serving only to lull critics to sleep. C is a C is a C, and the Affordable Care Act could end up being the Pied Piper that leads other carriers to deny mammography coverage for women in their 40s.

Again, the Task Force did not claim that women don't benefit from screening in their 40s, in spite of the many misquotes floating about in print and online. *They found the benefit to be statistically significant*, simply not enough to be worth the trouble. When you think about it, it would have been better if their meta-analysis had revealed no benefit at all (as seen in the CNBSS). By agreeing to a benefit, that is, saved lives, yet determining harms as "too great," the Task Force set themselves up for heated and persistent criticism. How many mammography call-backs or benign biopsies does it take to equal a young woman dying of breast cancer? Only the epidemiologists seem to know for sure.

## Screen Every 2 Years Instead of Every Year

This recommendation nearly generated the same degree of vitriol, but not quite. After all, ever since the Civil War, the National Cancer Institute guidelines have been: Screen every 1–2 years starting at age 40. But even more to the point, the most powerful benefit of screening mammography alone was seen in the prospective, randomized trial with the *longest* average interval—the Swedish Two-County trial where the interval ranged from 24 months (ages 40–49) to 33 months (ages 50 to 74).

This 33-month interval approximates the norm in the U.K. where women are invited to screen every 36 months. It was always a curiosity to me why the U.K. opted to go with every 3 years, generating a very long interval between screens, making length bias worse, effectively selecting only the slowest growing tumors. In an interview with a U.K. official, I heard the reasoning: "We felt that it would be much easier to shorten the interval if future data so indicated, as opposed to lengthening the interval."

The U.K. was prophetic in this regard. The public outcry in the U.S. when "every 2 years" was proposed by the Task Force was unimaginable to those in longstanding comfort with yearly mammography. Had we been shifting from every 3 years to every 2, there might have been some groaning about the interval being "too often," but nothing compared to the backlash from those accustomed to annual screens. It was the combination of "against routine screening under 50" coupled with the "two-year interval" that prompted Dr. Kopans to reach the breaking point when he was quoted in the *Washington Post*, shortly after the 2009 Task Force announcement: "Tens of thousands of lives are being saved by mammography screening, and these idiots want to do away with it. It's crazy—unethical, really."

Let's understand from the beginning that there has never been a study that compared intervals—every year vs. every 2 years. Why not? Look at the staggering number of women that had to enroll in the original trials where, even then, the number of breast cancer deaths is so low that statistical significance is hard to achieve. Now imagine both limbs of a trial (every year vs. every 2 years) where there is benefit to all participants, such that only a small difference is theorized. It would require a clinical trial involving perhaps a million women to make a distinction. The expense would be staggering, not to mention the technology obsolete by the time results were available.

This is also why you don't see mortality reduction as an endpoint when it comes to screening with other modalities, either alone or added to mammography. Instead, researchers study "cancer yields" with various approaches, then the mortality reduction must be theorized through mathematical modeling. One problem—without prospective mortality reductions demonstrated after randomization, the armchair think tanks can shrug off the newer approaches as "insufficient evidence." And this is what the Task Force has done with breast MRI, screening ultrasound, and now tomosynthesis, in spite of very impressive data.

This is where evidence-based medicine, or empiricism, starts to blur lines with rational thought. Mathematics—not statistics per se—but classical math is derived "from within," that is, pure rational thought (remember Descartes—"I think, therefore I am"—who believed everything came from within). One can mathematically model outcomes based on reliable data, and to my view, be quite accurate. We tend to think of risk assessment as a service for individuals. However, applying risk to populations and calculating disease "prevalence," one can plug in the Sensitivity of the screening tool and generate "cancer yields," or CDRs (cancer detection rates), a practical surrogate for mortality reduction (caveats, yes). Then, these comparative cancer yields can be confirmed in clinical trials, using various imaging methods. We are never going to have the luxury of prospective RCTs to answer all the questions in medicine, so we need to use our brains to the best of our ability, asking, "What if?"

And this is exactly what the 2009 Task Force did in their recommendation to switch to every 2 years. In the absence of prospective RCTs comparing screening intervals, they calculated benefits and harms, using every year, every 2 years, and every 3 years, in a scheme of mathematical modeling that I can't criticize (they even included compliance), coming to the conclusion that *most* of the benefit was maintained by screening every 2 years. At the same time, harms (and costs) were cut nearly in half.

But what does "most" mean? What is "most of the benefit was maintained"? In fact, they calculated 81% as the definition of "most." 81% of the benefit was maintained. I'm going to ignore the fact that different models were used for each of the intervals, and there was a wide range, but they settled on the 81% as representative of the "every 2 years" approach.

So now let's make some sense of this number. The 81% has to be applied to a baseline benefit from annual screening. If we say that a relative mortality reduction of 30% is achieved with yearly screening in women over 50, then 81% of the 30% is 24%. Thus, if you screen every year, and your expected benefit is a 30% relative mortality reduction, then if you switch to every 2 years, the expected mortality reduction is 24%.

But remember, these are *relative* risk reductions. Recall how the absolute numbers are much smaller. In fact, if we start from a 3% absolute lifetime risk of dying from breast cancer, then yearly mammography will reduce that by a relative 30%, or from 3% to 2%. So, using a 24% mortality reduction instead of 30% makes a negligible difference in the individual patient. To be painfully compulsive, a 30% reduction in 3% is actually a 0.9% reduction to 2.1%; a 24% reduction in 3% is 0.72% reduction to 2.28%. One could claim that the lifetime risk of dying of breast cancer is converted from 3% to 2.1% with annual screening, and from 3% to 2.28% with biennial screening.

At the individual level, this is barely measurable, so one woman is very likely going to be fine with biennial screening. But recall the tricks we learned in the Chapter 8, The Number Games. If you want to minimize an effect, talk about one patient. If you want to maximize the effect, talk about the general population. If we apply the every 2 years plan to the general population, we are going to have *several thousand* more breast cancer deaths every year.

Modeling exact numbers is tricky as it depends on compliance levels. Given only fair compliance in the United States with mammography in the first place (it's not quite the "religion" here as it is in Sweden), then switching to every 2 years will only impact those who were rigidly compliant with annual screens. This is why estimates of effect vary widely and are highly dependent on the definition of compliance over time.

Notably, the Task Force considered *every 3 years* as a possible recommendation, in line with the U.K., but felt they would be giving up too much benefit to go that route. The important thing to remember is that there is a vast chasm between the benefit at the individual level vs. the entire population. And this is what's so peculiar about the anti-screening sentiment that points out the negligible benefit to individuals when the very premise of epidemiology, biostatistics, public health and preventive medicine is to think in terms of the entire population.

And, once again, the Task Force is routinely misquoted on this issue. The Task Force did not say that every 2 years for screening was *equal* to every year, as some have claimed. They quite specifically made this point, revealing that, with every 2 year screens, "most of the benefit is maintained." The alternative phrasing, of course, is that "some of the benefit of mammography will be lost."

Within 24 hours, anti-screeners began piling on, booking TV appearances to endorse the Task Force by approving things that the Task Force never said, spouting the same to all forms of media and thoughtless print articles, saying, "We've been telling you for years that the 2-year interval makes no difference." The Cochrane group joined in the fray with "We've been saying biennial is as good as annual all along," a remarkable statement coming from an evidence-based think tank, grossly distorting what the Task Force had said.

The media quotes were sometimes entertaining. One CEO of an insurance giant endorsed the Task Force whole-heartedly, even summoning pretentious patient concern: "We must pay attention to our scientists … we've been concerned a long time about damaging radiation." Where did that come from? Were radiation doses calculated from the old BCDDP where some of the equipment misfired, dramatically? Or the HIP plan of 40 years ago when women glowed in the dark after mammography? Well, the Task Force did address the potential harm of radiation, opting to use the highest imaginable numbers that we will address later in the book. Oddly, for a think tank devoted to evidence-based medicine, the Task Force chose to amplify this harm without any direct evidence, all harms being theoretical.

Radiation exposure today with digital mammography is so low that it adds next-to-nothing when considering the background radiation. Living on planet Earth exposes all of us to radiation equivalent to a mammogram every 3 months or less, depending on location (radon levels) and altitude (cosmic radiation). So I say to my patients, "Unwittingly, men get 4 mammograms every year, while women get 5." And to boot, even high levels of radiation have little impact on breast tissue after the age of 40, fitting nicely with the recommended start time for mammography.

The firestorm of Task Force controversy sent the secretary of Health and Human Services scrambling for safety, stating that the advice of the Task Force would not alter anything (at least, for the moment). In contrast, the American Academy of Family Physicians (AAFP) was in a bind, having long endorsed the Task Force in their many recommendations. In fact, its membership had served as participants, with family practice increasingly focused on public health. Here, the devotion to its rising star won out, and the AAFP chose to ignore the guidelines of all oncology-based organizations, instead, pledging allegiance to the volunteer Task Force. The American College of Physicians (internal medicine) chose to walk on slightly thicker ice by acknowledging the need to discuss options with patients and include individual risk levels in this personalized approach. As sugar-coated as that might seem, the horrible taste remaining is this: "If, after the ideal discussion of options, a patient decides to proceed at age 40 with screening.... Will those mammograms be covered by insurance?"

Meanwhile, breast radiologists, and many breast experts, sat in stunned silence while the following organizations that endorsed annual screening at 40 were ignored: American Cancer Society, National Comprehensive Cancer Network, National Cancer Institute (1–2-year intervals), American Medical Association, American Congress of Obstetricians and Gynecologists (1–2-year intervals), American College of Surgeons, American College of Radiology, Society of Breast Imaging, and the American Society of Breast Disease (merged into the NCBC—National Consortium of Breast Centers).

Other expert radiologists went on the offensive, most notably using the Task Force raw data, including CISNET, and re-calculating with vastly different outcomes and conclusions. Most notably, Drs. Hendrick and Helvie led the charge here,[2] showing how soft and malleable the data can be, fit for any agenda. Among their many projections drawn from re-visiting the six CISNET models, they pointed out that the most aggressive model (annual mammography from age 40 to 84) would result in a 40% mortality reduction, which would be saving (relatively) 71% more lives than the CISNET model chosen by the Task Force where the mortality reduction was only 23%.

But what pro-screeners grabbed onto was this conclusion from Hendrick and Helvie in the discussion of actual number of lives saved: "For U.S. women currently 30–39 years old, annual screening mammography from ages 40–84 years *would save 99,829 more lives* than the Task Force recommendations if all women comply, and 64,889 more lives with the current 65% compliance rate." These numbers underwent a nuanced shift by pro-screening forces and were quoted by some as "100,000 women are going to die if we follow Task Force guidelines." But no matter how you spin it, the number of lives lost doesn't look good. When you strip away the propaganda coming from both sides, more women are still going to die of breast cancer with Task Force guidelines.

The Task Force Grade for *biennial* screening starting at *age 50* was a B—that is, "recommended, but with only moderate certainty or moderate benefit."

Misquoting the Task Force seemed to evolve into a recreational sport. And this went for their other positions as well.

## Other Task Force Recommendations for Breast Cancer Screening

The only other measure where the 2009 Task Force passed judgment was in the teaching of breast self-examination where they issued a D—don't do it. This aroused considerable ire, largely because the word "teaching" was another word lost in translation. The condemnation didn't apply to *performing* self-exam (where, more than likely, they would have generated an "I" for "insufficient evidence"). The ruling pertained specifically to two prospective, randomized trials (China and Russia) where formal teaching programs were evaluated. In the groups where self-exam was "taught," the breast cancer mortality rate was unchanged, but the false alarm rate was significantly higher, with extra imaging and biopsies performed.

I have trouble getting excited about this D Grade. Self-exam has always been treated with some sort of reverence that I never fully understood, given that cancers found in this fashion are much more likely to be larger (average size 2.0–2.5 cm) and with positive nodes. Due to promotional efforts on self-exam, ignoring the exacting techniques that make women feel they might be doing it "wrong," I think many people equate the benefit of self-exam to screening mammography. This is not the case. The two approaches are not equivalent. Breast cancers discovered on self-exam are skewed toward Stage II and III, while mammographic cancers are skewed toward Stage I, average size 1.0 cm. Granted, when tumors are close to the skin surface, and depending on breast size, there will be Stage I cancers found on self-exam. But the question at hand surrounds the benefit of formal teaching programs. As I tell my patients in an advanced screening program, our intent is to find breast cancer *before* it can be felt.

All other Task Force positions were given Grade "I" for "insufficient evidence." And when your criteria for "Sufficiency" is limited to prospective, randomized trials that reveal a statistically significant mortality reduction, there are going to be precious few improvements in screening endorsed by the Task Force. As noted above, from here on, those of us trying to effect improvements are going to have to live with "cancer yields," interval cancer rates and tumor stage/biology, and the stage/biology of those tumors discovered through screening. To demand prospective RCTs for each new development in technology is only going to result in the "insufficient evidence" list getting longer and longer.

Here are the 2009 recipients of the "I" Grades:

Screening women aged 75 and older
The benefit of clinical exam in addition to screening mammography in women 40 and
    older
The additional benefit of either digital mammography or breast MRI over film screen
    mammography

As for women over 75, yes, there is insufficient data. No one argues that point. The prospective clinical trials had entry ages younger than 75, though some data can be extracted from those who turned 75 during the study (as in the Swedish Two-County). The findings generally show a 20% mortality reduction that does not reach statistical significance. The problem with screening older women is competing mortality. The same tumor in a 75-year-old may not have time to manifest itself as it would in a 45-year-old. "Overdiagnosis" (pejorative for length bias that doesn't have time to reveal itself) increases as a probability with advancing age. Importantly, it's not that screening doesn't work in older women. Sometimes, it simply doesn't have time for its work to be unveiled. Some 75-year-olds, however, will live another 25 years, so we assume the role of Providence when we deny screening on the basis of average life expectancy determined by actuarial tables.

And don't fall into the trap of believing that older women newly diagnosed with breast cancer routinely have low grade biology, i.e., less aggressive tumors. While some do have low grade tumors, there are plenty of high-grade aggressive tumors discovered in this age group. Furthermore, recall that screening efficacy gains momentum through the decades. Far and away, the greatest benefit is demonstrated during the decade of the 60s. Are we to believe that this momentum comes to an abrupt end on the 70th birthday?

As for the efficacy of clinical breast exam alone, does a prospective RCT seem warranted to settle this issue? Again, it would require randomization to a "no mammography/no clinical exam" control group. This has been suggested to address the over-75 controversy, perhaps placing clinical exam head-to-head vs. mammography, avoiding the "no screening" control group, but this approach includes many uncontrollable variables, such as the examiner's expertise. Even the Canadian NBSS failed to show any benefit through scheduled clinical exams, remembering that this was a trial that, first of all included palpable lumps at the time of enrollment, and then focused on subsequent clinical exams by health care providers.[3] It remains a conundrum as to how the CNBSS has extolled the virtues of clinical exam to the exclusion of mammography for decades when, in fact, their own data does not support formal clinical exams. Additionally, should we submit every step in the classical, thorough physical exam to prospective RCTs? (Indeed, some are proposing an end to the classical physical exam, of course, due to the "lack of evidence.")

Lastly, the Task Force graded digital mammography and breast MRI with an "I." This passive endorsement of the older film screen technique demonstrates the problem of advancing technology—during this interval between the 2009 Task Force and the 2016 update, digital mammography replaced film screen mammography nationwide. And now, 2-D digital is already on its way to obsolescence as 3-D tomosynthesis has hit the market running. Although there was plenty of data to review for digital mammography, the lack of a prospective RCT with mortality as its endpoint paralyzed the Task Force in its assessment. They will never render an opinion on routine digital 2-D mammograms as the technology will have come and gone without the required RCTs for their brand of evidence-based medicine. In 2016, they quietly dropped the issue of digital vs. film screen.

Remarkably (but consistent with their mandate for RCTs), the Task Force also claimed insufficient evidence to comment on breast MRI for screening, a tool with vastly superior sensitivity to mammography, demonstrated in multiple international clinical trials (albeit none of them designed with mortality as an endpoint). Mortality reduction, however, has been mathematically modeled (as CISNET did for the Task Force) in BRCA gene-mutation carriers who undergo annual MRI screening, with clinical support of actual mortality reduction now emerging. Both the American Cancer Society and the National Comprehensive Cancer Network (NCCN) endorsed MRI screening in high risk patients, begun in 2007 after review of considerable published data on cancer yields in head-to-head comparisons of mammography and MRI, *two years* before the Task Force rendered their opinion of "insufficient data."

If one can condemn through faint praise, what does it mean if you offer no praise, or "insufficient evidence"? For many physicians, the "insufficient evidence" meant outright condemnation (a D grade), and it took less than 24 hours for me to hear, "Did you hear that the Task Force ruled against breast MRI for screening?" That was not the case.

In 2015, the Task Force drafted a new set of recommendations and announced their proposed guidelines in April as being open to public feedback. This gesture allowed the draft to compost, attracting the flies of condemnation until the official proclamation of those guidelines on January 12, 2016.[4] Public response was ample and largely critical, and in their official 2016 publication, the Task Force addressed criticisms with remarkable diplomacy, transparency, and total inflexibility.

The Big Two remained unchanged from 2009: (1) start at 50, and (2) screen every two years. Calculations were slightly different across the board, regarding both benefits and harms, but not enough to alter 2009 recommendations. Notably, during the 6-year interval following the 2009 report and the American Academy of Family Physicians endorsement, no additional physician groups or cancer organizations adopted Task Force guidelines.

The 2009 statements about teaching self-exam and clinical breast exam simply dropped out of sight in 2016. No mention was made. Instead, the "I's" have it. Women 75 or older = I. 3-D tomosynthesis for screening = I. Women having dense breasts with regard to any type of multi-modality imaging (including ultrasound, tomosynthesis, or MRI) = I.

Unstated, 2-D digital mammography came and went, while the Task Force stood on the sidelines. Film screen vs. digital mammography is not addressed in 2016, as it's no longer an issue. Now playing catch-up with tomosynthesis, the Task Force admitted in 2016 that 3-D appears to increase cancer detection rates and to decrease false-positives (a call-back for additional views qualifies as a false-positive, even if no biopsy is required). However, the data remains insufficient, which may well be true in January 2016, but the tomosynthesis flood of data is underway, with *consistently* favorable outcomes, and will become the standard of care long before the Task Force brings itself to an opinion (if they *ever* render an opinion).

As for breast MRI screening, though, the 2016 Task Force altered its approach from 2009 by limiting the discussion to women with dense breasts (addressing *all* forms of accessory imaging modalities), stating "insufficient evidence" with regard to *this indication only*. Most breast radiologists disagree, pointing out that ample evidence exists for multi-modality imaging for women with extremely dense breasts. And, in fact, the American College of Radiology and Society of Breast Imaging have already stated such, offering screening ultrasound as the adjunct of choice for women without major risks other than the density itself.

That aside, however, the tricky rhetoric in 2016 completely evades the topic of *high-risk* multi-modality screening, unrelated to density, rendered as "insufficient" in 2009. A footnote states that the new 2016 Task Force recommendations overall apply only to asymptomatic women age 40 and older "who do not have pre-existing breast cancer or a previously high-risk breast lesion and who are not at high risk for breast cancer because of a known underlying genetic mutation (such as a BRCA mutation or other familial breast cancer syndrome) or a history of chest radiation at a young age." Rather than endorse MRI screening in this very group described above, as has long been the policy of the ACS and NCCN, the Task Force simply stated that their general 2016 recommendations—Grades B, C, I, I and I—do not apply to these high-risk women.

So what are these excluded high-risk women to do? The 2016 Task Force didn't say. Did they pull a fast one here? Are they passively endorsing high-risk screening without saying so? They don't mention specific modalities for high-risk patients, so it's very hard to call it an endorsement, passive or not. In fact, they are simply providing screening recommendations for the average risk patient, then stating that their latest recommendations don't apply to high-risk women. It's another example where the world has passed them by. Multi-modality screening for high-risk women is now an established standard of care, with insurance coverage when patients meet certain qualifications. Just as digital mammography flashed by while the Task Force contemplated data, the same is true for high-risk screening, specifically using breast MRI.

When the 2015 draft and 2016 recommendations were released, the shock value of 2009 was gone. Those of us who "practice what we preach" barely took note of the Task Force update. As with all societal changes, good and bad, we had gradually grown accustomed to the anomaly of the Task Force. Few pendulums in science stop at the perfect place, so the hope was that this "overcorrection" by the Task Force would swing back to acceptability someday.

A few years ago, I was giving a tour of our breast center to a new family physician, fresh out of training, and I was describing our high-risk screening program as well as the research that went with it. Somehow, we moved toward a discussion of our policy of annual mammograms starting at age 40, continuing through good health, in line with the majority of organizations. He was startled to learn that *anyone* was recommending annual mammography, much less that it begin at age 40. He had been trained as though there were only one set of guidelines in the universe, that of course being the U.S. Preventive Services Task Force. When I explained that the Task Force actually holds the minority opinion when it comes to breast cancer specialists involved in screening and diagnosis, he was taken aback. His reply: "Well, I'm certainly not going to answer it that way when I take my Boards."

And that's how you change physician behavior. The old guard dies off, and the new guard takes over. Fads and fashions, we are not immune in medicine.

The new guard is responding to shrinking budgets and limited resources, doing everything they can to put a lid on it. However, as an individual contemplating mammograms and screening for cancer, you want to make sure that they're not talking about the lid to your coffin.

# 15

# The Zombies Among Us

"New Study Casts Doubt on the Benefits of Mammography!"

In 2014, rising from the dead once again after repeated annihilations, the Canadian NBSS offered their 25-year follow-up in the February 11, 2014, issue of the *British Medical Journal*.[1] Because there had been no benefit to mammography in either the NBSS-1 (40–49) or the NBSS-2 (50–59) trials, this long-term follow-up study lumped the CNBSS into a single entity.

Health and science journalists, including several who have followed this story from its beginning, gushed with enthusiasm, anointing the CNBSS as the most scientifically valid of them all. Some could barely contain themselves as they called it the "one of the largest" screening trials ever, a reckoning force.

As we've noted, sample size was rather average. Even with both NBSS-1 and NBSS-2 combined, the nearly 90,000 participants fall shy of the 130,000-plus in the Swedish Two-County trial. But the slanted rhetoric traveled well beyond mere size.

The CNBSS is hardly "new." The *most recent* mammogram taken as part of the CNBSS was in *1985*, 13 years before Canada instituted measures to assure mammographic quality through steps analogous to the 1992 Mammography Quality Standards Act in the U.S., implemented in 1994. Even for state-of-the art mammography in the early 1980s, the CNBSS mammograms were grossly unacceptable as we have already seen. Second hand machines (to save money), no grids to reduce scatter and sharpen the image, poor interpretive skills allowing missed cancers, often no biopsy performed after recommendation, no MLO views (until the final few years) such that the most likely area of the breast to harbor malignancy was not included on the X-ray plate, and on and on.

Yes, we have previously hammered the quality issues into a flat sheet of tin, and we have also wondered repeatedly how such a corrupted randomization process at the beginning of the trial could be ignored today. Yet, it seems, history has been on the side of the CNBSS. Why? For one thing, so much time has passed that the historical revisionists are having a field day: "What randomization problem?" "What quality problem?"

Recall that, in 2002, the World Health Organization (WHO) *excluded the CNBSS from analysis of the impact of screening mammography on mortality from breast cancer*, exactly as Robert E. Tarone, PhD, National Cancer Institute, had recommended in 1995 after discovering the statistically significant error in randomization in the CNBSS, with excess advanced cancers placed into the mammography limb.[2] Yes, forget that. Instead, the CNBSS has been embraced by the anti-screening contingency, such that our flat sheet of tin is now molded onto a calf that is anything but golden.

"The Canadian trials showed that early diagnosis doesn't save lives. The tumors in the mammography arm were statistically smaller, yet no lives were saved."

It makes you want to cry. The above quote came from a talking head, a physician on one of the online medical education sites who would probably be shocked to learn the whole story. Admittedly, our impish friend, the arbitrary and much-abused p-value ($p = 0.01$ in this case), indicated that the average size of cancers in the mammography limb was statistically smaller at 1.9 cm, compared to the no-mammography limb where the average tumor size was— get ready—2.1 cm. Two *millimeters* smaller? Who takes this seriously? Check your ruler as a reminder—this is 2 mm (millimeters), not cm (centimeters). This proves nothing about early diagnosis other than confirmation that the mammograms were as wretched as claimed by a host of expert radiologists. A measurement of 1.9 cm is *not* early diagnosis. It is the threshold where you can *feel* breast cancer. The CNBSS is not a trial of mammographic screening—it's palpating with style.[3]

The average tumor size discovered by screening mammography hovers around 1.0 cm, a worthy goal, given the evidence that a watershed size for prognosis seems to be around 1.5 cm. In fact, if you read the fine print of the CNBSS, for those tumors that were discovered by mammography alone, the average tumor size was 1.4 cm, more in line with what would be expected. The problem, however, is that only a small number of cancers (32%) were detected through mammography in the so-called mammography limb. *Two-thirds of cancers in the mammography group were palpable!* This is not high quality mammographic screening. This is a complete flip-flop of what is found in other screening trials, where the reverse is true—⅔ found by mammography, ⅓ by palpation. In fact, many breast centers today boast 80% or higher detection rates by mammography alone in their screening population. 32% is pitiful.

Keep in mind the CNBSS is not a trial endorsed by Canadian breast radiologists. Most are frankly embarrassed by it. The CNBSS is a trial commandeered by epidemiologists, most notably Drs. Anthony Miller and Cornelia Baines, who were skeptical of mammographic screening long before any results emerged from their study. They blatantly ignored recommendations for quality mammography from a series of world class experts, only some of whom I've mentioned in this book. Recall Dr. Wende Logan-Young's early participation where she was not allowed to look at actual X-ray images. Dr. László Tabár had the opportunity to see actual mammograms, which turned out to be more troublesome than not looking at all. Asked to review 50 cases, he flunked the first 15 in a row, and he was out. Stephen Feig, M.D., was incredulous that the MLO view was not being utilized, resigning in protest over the poor quality, and on and on.

And while CNBSS enthusiasts, including the science writers, swoon over the unique prospective designation of age groups as the powerful advantage of the trial, it must be understood that if the mammograms stink, trial design means nothing. If the breast cancer to be diagnosed is not even on the X-ray plate due to the ML view instead of the MLO, then prospectively designating age 40–49 means nothing. Recall the only two essential things for effective screening—(1) a vulnerable biology, and (2) the Sensitivity of the screening tool. X + Y = Z. Trial design is a measure to control the 4 biases, but *the most important thing we must address* (since we can't change biology) is the *Sensitivity of the screening tool*. Trial design, not included in this core equation, cannot overcome poor Sensitivity.

Be it out of ignorance regarding mammographic technology and interpretations, or be it out of intent, the CNBSS and its comrades-in-arms have been both casual and dismissive regarding the most important issue in screening for which we have a measure of control— Sensitivity—that is, the percentage of cancers that will be detected by the screening tool.

Paula Gordon, OBC, M.D., FRCPC, is the medical director of the Sadie Diamond Breast Program at the British Columbia Women's Hospital and a recognized expert in breast radiology. She responded to the latest iteration of the CNBSS with gloves off, stating that the journalists who have reported on this trial "*uncritically* will have blood on their hands." Not right away, she reminds us, "but if women heed the bad advice of these authors, we will see, in the next 5 years, the average size of breast cancers and the rate of spread to the lymph nodes increase. I will continue to have annual mammograms."[4]

Note she is not castigating the investigators of the CNBSS, rather, the self-styled science journalists who repeatedly endorse the CNBSS with mindless disregard for the facts.

Dr. Gordon points out that, in British Columbia, 65% of cancers detected at screening are less than or equal to the watershed 1.5 cm, and node-negativity is more common as well. Both of these parameters were monitored in all clinical trials and with better outcomes than the CNBSS.

At the April 2015 meeting of the American Roentgen Ray Society, in a face-to-face debate with the CNBSS leadership, Drs. Miller and Baines, Dr. Gordon said, "I contend that the NBSS was seriously flawed and the results should not influence policy. Fortunately, Canadian women have ignored the results of the NBSS, and their wisdom is supported by the Pan-Canadian study published last year by Dr. Coldman and colleagues ... which showed a 40% mortality reduction among screened women."[5]

Do these small differences in size at detection really matter?

Recall the odd relationship between tumor diameter and tumor volume. There's a huge difference. Volume = $4/3\pi r^3$. A 2.0cm tumor is not "twice as large as a 1.0cm tumor." It may have twice the diameter, but when it comes to the number of malignant cells it contains, volume rules, not diameter. The volume of a 2.0cm tumor is 4.188 cubic centimeters, while the volume of a 1.0cm tumor is 0.524 cubic centimeters. Thus, a 2.0cm diameter tumor has approximately 8 *times* the volume of a 1.0cm tumor. So the "early detection" in the mammography limb of the CNBSS yielded tumors averaging 1.9cm in size (recalling that two-thirds were palpated), 8 times the volume of the average mammographically-discovered cancer.

Unlike the WHO, the U.S. Preventive Services Task Force included the CNBSS, so we have a significant dilution of the benefit of mammographic screening in the Task Force recommendations. Take away the CNBSS, and one wonders how the Task Force would handle the shift toward benefit over harms. This is why your friendly breast radiologist goes slightly berserk if you say you are going to follow Task Force guidelines—it is, in fact, an indirect endorsement of the Canadian NBSS in all its tainted glory.

And while the American Academy of Family Physicians traditionally endorses the Task Force, there has been some breaking in the ranks when it comes to the CNBSS. Therese B. Bevers, M.D., professor, Department of Clinical Cancer Prevention at the University of Texas MD Anderson Cancer Center, is a Fellow of the American Academy of Family Physicians. She has been quoted previously in this book, and I offer this summary statement as well: "The strengths of the CNBSS are contrasted by a vast collection of flaws that render any findings, past or present, meaningless."

Throw it out! Again, it's not so much the fact that advanced cancers were randomized to the mammography limb, it's the fact that palpable tumors were allowed in the trial at all! It is a gross violation of the very definition of asymptomatic screening to include women with diagnostic problems. Add the horrific quality of the mammograms, and why are we even discussing the CNBSS after all these years? Why would educated, highly intelligent individuals cling to the CNBSS when it is clearly an outlier? Why would our talking head, who was so enthusiastic about finding 1.9cm tumors casually mention that "there were some minor problems with randomization in this trial early on, but those were all worked out."

Disregarding the fact that intelligence is poorly correlated to wisdom, I have a theory as to why anti-screeners can't let go of the CNBSS, beyond the zero benefit of mammography. I don't believe it necessarily relates to Fisher Theory, but recall, if that theory is true in its purest form, then early diagnosis through any means cannot alter outcomes. All breast cancers are predestined in their behavior from the beginning, according to pre-mammography-era Fisher.

But anti-screeners and CNBSS-lovers may not be delving that deep. Human bias is powerful, often mysterious in its origins. I believe the reason goes back to the bugaboos we've already covered—the "identical cousins" of length bias and overdiagnosis. Recall that length bias is where slow-growing tumors are preferentially identified by screening that is hampered by the chosen interval (with faster-growing tumors appearing between screens). Then, in its simplest definition, overdiagnosis is length bias interrupted by death.

Nearly everyone agrees that both length bias and overdiagnosis bias are inevitable by-products of screening. They are not theoretical in nature, but fact. The challenge is in trying to determine the power, that is, to quantify the effect. In those clinical trials where a mortality reduction is demonstrated through screening, the length bias is largely "controlled," but not absent. It would be more accurate to say that the benefit of screening goes beyond the impact of length bias/overdiagnosis, that is, these biases are overshadowed by the mortality reduction.

But what do we get from the CNBSS? All other trials show some degree of benefit for women in their 50s and nearly all for women in their 40s, p-values acceptable or not. Instead, in the CNBSS trials, neither group requires a statistician when it comes to mortality reduction. There is nothing to twist or turn. The same number of deaths occurred in both limbs in both trials. And here's where the anti-screeners begin to salivate, not from the lack of a benefit, but from the opportunity to see, for the first time, length bias and overdiagnosis in full magnification. Previously, the CNBSS had not specifically tackled length bias and overdiagnosis, given that long follow-up is required. This is why, I believe, the CNBSS has been reanimated as a zombie.

You see, in spite of zero benefit overall to mammography, if one looks only at those tumors diagnosed through mammography alone, *there is an apparent improved survival at 25 years* (80% survival compared to 66.3% in the mammography group and 62.8% in the no-mammography group). Forget that we don't like to use "survival benefits" as it allows *lead* time bias, but I'm regurgitating the CNBSS argument at this point. So, given that the *overall* survival is not impacted by mammography, this sub-group survival benefit seen in the mammographically-discovered cancers is artificial and entirely attributable to length bias. Mammograms are simply plucking out the slow-growing tumors rendering the illusion that lives are being saved.

This demonstration of length bias is accompanied by its co-worker, overdiagnosis. When the CNBSS was tallied in the end, more cancers were found in the mammography group than in the no mammography group, to the tune of 142 during the screening period, something that would be expected to correct over time. Yet there was only partial correction, a persistent excess of 106 cancers at 15 years after enrollment, seeming to stabilize at that level. To keep this in perspective, more than 6,000 cancers were diagnosed in 90,000 women over the course of the CNBSS and its 25-year follow-up.

From these excess cancers, the calculation was made, for the first time in the CNBSS, that the overdiagnosis rate for invasive cancer was 22%. Furthermore, remembering that mammograms alone detected only 32% of the cancers, and if one presumes that all overdiagnosis occurs in the mammographically-discovered group, then the overdiagnosis rate becomes a whopping 50%. This bloated number is difficult to reconcile when one considers the 1% disease reservoir in autopsy studies for invasive breast cancer. Without mammographic screening, a true 50% overdiagnosis rate would translate into a large percentage of women who die with undiagnosed invasive breast cancer. Yet, as we've seen already, this number is only 1%.

Drs. H. Gilbert Welch and Peter Gøtzsche and the other iconoclasts now had tremendous fodder to add to their Powerpoint presentations. They had been vindicated! Previously neutral physicians were sent scrambling for explanations which, unfortunately, are not easy to understand. Welch et al had performed similar calculations in other trials where there are always more cancers in the screened group, but it's hard to sway audiences when that darned mortality reduction keeps getting in the way. Not so for CNBSS where one can see in crystalline purity the full beauty of overdiagnosis without lives being saved.

The counter-explanation to this high rate of overdiagnosis is fairly straightforward, but at the same time, hard to appreciate with intuition alone. A vocal minority of pro-screening epidemiologists have been saying all along regarding the inflated overdiagnosis numbers—*you must correct for lead time at the end of a study* (not length bias, but lead time). We have covered this already, but it's amazing how little attention it gets. To completely eradicate lead time bias, you must stop screening in both limbs and observe patients for the rest of their lives. Given this impossibility, "no screening for 10 or so years" in either limb is reasonable. But even that doesn't happen. Screening choices at the end of a trial are random, with crossover in both directions. If women assigned originally to the mammography group continue to get regular mammograms after the official screening phase of the study has ended, *the control group will never "catch up."*

Those who simply read abstracts, or just the concluding statement within an abstract[6] have grabbed onto the "22% overdiagnosis" number from the CNBSS, conveniently mid-way between the alleged (and absurd) range of 0 to 50%. Yet, in those journals where pro-screeners are still welcome, authors have pointed out that with lead time correction, overdiagnosis numbers drop precipitously. As noted above, the CNBSS noted a persistent excess of 106 cancers that "seemed to stabilize" at 15 years. Yet lead epidemiologist for the American Cancer Society Robert A. Smith, PhD, has published his perspective[7] of the graphs used in the 2014 CNBSS update, where instead of 15 years, if one draws the line at 25 years, as the title of the article states, the overdiagnosis rate would only be 3.7%. He further states: "the midpoint estimate (15 years) is biased for reasons noted earlier: women diagnosed in the last year of the trial would have had only 7 years of follow-up, and the incidence in both arms was influenced by the introduction of service screening in the provinces."

The calculation of overdiagnosis is always through indirect analysis and reasoning, and it should be obvious by now that the proposed numbers are made of putty. That does not keep the screening minimalists from plastering "20–30% overdiagnosis" into their informed consents as though it were gospel.

The anti-screeners have seized the misleading information from the Canadian NBSS, while the casual observers have fallen prey to the lure of headlines written by the uninformed. No longer can one sit in a breast cancer scientific meeting, knowing that nearly everyone is on the same page when it comes to screening for early diagnosis. Ten years ago, attendees could look to their left and look to their right, enjoying the comfort of like minds. Today, zombies stagger with superhuman persistence. Look to your left, look to your right, and one of the two is likely an anti-screener or, at a minimum, a minimalist.

The proposed "informed consents" for screening that claim an overdiagnosis rate of 30% are disturbing. If doctors don't understand the meaning and origin of this number, why do we fling it in the face of our patients? This number is highly misleading because many incorrectly interpret the 30% to mean "If you accept lifetime mammographic screening, you will have a 30% probability of being overdiagnosed." Again, the "overselling" of mammography is, today, being countered by the "overbashing" of mammography. The correct wording (though 30% is still inflated) should be *If you are diagnosed with breast cancer*, then there will be a 30% chance of overdiagnosis." But even the 30% is wrong when talking about invasive breast cancer. Correct for lead time, and we're looking at something in the vicinity of 5%, something we've already covered.

But what if we include DCIS? While DCIS is beyond the scope of this book, all would agree that the overdiagnosis issue here is more substantial. 30% of DCIS an overdiagnosis? Maybe, but DCIS is only about 25% of the overall diagnoses made at a breast screening center. An entire text has been written about DCIS[8] and its editor, Dr. Mel Silverstein, and associate editor, Dr. Michael Lagios, have devoted substantial portions of their careers to the identification of women who can be treated for DCIS with excision alone (no radiation, no mastectomy). The hazard of overdiagnosis is overtreatment. Take away the overtreatment of DCIS, and overdiagnosis is not going to be the same problem.

Semantics, syntax distortion, deletion of key facts, twisting of available data, out-of-context quotes, the whole bastion of baloney fills my files with regard to the bizarre efforts to hamper screening. Studies have been performed, complete with p-values, to prove that a benign breast biopsy (under local anesthesia in the office) prompted by screening, results in permanent psychologic damage. While this can certainly occur in a small minority, casting the whole of womandom in this light seems remarkably demeaning, yet often, articles in this vein are written by women about women. Yes, a benign biopsy, even when the cancer fear proves short-lived, is a traumatic event. But it's not even on the same scale with the trauma of a delayed diagnosis of breast cancer, and you can bet your last p-value on that.

Those dedicated to the pursuit of "truly informing" women about the hazards of screening seem to have no limits. I've seen articles where the randomization process in the Swedish Two-County trial was attacked with nary a word about the gross corruption of the CNBSS randomization. Here, I have to invoke Dr. Paula Gordon's rhetoric—these authors will have "blood on their hands." Screening less means more deaths. Even the Task Force admits that "most of the benefit is maintained" when the screening interval is extended from one to two years, which is alternatively stated as, "some of the benefit is lost." "Benefit," of course, is the privilege of being alive.

The CNBSS is *not simply an outlier* that is disregarded by those in the know, embraced by those in the know-it-all. The CNBSS is the standard-bearer for length bias and overdiagnosis, to the point that the true believer in the futility of screening—and this is already in print—will state that the CNBSS confirms that *all attempts to improve upon mammography through other modalities such as ultrasound and MRI will only worsen the problems of length bias and overdiagnosis.* That's the real threat. This warped circular reasoning is the true danger—that is, the acceptance of the CNBSS length bias and the 22% rate of overdiagnosis (deduced as closer to 50%) at face value and the *extrapolation into other technologies and the future.*

One of the justifications for this book is to lay the groundwork to discuss improvements in screening. Yet, the anti-screeners, now emboldened by the 25-year update from the CNBSS, completely ignoring the reduction in advanced stage disease and proven mortality reduction in the 29-year update from the Swedish Two County study, squawk to no end about the obvious length bias and horrific overdiagnosis problem that accompany mammographic screening.

I hope you understand now why the CNBSS study is so critical to this debate. The arguments against its acceptance were appreciated by the World Health Organization, but in spite of the rejection by WHO, those now carrying the CNBSS banner are increasing in number as fewer and fewer understand the whole story. Oh, yes, did I mention that when the WHO's International Agency for Research on Cancer rejected inclusion of the CNBSS at its workshop in 2002, the meeting was chaired by none other than Dr. Anthony Miller, head of the CNBSS? What incredible irony. The chairman was overruled. His baby was tossed out the window, while he chaired the very committee that did the tossing. At that point, and for the second time, we thought the CNBSS was dead. No longer would it influence and dilute the benefit of screening mammography as demonstrated in other trials, rendering meta-analyses in limp support of mammography. My choice of the zombie metaphor might seem more apropos now.[9]

The CNBSS results can get beneath your skin like a bad tattoo. For the casual observer, the CNBSS can be disturbing and can shake one's faith in screening. For those who understand its odd place in history and its flaky foundation, I doubt it has the same effect. If it were only an outlier, we would ignore it. But it's so much more—it is the ill-chosen basis upon which to condemn all efforts to improve screening. Thus, the CNBSS will return again and again in the headlines, no matter how lifeless, no matter how shabby the zombies appear, no matter how many stumbling steps they take, and no matter how fictional it may be, the study and its advocates will always be with us, the calling card for those who have dedicated their lives in the fight against the early diagnosis of breast cancer.

# 16

# Circumstantial Evidence-Based Medicine

Long before Pythagoras ever squared his first hypotenuse, extending through today's numerologists, humankind has been captivated by numbers, sometimes to the point of worship. Probability theory, however, is a relatively new development. Initially, there was simply the collection of raw data (descriptive statistics) by nation-states, generating the term "statistics." Later, interpretations were drawn from this raw data (statistical inference). But where statistics really soared was when they were applied to future events, thus the term *probability theory*, which is separate from, but related to, general statistics.

The motivation for developing probability theory in the 1500s and 1600s should be no surprise—games of chance, with a special emphasis on tossing dice. Today, we use statistics in science both for interpretation of data as well as predicting future outcomes. However, recall our "double-negative" approach, consistent with the prevailing philosophy of Karl Popper that claims we can never prove anything as true with absolute certainty, that there are merely increasing degrees of falsifiability. Thus, under this construct, we are only "allowed" to reject null hypotheses (no difference between study groups) to a certain level of probability. That probability might be 99.99999%, but it's never 100%.

Today, we claim to be in the new era of evidence-based medicine. But make no mistake about it—a more accurate description is the era of *statistical-based medicine*. Regardless, it is a welcome advance, a shiny new development, a worthy goal, a true cornucopia of clichés. At the same time, it can be disastrous when clinicians huddle around the altar of p-values and surrender their brains to biostatisticians. "The numbers don't lie" is a battle-cry we often hear today in science and medicine. And this is true in the Platonic sense, in that Reality is reflected in the most rational of all mental disciplines—mathematics. No, the numbers don't lie, but the people who know how to manipulate them do. But intentional deceit is relatively rare. The problem, as we have seen, is that human bias is reflected in number management. Indeed, numbers are more closely related to clay than they are to statues of certainty.

Fifty years ago, when the rules of prospective randomized trials and statistical analysis were in the formative stage, clinicians involved in research could self-teach the basic mathematics and principles of epidemiology. No longer true. Not even a formal course in statistics or reading a book will suffice. The discipline is enjoying exponential growth with its complexity fueled by software developments. Today, advances in medicine are shepherded by individuals far removed from medical school.

Statistics were once the cart that followed the horse of the physician-scientist. Clinicians would perform experiments or clinical trials, and then dump the data into the lap of their statistician for analysis. Today, the statistician must be involved in the first step of study design. All is good so far. The cautionary tale here is that we tend to forget that statisticians have their own camps, and that numbers are always open to different methods of analysis and interpretation, a subjective call. Meanwhile, the clinical experts are placed on the back burner, to the point that some organized think tanks have no interest in what these experts have to say. "The truth is in the numbers, and the numbers speak for themselves." No caveats, no nuance, no wisdom. Total faith in numbers. Thus, we must ask the question "When are we dealing with scientific truth and when are we practicing sophisticated numerology?"

To their credit, think tanks have rows of notches in their belts, demonstrating how off-base clinicians can be in their practices and beliefs. The Cochrane Collaboration is one of the best-known organizations dedicated to "systematic reviews of the literature to improve health care." Even their logo includes a graph called a "forest plot," depicting disparate outcomes from several clinical trials, meant to reflect their historic victory in a formal review of literature—specifically, individual studies showed no benefit to corticosteroids for women about to give birth prematurely, but a combined analysis confirmed that newborn lives are saved. These lives became a logo.

But what if the individual trials that are combined into the gold standard of evidence-based medicine—the meta-analysis—are flawed? Is this GIGO—garbage in, garbage out? Indeed, a large, well-designed prospective randomized trial can single-handedly come closer to Reality than a meta-analysis composed of small, flawed trials.

Here's where things get tricky. The reverence for the prospective randomized trial, and its ultimate incorporation into a systematic review or meta-analysis, has become so great in statistical-based medicine, that "lesser" quality evidence is sometimes ignored entirely to the point of intentional exclusion, no matter how defective the available prospective RCTs might be. Thus, the very name "evidence-based" medicine can be considered Orwellian when it is used to suppress evidence. In its extreme form, once again, this is pure empiricism to the exclusion of rational thought.

To be fair, "evidence-based medicine" simply *ranks the evidence according to quality* into a hierarchy, with meta-analyses and systematic reviews at the top, the individual prospective RCT next, then observational studies (the subject of this chapter), and lowest on the list is expert opinion. This is a perfectly valid approach and cannot be criticized, if only we weren't forced to ignore the lower levels of evidence. On any given day, a lower level athletic team can knock off the top-ranked team, and so it is with observational evidence.

The best analogy, however, comes not from sports but from our legal system where evidence submitted for a verdict can come in two forms: direct evidence or circumstantial evidence. Yes, an eyewitness account of a murder is held with higher credibility than blood splatter patterns and the forensic experts who describe them, but aren't we all familiar now with the astonishing errors that occur with direct evidence? Eyewitnesses routinely miss the mark. Mark Twain described it like this: "You can't depend on your eyes when your imagination is out of focus." Sometimes, circumstantial evidence ends up being of great importance in the goal of jurisprudence.

Not so, it seems, for some evidence-based think tanks, such as the U.S. Preventive Services Task Force, where the observational (circumstantial) evidence for mammographic screening is given only a condescending nod. The Task Force denies this, by the way, in their 2016 response to public criticism, claiming that 200 observational studies were reviewed, "including 83 that specifically evaluated the benefits of screening mammography." The Task Force admits that the mortality reduction is greater in these studies, possibly reflecting modern equipment, yet at the same time, cannot be confirmed due to the limitations imposed by the standard biases of non-randomized trials. Thus, the newer observational data could not actually be incorporated into the "benefit column" of their system of weights and measures. Strictly speaking, the observational evidence was not *excluded* as many Task Force critics believe, it was duly noted, for the record.

If the available prospective RCTs on mammographic screening, churned into meta-analyses, were all pristine and employed modern technology, then the Task Force approach makes good sense. But from what you know now as a reader, it is absurd to think that the historical clinical trials for screening mammography are reflective of what is done today when it comes to breast cancer screening.

Statistical-based medicine rests on a foundation of theoretical cement, but in practicality, is largely sand. Recall how few can accurately define the meaning of a p-value, and that includes some statisticians. Yet that's not the worst thing about p-values—recall that the threshold of "statistical significance" ($p = 0.05$) is arbitrary, turning biologic continuums into false dichotomies. And I'm just getting started.

The problem is human bias, conscious or unconscious, and while evidence-based medicine is the attempt to get human bias out of the picture, it really just transfers the source. Bias can be programmed into the design of a clinical trial, and can certainly be used to manipulate the data in whatever direction is desired. Consider how many of the controversies in this book revolve around fixed historical data for which there are two strongly opposed camps that interpret the same data in different fashions. This is the origin of the old truism "You can use statistics to prove anything," a claim that makes statisticians cringe, but is not too far off base.

How do the biases of statisticians play out? First, the calculated numbers can simply be incorrect, yet go unnoticed. Periodically, statisticians will publish their own house-cleaning reviews, and the results are disarming, with lousy stats published even in the most prestigious journals. Independent reviews have exposed the lack of statistical monitoring in scientific publications, even when research is generated at the top tier medical centers. The September 2011 issue of *The Economist* contains an article entitled "Misconduct in Science: An Array of Errors" with the subtitle "Investigations Into a Case of Alleged Scientific Misconduct Have Revealed Numerous Holes in the Oversight of Science and Scientific Publishing." The concern is not the occasional renegade; instead, it's the current lack of oversight with shaky statistics generated from inaccessible raw data.

But there's so much more that casts doubt on the royal hierarchy of quality evidence. Take the final step in the scientific method—reproducibility. One study reviewed papers on research trials that were highly cited by other authors (more than 1,000 times), attempting to document how often the results were reproduced.[1] In one-third of the studies, results had been contradicted in subsequent trials or had at least been exaggerated. Only 44% were ever replicated, while 24% remained unchallenged. The author concluded, "Controversies are most common with highly cited nonrandomized studies, but even the most highly cited randomized trials may be challenged and refuted over time, especially small ones." This should be no surprise. Who has the time or motivation to repeat what someone else has done, unless there's a drive to disprove earlier results (and note the pre-fab bias built into that attitude).

Furthermore, clinical trials with negative outcomes are often not reported, even though the lack of benefit is important in and of itself. Sometimes, this is the fault of journal editors trying to pump up their "impact score," but sometimes it's the investigators themselves who say, "Why bother?" A variant of this is *file drawer bias*, where I'm as guilty as anyone. I could easily generate 20 or more papers from the data on breast MRI that I've accumulated over the years, yet will never have time to publish. High quality data is sitting there, every bit as important as much of what is already in print, but most of it will remain in the file cabinet.

Another source of hidden data that keeps us from accessing Reality is proprietary information that cannot be shared until patents are secured and the product ready to go. The list of biases is actually longer than the 4 Horsemen that I presented earlier.

The message here is cautionary—evidence-based medicine has a tendency to surrender clinical wisdom to the statisticians and epidemiologists who, once concerned with populations, are now practicing medicine at the individual level. Numbers are being generated that apply to patients one at a time. Guidelines are administered one patient at a time. A health care provider counsels one patient at a time.

The scientific method sounds straightforward until you actually try to do it. Fortunately, my criticisms above are being addressed by those devoted to quality research. P-values are giving way to confidence intervals, statisticians are being included early in the design of clinical trials, checklists from journals are being required of authors to help assure low-bias reporting, leading journals have begun offering statistical support for an impartial review of data prior to publication, open access journals allow peer-reviewed publications giving hidden data a new outlet, and advances are being made in statistical education and the software that goes with it. The problem of bias is being addressed on many fronts and many angles.

But rest assured, human behavior will always find an escape route.

The problem for us, in addressing mammographic screening, is that *none* of these ongoing improvements in scientific method and reporting will help us analyze studies that are now 30 to 40 years old. These trials have one unique redeeming feature that will never be repeated—they were conducted in the era prior to adjuvant systemic therapy, so this influence is one less confounding variable. Beyond that, however, they are hardly solid evidence. Does this mean that the trials that show benefit are flawed, too? Yes, they are flawed by today's standards, so the question is submitted for your consideration—do those trials that showed benefit for screening mammography overestimate or underestimate the effect of screening? Bias can work in both directions. And for the rest of this book, you will be encountering my personal bias in that the historical trials *underestimate* the benefit of screening. So let's examine the circumstantial evidence that seems to support this contention.

The exclusion of observational data is only acceptable when prospective RCTs are high quality. When RCTs are poor or outdated (or non-existent), this is precisely when you slip down the hierarchy into the murky world of observational studies. We are greeted in this underworld by the Four Horsemen of Bias—Selection Bias, Lead Time Bias, Length Bias and Overdiagnosis Bias—and some additional biases as well. Yet, if we know they are present, we can always carry with us a protective grain of salt.

Another of these additional biases is *reporting bias*, true for high quality clinical trials as well, but more prevalent in observational studies. Reporting bias is the phenomenon where positive studies are published far more often than negative studies. So what does our grain of salt tell us about mammographic screening? First of all, this topic is so contentious, with strong backers of the negative stance, reporting bias is held to a minimum. A negative study stands a very good chance of being published in today's climate on this topic.

Some of these observational studies involve over a million women, so if a large team of researchers spends years in their review only to discover that there was no benefit to mammography, we'd definitely hear about it. Too, there are many epidemiologists highly motivated to minimize the impact of screening, yet rather than generate new data confirming their negative belief (no benefit), their effort is spent attacking those historical trials where a mortality reduction was documented. Still, we have to admit the ever-present possibility of reporting bias in observational studies.

What exactly are the observational studies? Here's a list that reflects the wide variety, though we will not tarry with examples of each:

Case-control studies
Cohort studies
Population-based mortality reductions
Reductions in advanced stages of cancer
Detection rates
Cancer yields in a screened population
Stage/Grade/Biology of screen-detected cancers
Interval cancer rates and tumor biology of interval cancers
Studies of biology as related to lead times/sojourn times

In the great hierarchy of evidence, none of these approaches will equal the level of evidence achieved through a prospective, randomized trial. Yet are they to be dismissed entirely? If so, why did investigators bother doing the research in the first place? And, just as meta-analyses of prospective RCTs can claim many notches for its belt, there are notches for the observational studies as well. For instance, it was a case-control study that first demonstrated the link between tobacco smoking and lung cancer.

In a case-control study, one group with a "condition or treatment" is compared to a "hand-picked" group that is intended as comparable in all respects, but without the "condition or treatment." When the measured outcome in a case-control study is death rate (as opposed to survival rate) one actually circumvents *three* of the Four Horsemen: Lead Time Bias, Length Bias and Overdiagnosis. The remaining weakness is *selection bias*. That is, how was the control group selected and how do the participants match up to those in the treatment group? Some case-control studies will use larger numbers in their control group than their treatment group, or even use two or more control groups, to bolster claims of validity. In truth, however, only the randomization process throttles selection bias.

There is often a temporal aspect to observational studies as well, in that they are sometimes performed as a prelude to prospective RCTs, serving as the theoretical basis upon which a prospective randomized trial is justified, organized, and funded. It is impossible, however, to perform prospective RCTs for everything we do in medicine, so observational studies, or circumstantial evidence, is all we'll ever have for most of what we do.

There are hundreds and hundreds of these observational studies related to mammographic screening and the early detection of breast cancer. It requires much of a lifelong career to assimilate the information. Is it any wonder that the Task Force relegates them to a cursory afterthought, given that this same Task Force is trying to keep up with nearly 100 other preventive health measures?

In this battle over screening mammography, the weaponry is based in numbers. These numbers may appear to have been forged into the tempered steel of sophisticated statistical analysis, but they are more accurately described as plastic. Recall how MD Anderson's emeritus professor of radiology, the late Dr. Gerald Dodd, Jr., warned us about the encroachment of non-clinical forces into the practice of medicine? Today, we are at the mercy of our non-clinical colleagues who toy with the numbers on their fingertips. Task Force members, by the way, are mostly clinicians who have a special interest and training in epidemiology and public health. But even the Task Force will outsource much of the number games to biostatisticians. So an important question to ask is "Who pays the biostatisticians, those who torture the data until it talks?"

Of the biases other than the Four Horsemen, one that gets the spotlight today is *financial bias*. Clinicians who present their papers at scientific meetings are now required to give a confessional testimony at the start of every presentation outlining their financial conflicts of interest. Often, these flash cards include many names and many conflicts that appear on the screen for about a millisecond. Some have recognized that, while this is an important source of bias, it is hardly comprehensive, nor is everyone honest in listing their conflicts. As with most trends, they just keep trending, and we're now at the beginning of new era of recording and reporting more potential bias—researchers are being asked to reveal any and all relationships, *personal* and professional, that could impact study results. "Well, gee, my kids play soccer with Dr. X's kids, so this personal relationship could color my views." It will be fascinating to watch where this pendulum comes to rest.

Returning to our circumstantial evidence in observational studies, I'm going to select only a few to make the point. And to begin, not all such studies are in strong support of mammographic screening.

In 2010, the media swarmed over a paper from Norway published in the *New England Journal of Medicine*[2] that minimized the importance of mammography. With results given mostly as "deaths per 100,000 person-years," it is not as easily interpreted as most, but the bottom line was a modest 10% reduction in mortality through screening, with the bulk of improved mortality reduction coming through systemic therapies. Critics of the study had much to talk about, though few were ever heard. Far and away, the most common criticism was the shockingly short mean follow-up period of *2.2 years* wherein a benefit to screening is nearly impossible to measure.

In contrast, a 2011 case-control study from Nijmegen, the Netherlands,[3] 55,529 women were invited to mammographic screening between 1975 and 2008. A relative mortality reduction of 35% was statistically significant. For the first half of the *32-year* study, mortality reduction was 28%, while the last 16 years revealed the remarkable mortality reduction of 65%, this increasing benefit likely due to improvements in mammographic technology between the start date of 1975 and 2008. The media found very little interest in this pro-screening study, by the way.

A massive study out of Sweden[4] once again visited the 40–49 controversy in a cohort called "SCRY," or Screening of Younger Women, that included all Swedish counties. During the study period, there were 803 breast cancer deaths in the study group (7.3 million person-years) and 1,238 in the control group (8.8 million person-years), with an average follow-up of 16 years. The relative reduction in breast cancer mortality for those who attended screening was 29%, double the benefit seen in the prospective RCTs.

Upon publication of this massive study, Dr. Kopans was quoted as saying that it should "end the debate" about screening younger women. Later, he would claim that his words were taken out of context, but not until epidemiologists poked the bear, attacking Dr. Kopans' apparent lack of understanding that this was only an observational study. To wit, Dr. Kopans was fully aware of this fact, but too late—the epidemiologists returned to their respective caves while Dr. Kopans returned to researching new technologies to improve the accuracy of mammography.

The IMPACT Working Group in Florence, Italy, reported on 1,750 breast cancer deaths compared to 7,000 controls.[5] Invitation to screen resulted in a 25% relative reduction in breast cancer mortality. However, among those actually screened, mortality was reduced by 54%, adjusted to 45% after correction for self-selection. Again, a greater benefit than what was seen in the prospective RCTs.

From the United Kingdom, service screening performed in East Anglia reduced breast cancer mortality by 35% among those invited to screen and by 48% in those who actually attended screening.[6] Some of these investigators applied the same method to a case-control study in Wales, where the mortality reduction was 38%, and with bias corrected was 25%.[7]

And in the last chapter we saw a remarkable difference between the negative outcome of the Canadian NBSS vs. what actually happens in Canadian practice. The Pan-Canadian study of service screening included 2,796,472 screening participants from 7 of 12 programs that represented 85% of the Canadian population.[8] Age at entry into breast cancer screening had minimal impact on the magnitude of mortality reduction, ranging from 35% to 44%.

Given what we have learned in this book, it should be no surprise that dueling epidemiologists see data differently, and there are critics who have taken these studies to task, just as the pro-screening epidemiologists defend their positions. All publications prompt a debate as to methodology. I've barely scratched the surface here with case-control studies, and not bothered with the many other types of observational studies.

Also, I've not given fair attention to one of the more troublesome claims made by screening minimalists and anti-screeners—the fact that the number of advanced breast cancers has not declined in tandem with the increase in early detection, with the implication being overdiagnosis. The graphs are simple and convincing. The counter-explanation is convoluted and complex. Again relying on Dr. Tabár's data from Sweden, where actual chart reviews were performed rather than crunching Big Data, there is, in fact, a concomitant decline in advanced breast cancer cases to complement the rise in early detection.

Let me conclude with a unique study out of Harvard/Massachusetts General,[9] home to Dr. Kopans and other highly respected clinicians in breast medicine. This study was billed in the media as a "reverse randomized trial," starting with breast cancer deaths and working backward. However, in the strict sense, it's a case-control study, minimizing lead time bias, length bias, and overdiagnosis bias. But this is where it departs from the usual case-control study with inherent selection bias as the major flaw—in this particular instance, where both screened and unscreened patients died of breast cancer, there was *no selection bias*. This is why the study caught the eye of so many—although non-randomized, the Four Horsemen of Biases were not the same problem as seen in other observational studies. Take away these biases, and the non-randomized findings might be every bit as valid as a prospective, randomized controlled trial.

In contrast to the Big Data papers without chart reviews, these investigators closely reviewed 7,301 medical records of women diagnosed with breast cancer between 1990 and 1999, with 1,705 documented deaths, 609 due to breast cancer. Among these 609 breast cancer deaths, 29% were among women who had been screened with mammograms, whereas 71% of the deaths were among unscreened women, most of whom had *never* had a mammogram (a small fraction had undergone mammography more than 2 years prior). It was a simple conclusion: *"Most deaths from breast cancer occur in unscreened women."* And if there is a single takeaway from this chapter, or even this book, that would be it, taken from a study where the 4 Horsemen were tethered, if not bound.

If one includes commentaries and letters and counterpoints made in the literature, there are over a thousand articles written about mammographic screening. And, across the board, observational outcomes, where there is a control group, indicate similar benefit (clustering around a 30–40% mortality reduction overall; and, 20–25% mortality reduction for women in their 40s). While this benefit is greater than what is seen in the prospective, randomized trials, recall that the prospective trials include many women who were not compliant. And while the official results from these RCTs include these women in the group to which they were originally assigned, compliant patient outcomes are often tabulated secondarily. And it is fascinating to note that the benefit seen in this compliance data of RCTs matches the benefit seen in the observational case-control studies. In a word, *this consistent level of mortality reduction seen in both the compliant patients in RCTs and the observational studies explains my personal bias.*

Given the antiquated nature of the prospective randomized trials, especially noting the substandard epidemiology and outdated technology of the day, you would think someone might stand up and shout, "Wait a minute! Observational data is not simply desirable in the evaluation of screening, but perhaps modern screening data should be considered *preferentially* over the highly limited and archaic mammographic prospective screening trials."

In fact, the statement has been made. Dr. Stephen Feig, expert breast radiologist who has been fighting alongside Dr. Kopans for decades now, made this statement in an editorial[10]: "In general, results from service screening studies demonstrate substantially greater mortality reduction among screened women than among women offered screening in RCTs where calculated benefits reflect dilution with women who do not accept screening and comparison with a control group in which some women obtain screening outside the trial. Thus, service screening studies provide a more realistic estimate of the actual benefit from screening."

What would the U.S. Preventive Services Task Force think about this chapter on circumstantial evidence? What would other evidence-based think tanks think? For the most part, they would not consider this chapter at all. It simply would not exist. Not even the critically important Harvard study where biases are taken to the mat, so to speak, with chilling conclusions for the unscreened. As for Dr. Feig's statement, the Task Force has made it clear that you cannot trust providers to set policy, under the mistaken belief that financial bias is the ruling bias. For the Think Tanks, only the unbiased purity of statistics and epidemiology can direct patient care.

So let me drag a statistical expert into this polemic, the lead epidemiologist for the American Cancer Society, an organization that has historically examined all evidence, fully understanding the hierarchy of quality. In a 2014 article[11] after discussing the balance of benefits and harms of mammography as varying widely according to different interpreters, Robert Smith, PhD, concludes with "*The strong evidence of benefit associated with exposure to modern mammography screening suggests that it is time to move beyond the randomized controlled trial estimates of benefit and consider policy decisions on the basis of benefits and harms estimated from the evaluation of current screening programs.*"

That remarkable statement went unpublicized, in spite of its revolutionary implications.

# 17

# The Social Tsunami of Anti-Screening

In the pre–Powerpoint era, I began my 35mm presentations on "population screening" by drawing an analogy to childhood immunizations. Admitting that screening for adult onset disease was not nearly as efficient as the gold standard in public health—vaccinations against epidemics—I never dreamed that social forces would take even the vaccine gold standard to task.

Society, right or wrong, is both fickle and malleable. Currently, we are sloshing about in self-imposed confusion over mammographic screening. Yet that trend goes well beyond screening, into breast cancer management in general, into medicine on the whole, into science and into our everyday lives. Call it "less is more," "do no harm," or a "kinder, gentler world," we are moving toward a new reality. Sadly, as I've stated before, the biology of breast cancer doesn't give a flip about our social trends.

Journalists and science writers today are skewed heavily toward "doing less" and questioning the value of mammography. Few authors write from the pro-screening angle, in spite of the evidence you have seen offered in this book so far. "Early detection saves lives" is old news. Who cares? It's nothing more than dog-bites-man. The edgy writers seek the man-bites-dog story, where the action is, where the editors are boosting circulation through controversy.

Another trend in the media is the effort to "undo the scare tactics" that have been used in the past to prompt mammography compliance, apparently an ill-conceived form of retrograde guilt in response to the "overselling of mammography." A prime example would be the side bar "facts" used in *TIME* magazine (October 12, 2015), wherein the cover story was "What If I Decide to Just Do Nothing?" (the ultimate "less is more"). While the inside article addresses overtreatment in breast cancer with legitimate points, the side bar "facts" are deeply disturbing: "1 in 800—the chances of a woman in the U.S. getting diagnosed with invasive breast cancer." And "1 in 4,566—the chances that a woman in the U.S. will die from breast cancer." Do these numbers look strange? They should. Especially, since "1 in 8" has been so thoroughly engrained in the public for many years now. A 100-fold difference? What gives?

Well, it has been declared that "1 in 8" was a scare tactic, often tossed into the public arena without the explanation that this was a *lifetime* risk, from age 0 to 90. So, to counter the old propaganda with new propaganda, it appears that "1 in 800" is going to be tossed into the same arena, again without explanation. *All absolute risk calculations are meaningless unless they are framed within a duration of time.* That said, the only way I can make "1 in 800" mean anything at all is if we limit the duration of time to *one year*. Even then, the "1 in 800" factoid is a lowball number, so it would be more accurate to say this: "If you are a woman *in your 40s*, then the chance of being diagnosed with breast cancer *during the next year* is 1 in 800." The same is true for the reckless misrepresentation of "1 in 4,566," a *1-year* probability, where the *lifetime* risk is actually "1 in 35."

Who is being served by these misrepresentations? For a woman age 40 trying to decide if she wants to begin screening in her 40s, the number she needs to know is "1 in 70"—that is, over the course of the *next 10 years*, that's the probability she will be diagnosed with breast cancer. As for "1 in 800" left dangling in the breeze without critical qualifiers, it is inexcusably misleading. Scaring women into good health is an ethically marginal, but defensible, position; "un-scaring" women into death is another thing entirely.

The times they are a-changin'. When the National Cancer Institute attempted to change the screening age to 50 in the 1990s, the counter-attack was swift and hard, and the majority of practicing doctors at the time barely noticed that a Civil War was in progress. Not true in 2009 when the U.S. Preventive Services Task Force made the same move. An agenda had emerged in the interim that called into question many preventive health practices, which on the whole, are inefficient. While many of us believed the Task Force recommendations would suffer the same fate as the NCI Advisory Panel, we were wrong. The Zeitgeist had shifted, and the anti-screeners and screening minimalists were gathering momentum. No longer was it a War on Cancer, but a War Against the Harms of Diagnosing and Treating Cancer.

Recall that the meta-analysis of the 2009 Task Force was identical to 2002 when it came to the benefits of screening women in their 40s, with a statistically significant mortality reduction of 15%. Using new methodology to calculate harms and the harm-to-benefit ratio, a policy reversal occurred, no longer endorsing screening for women in their 40s. The real change was not the science and claims that "new data" had prompted the reversal. No, the real change was in societal attitudes about preventive health measures, which are notoriously expensive. In effect, the 2009 Task Force stated, "Yes, lives are saved with screening women in their 40s, but it's not worth the cost and trouble for such a small gain."

What are these "harms" that keep pouring down like rain on this debate? Most famously, there's the harm of a call-back. You undergo your screening mammogram, then a few days later, you are called back for an extra study. This is unnerving for many, but not all, less so for those who have been through it before. However, in the tally books, this is called a "false positive." I have seen poorly informed journalists weigh in on this staggering "false-positive" rate, going on and on about how this results in unnecessary chemotherapy, surgery, and radiation. This is so far off base as to warrant disciplinary action, if there were such a thing.

Instead, this type of "false positive" is a callback for additional views and perhaps a targeted ultrasound, the majority of call-backs turning out to be nothing. Roughly 5–10% of women are called back routinely after a screening mammogram. Over the course of 10 years, more than half of the women in mammographic screening programs will experience a call-back.

Yes, it would be nice if all breast centers could proceed with the work-up at the same time as the screening study, and while a few try their best to do so, our two-step standard of care is a by-product of mass screening where a busy center might complete more than 100 screens in a day. Immediate interpretations and work-ups wreak havoc with efficiency at a busy center.[1] With a nod to the future, one of the benefits of the new tomosynthesis 3-D mammography is a reduction in the call-back rate.

In those anti-screening podium presentations that use a 1,000 square grid on a Power-point slide, showing what happens to 1,000 women in order to save one life, an impressive 100 squares or more will light up to demonstrate the call-back rate. And before that final square lights up in all its insignificant tininess, denoting a solitary saved life, we are treated to 25 squares that light up representing the "unnecessary" biopsies that are performed.[2]

Make no mistake—"unnecessary" is pejorative, intended to cast mammography in a bad light. "Unnecessary" is a status known only after the fact, retrospectively, when everyone is an expert. At the time when the biopsy is recommended, it is not "unnecessary." Quite the contrary, it is necessarily done in 5 or 6 women to properly find cancer in the one. If biopsies were restricted to only those patients where we are certain malignancy is present based on imaging (called a BIRADS Level 5), then we would miss many life-threatening cancers. That is, we would miss the Level 4 patients where the probability of cancer is in the 15–20% range. Nearly all Level 4 patients are biopsied, fully aware that the majority will be benign. And before suggesting that we tighten the reins, performing fewer biopsies, we need to address the problem of malpractice litigators who already have a field day suing radiologists for failure to diagnose breast cancer.

"Unnecessary" casts the image-guided needle biopsy (under local anesthesia) into the same garbage pile as "unnecessary surgery," with the deplorable implication of intent-to-deceive. The word itself is a key tool in anti-screening rhetoric.

Prior to 1995 or so, mammography-generated biopsies required a surgical excision, with the great paradox being that the smaller the lesion, the harder it was for the surgeon to find it, and more tissue might then be removed than someone with a palpable lump. Often these lesions, such as calcium clusters could not be felt, and had to be confirmed by performing X-rays of the specimen. This is still required today when surgically excising known malignancies, but most of our screen-generated biopsies back in the old days ended up being benign, with two, three, four or more pieces of tissue sometimes removed before the calcifications could be confirmed as "out of the patient" by their presence on the X-ray specimen. Later, when the benign diagnosis was rendered, one could only sigh. But today, image-guided core biopsies under local anesthesia in the office are the mainstay, and they have reduced costs and deformity by leaps and bounds. Only rarely is the target missed, at a rate no different than the old-fashioned surgical excision approach. Breast biopsy is thus a vastly improved process.

Yet, in keeping with human nature, we adjust to advances and take them for granted. The revolution in biopsy technique is now considered a serious harm, and the sport of mammography-bashing has taken delight in documenting just how injurious these biopsies really are, complete with permanent psychological damage.

Then there's the harm of overdiagnosis. We've covered this ad nauseam already, so I won't dwell on it here, other than to point out again that anti-screeners are trying to drag breast cancer into the depths of "festering cancers" as seen in the prostate gland, and it simply isn't true. What is the chance of a woman dying with an undiagnosed invasive breast cancer? Answer: 1%. What is the chance of an 80-year-old man dying with undiagnosed prostate cancer? Answer: 80%.

As for DCIS, in a nutshell, if you are diagnosed with this entity, ask your surgeon point blank: "Am I a candidate for wide excision alone, without any other treatment?" Guidelines are in place for this option, vaguely from the NCCN, and quite specifically using the Van Nuys protocol and scoring system. The only hazard of overdiagnosis is overtreatment. Wide excision alone takes away the harm of overtreatment, and could possibly save a life in the long run.

And, yes, there is a small chance of a genuine false-positive, that is, an error in pathology interpretation. It is always a good idea to get a second opinion after a diagnosis of breast cancer, especially for "in situ" disease. This is done quite often, and there should be no hesitancy for such a request.

A final "harm," or alleged harm, is often tossed into the mix as well—the danger of radiation exposure. Some academic radiologists and physicists have devoted much of their careers to dispelling the myths that hover about this issue. Yes, early mammograms had radiation exposure levels that today are considered unacceptable, especially since some women with risk factors began yearly studies in their 20s with high-dose technology. And yes, there are radiation doses high enough to induce cancer—the younger you are, the more likely it can occur—but if we limit the discussion to *proven* radiation-induced cancer, we're talking about doses immensely higher than what a lifetime of mammography delivers, high enough to treat Hodgkin's disease.

Today, the risk of radiation-induced breast cancer from mammography is so small for women who begin screening at age 40, that it cannot reliably be measured. In fact, even the high doses of Hodgkins' disease treatment don't seem to increase risk very much after age 40, if at all. There is some residual concern about annual mammograms starting at age 25 in the gene-positive patients, given that 15 sets of mammograms will be done prior to reaching the "safe zone" at 40 and beyond. Thus, we rely more heavily on ultrasound and MRI, where there is no radiation exposure, for these very young women.

One oft-quoted calculation for radiation-induced cancer risk with mammography is 1 breast cancer for every 100,000 mammograms. This, of course, would be impossible to prove. Contrast that to a 1 in 12,000 risk of being struck by lightning. As mentioned earlier, the way I usually explain this is in the context of our daily radiation exposure from a variety of sources, most notably radon and cosmic rays. If you choose not to undergo mammography out of fear of radiation-induced cancer, then you will be getting 4 mammograms every year anyway through background radiation, while the woman who opts for annual mammograms will be getting the radiation exposure of 5 mammograms every year. We'll return to some inflated risk of radiation numbers later in the book.

I have read some proposed informed consents for routine screening mammography that are frankly inexplicable. The emphasis on "overdiagnosis" is especially disheartening—the numbers are inflated and, too, what can we do about it with regard to invasive breast cancer? We don't know which tumors are going to kill and which ones are not. What purpose is served by this "information," especially when the numbers themselves are highly controversial with a ludicrous range from 0 to 50%?

Yes, in the past, there was no informed consent at all. So now, to make up for all those years, are we to punish ourselves and our patients with an exaggerated list of harms? Does retrograde guilt mandate such a negative perspective? How did we get to the point of casting a health measure that saves lives in the worst possible light? But that's the trend. It's a kinder, gentler world, and we don't want to cause angst in the process of saving lives.

Humankind is chronically dissatisfied. We fluff our pillows, but later on, that same pillow feels like a sandbag. And if we corrected all perceived societal ills today, tomorrow morning there would be new injustices calling for reform.

Perhaps it seems callous, but to my view, we're already in a "kinder, gentler" world of breast cancer management. My reference point, of course, is going to be vastly different than someone coming out of training today, or even within the past 10 years. I trained in the pre-mammography, pre-breast conservation, pre-tamoxifen era, when things were really rough.

If you've not seen a Halsted radical mastectomy outcome, then go online and do a search. You will find ribs barely covered by skin grafts, radiation ulcerations, and elephantiasis of the arm where extensive lymph node dissections were performed, not to mention a special type of sarcoma developing in that arm after years of massive lymphedema.

When I was a surgery resident in the pre-tamoxifen era, a common surgical procedure in patients with metastatic breast cancer was bilateral adrenalectomy (removal of both adrenal glands), with oophorectomy in premenopausal women, performed to eradicate all sources of hormones. This was an operation with high morbidity followed by tricky endocrine management since it wasn't only the sex hormones that were brought under control, but other steroidal hormones as well. All this in a patient who would inevitably die of breast cancer anyway.

Oh how thrilled we were when the neurosurgeons suggested the simple removal of the pituitary gland by scraping it out of it bony nest at the base of the brain through an approach via the sinuses comparable to a prefrontal lobotomy, only a different target. Of course, the endocrine management here was even trickier, once the "master gland" had been removed.

Yes, "kinder, gentler" is a relative term. Today, women take an "anti-estrogen" pill that can accomplish the same effect as bilateral adrenalectomy or removal of the pituitary gland.

We are advised nowadays not to frighten patients by using words like "cancer" unless we really mean it. Instead, new terms have been proposed for precancerous states that sound so bland that the diagnosis sounds like a normal finding. IDLE (indolent lesions of epithelial origin) sounds sort of fun, something you might want to do on a vacation, if it weren't for *the fact that some of these lesions are going to become invasive cancer and a small percentage are going to kill people if untreated.*[3]

The "kinder, gentler" approach is everywhere, though. Even the epidemiologists have gotten in the act. The old traditional "case-control" terminology has been called politically incorrect, the word "control" having more power than it deserves. After all, it's *not* to be confused with a randomized, *controlled* trial, so we shouldn't be giving it undue credibility when the control group is not that well controlled. The replacement? Case-referent. (Ah, that's much better.)

It starts early. The tsunami is set in motion as early as the MCAT, the Medical College Admissions Test, overhauled in 2015 for the first time since 1991. A new section has been added "due to the rapid and massive demographic changes taking place in America, such that becoming an MD these days requires skills that physicians of former generations never needed," according to one online peddler of a study guide. That new section is called "Psychological, Social, and Biologic Foundations of Behavior," with 95 minutes to complete 59 questions. After reading sample questions, I could feel the undertow of the tsunami, weeding out those that couldn't think in terms of society as a whole. In my day, we had a section called "General Knowledge," prompting us to memorize trivia such as the names of the three major pyramids at Giza, which is of no relevance whatsoever to being a good doctor. Nevertheless, there was no agenda in learning the names the pyramids either.

But I digress. The point is that, after 40 years of mass population screening, this public health measure is falling out of favor by the specialists in public health. Perhaps not to the extreme of the total anti-screeners, i.e., the screening nihilists, but to a compromise position, that is, less screening. The point I will make before we're done is that compromise is not the answer. That, in fact, there is plenty of room to improve what we do, saving even more lives than what is currently done, and in a cost-effective fashion. But these advances will never take place if we listen to voices of doom and harm in describing a measure that saves lives.[4]

I've mentioned several times how different sets of eyes interpret the same data differently. This is true for evaluating the harms of screening as well. Do those of us who practice medicine in a screening facility grow hard to call-backs and biopsies? Perhaps to a degree, though my administrative assistant and I still draw straws to determine who calls the patient for a return work-up. And, yes, we cringe when those rare casualties of screening get caught in a vicious cycle of radiologic and pathologic snafus, dropping out of screening programs entirely.

But imagine this—saving lives *is also routine*. While anti-screeners and screening minimalists are spouting their positions from the blood-free offices of the epidemiologist, a typical breast screening center performing 100 mammograms a day, will save one life every 10 working *days* (if we use the NNS = 1,000 for all age groups). And if you want to use numbers in the Task Force range, then breast radiologists *only* save one life every 20 days. There are thousands and thousands of breast centers around the world doing just that.

It shocks newbies to see "number needed to screen to save one life," as it reeks of inefficiency at 1,000 to 2,000, but these NNS and NNI numbers are not new. We've known the rough estimates for decades. But today, these estimates are presented often and with unwarranted precision, intended to cast the concept of screening into question. Screening is different than treatment. It's much harder to make screening efficient and cost-effective. Like most public health measures, be it seat belts or mammography, the intervention touches many more lives than it saves.

"Do no harm" is one of the most vacuous phrases in all of medicine, often expressed in Latin in order to add gravitas to a "don't do it" stance by someone about something. It is attributed to the Hippocratic Oath, which is a stretch. "Do no *needless* harm" would be more appropriate because *everything we do in medicine carries the potential of harm*. One of my old surgery professors used to say, "There's a mortality rate associated with everything in medicine, and that includes drawing a blood sample." (Years later, I had a patient faint and injure herself after a blood draw. Fortunately, she survived, so I did not fulfill the prophecy of Dr. John Schilling.)

Harm comes with the territory in medicine. I believe a self-selection process is at work, where many of the women who do not routinely get mammograms have already weighed the evidence, and decided against mammography for whatever reason. Many times these reasons are without basis (no risk factors, radiation exposure from the mammogram, etc.), but in the minds of these women, the harms definitely outweigh the benefits. But if we're going to inform patients to the hilt, whether they want to hear us or not, then why is there so little effort to inform patients who are not complying with mammography and putting their lives at risk? Don't they deserve the same attention as those already getting mammograms? Instead, we're supposed to offer extensive informed consents with a decidedly negative slant only to those women already getting mammograms, in effect, to get them to back off.

One thing about a tsunami—if you're standing on the beach, you're the last to know that it's about to hit. And, if you don't believe a social tsunami is in progress, I'm going to list a number of strong positions taken in breast cancer today, some of which I thoroughly support, some I'm neutral, and some I oppose. The point is that such a list exists.

Lobular carcinoma in situ is not cancer.
Ductal carcinoma in situ is not cancer.
One-third or more of invasive breast cancers are no threat to a woman's life.
Margin status and lumpectomy recurrences don't matter.
Partial breast radiation is all that is needed after lumpectomy.
Intra-operative radiation will suffice, or no radiation at all after lumpectomy.
Positive axillary nodes missed by sentinel node biopsy don't matter.
Contralateral cancers discovered through multi-modality imaging don't matter.
Contralateral preventive mastectomies are never indicated for unilateral cancer.
Pre-operative MRI staging doesn't help surgical management.
MRI-discovered and Ultrasound-discovered cancers only make overdiagnosis worse.
We can screen for breast cancer less often and only in women over 50.

I call this list, in its totality, the Zen approach to breast cancer, or "Embrace Your Inner Malignancy."

The point is not whether each item is true or false. The point is that we're in the middle of a social tsunami to do less. "Less is more." And, while some of the claims above are quite valid, and the goal of a "kinder, gentler" approach to breast cancer is indeed admirable, keep this one thing in mind: *Not a single additional life will be saved by anything on the list above.*

Indeed, for some, ground will be lost. These are not advances in the battle against breast cancer; they are measures to keep a cease-fire in place and thus, spare the ammunition. Some are measures that benefit society, while ignoring the individual.

It's a tough call when it comes to the "society vs. individual" debate. I suspect that if one combined all the arid academic departments of philosophy from 50 universities, we would not advance any further than *Star Trek*. Spock and Captain Kirk argued this point throughout a number of films wherein Spock insisted that "the needs of many outweigh the needs of one," and that anything else was "illogical." Yet, time and again, the "many" put themselves in harm's way to save one person or one alien as the case may be (including Spock on occasion). The debate went to and fro over the years and through several blockbusters, but was finally resolved in *The Voyage Home* (1986) when Spock insisted that the crew combine their efforts to save crewman Chekov, even at the risk of jeopardizing their vital mission to save Earth and everyone on it. Captain Kirk pointed out Spock's inconsistency (Spock is half-human, half–Vulcan) by asking, "Is this the logical thing to do?" Spock's answer? "No, but it is the human thing to do."

# 18

# The 2015 ACS Peace Accord—
# Science or Societal Pressure?

Throughout the turbulent years of this mammography controversy, first with the Civil War, then the brouhaha launched by the Task Force, one obvious champion was left standing, defending its recommendation of "annual mammography starting at age 40"—the American Cancer Society. And while many would refrain from calling this organization "neutral," it is relied upon by many as the most authoritative source when it comes to breast cancer screening. Certainly, it can be considered closer to a neutral corner than the much-maligned "biased providers" that make up the specialty organizations. For many of us, the ACS became our go-to source, avoiding protracted arguments about mammographic screening by simply responding, "We follow American Cancer Society guidelines."

After the 2009 Task Force announcement and its semi-radical departure from the standard of the day, the ACS came to the rescue and held their ground. Although ACS Chief Medical Officer Otis Brawley admitted that mammograms may have been oversold to the public, he also said that the ACS had carefully reviewed the data, including observational studies, and that they would be sticking with age 40.

But societal pressures can be relentless. In fact, they can be more powerful than scientific truth. One can look at data at a certain point in time, and 10 years later, looking at the same data, it somehow appears different. A new conclusion is drawn within a new context. For breast cancer screening, that shift occurred when the minimalists and nihilists became more concerned about the harms of screening mammography than the fact that it saves lives.

On October 27, 2015, the American Cancer Society issued new screening guidelines that marked the most sweeping changes since their original recommendation in 1976 at the dawn of mammography. Their last official update had been in 2003, but "annual starting at 40" had been in place since 1997, and before that, dating back to 1983, it had been "every 1–2 years starting at 40, then annual after 50." As an aside, many may recall the "baseline mammogram at 35–39" recommendation that appeared in 1980, ending in 1992.

The "all meat no potatoes" version of the new 2015 guidelines are touted as "Begin annual screening at 45, then switch to biennial screening (every 2 years) at 55." But let's take a look at the potatoes, and then have some dessert.

When I heard the ACS announcement, my first reaction was this: "Well, they finally caved. And they've chosen a 'compromise' position, halfway between the Task Force and the American College of Radiology (and other specialty societies), with the hope that we can end this longstanding schism. After all, what better way to settle the 40 vs. 50 debate than to split the difference at 45?" My supposition was that the data would be the same as always, but now viewed in the new light of "less is more." One thing about a massive database is that it becomes so willing to be manipulated. The bigger the better.

The new American Cancer Society guidelines, *applicable only to women at "average risk,"* are as follows[1]:

**Strong Recommendation:**
Start mammographic screening at 45

**Qualified Recommendations:**
Annual screening at first (that is, at age 45)
Women 55 and older should transition to biennial screening (every 2 years) or have the opportunity to continue screening annually.
Women should have the opportunity to begin annual screening between the ages of 40 and 44.
Continue screening as long as overall health is good and life expectancy is ≥10 years.
No clinical exam for women at average risk.

What's the difference between "strong" and "qualified" recommendations? Well, there are separate definitions, depending on whether you are a physician or patient, based on a handbook published online by the Grade Working Group in 2013—GRADE (Grades of Recommendation, Assessment, Development, and Evaluation).

*Strong Recommendation:*
*Patients*—Most individuals in this situation would want the recommended course of action, and only a small proportion would not.
*Physicians*—Most individuals should receive the recommended course of action. Adherence to this recommendation according to the guideline could be used as a quality criterion or performance indicator.

*Qualified Recommendation:*
*Patients*—The majority of individuals in this situation would want the suggested course of action, but many would not. Patient preferences and informed decision are desirable for making decisions (their words, not mine).
*Physicians*—Clinicians should acknowledge that different choices will be appropriate for different patients and that clinicians must help each patient arrive at a management decision consistent with her or his values and preferences. Decision aids may be useful to help individuals in making decisions consistent with their values and preferences. Clinicians should expect to spend more time with patients when working toward a decision.

Note: there is only one "Strong" recommendation: Start at 45. Everything else is "Qualified." Furthermore, the old recommendations are embedded in the new! And the option of sticking to old guidelines has no asterisk, nor is it small font buried deep in the article; instead, the "old" approach is up front in the Abstract and an inherent part of the formal recommendations—Women should have the opportunity ... to start at 40 and continue annually. Yet this option was stripped from all coverage of the new guidelines within seconds of its release.

And therein lies the potatoes. Yes, the old recommendations are given secondary status by virtue of the syntax and accompanying data, but the old guidelines are still there.

The ACS didn't blindside us, by the way. They telegraphed what was brewing in 2011 in *JAMA*[2] where the ACS made the announcement that they had adopted the Institute of Medicine's protocol for guideline development. When that announcement was released, my first response, considering the anti-screening tsunami, was "Uh-oh." A cornerstone of formulating guidelines in evidence-based medicine is "You can't have providers establishing the guidelines."

Yet, in contrast to the "limited or no expert testimony" policies of the U.S. Preventive Services Task Force, the American Cancer Society went to extraordinary lengths for advice—inviting, prior to publication, external review by 22 expert advisors and 26 relevant outside organizations. Incidentally, both the Society of Breast Imaging and the U.S. Preventive Services Task Force were among the 26, so it's clear that outsiders had no veto power, though we don't have details as to specific contributions that external review allowed.

In fact, from the start, the ACS approach was far superior to the Task Force. Initially, the ACS Guideline Development Group (GDG) sent out requests for proposals, eventually selecting the Duke University Evidence Synthesis Group to perform a systematic review of the breast cancer screening literature. The ACS also commissioned the Breast Cancer Surveillance Consortium to update previously published analyses related to screening intervals and outcomes, with specific reference to tumor size and stage with varying intervals (recall, this is the "X" of our X + Y = Z equation, given that our only control over biology is adjusting the interval of the screen). It doesn't stop there, but you get the point.

The working group (GDG) was composed of 4 clinicians, 2 biostatisticians, 2 epidemiologists, 2 patient representatives, and an economist. This panel tried to achieve 100% agreement whenever possible, but 75% agreement was considered acceptable. All participants in the guideline process had to disclose all financial relationships, as well as non-financial relationships, i.e., personal, intellectual, practice-related, that might be perceived as a conflict of interest in the development of breast cancer screening guidelines.

But the point I want to make here—distinguishing the ACS from the Task Force approach—is the fact that the ACS considered observational data ("circumstantial evidence") as having an important role in addition to the historic prospective randomized clinical trials. Why? Because the findings in those case-control and incidence-based mortality studies are consistent with, and supportive of, findings in the prospective RCTs. To be exact, the observational studies show a greater benefit to mammography than the RCTs, up to a 48% mortality reduction in one meta-analysis (EUROSCREEN Working Group).[3]

As a point of interest, the Task Force has settled more conservatively on a range between 25–31% mortality reduction in the observational studies (greater than the 19–22% mortality reduction in the prospective RCTs, counting Canada, of course, but still well below the 48% mortality reduction of EUROSCREEN). The Task Force has noted that these better outcomes in the observational studies may be due to the use of modern technology and high patient compliance (compared to "invitation to screen"), or could simply be the epidemiologic biases at work, or a combination of both—true benefit reflecting current technique, stretched a bit by the Big 4 biases.

In a companion article to the 2015 ACS recommendations in the same *JAMA* issue,[4] this one from the Duke research team that served up the plate for the ACS, the point is made that their exhaustive review of the observational data was performed at the request of the ACS working group. Maybe I'm reading too much into this, but I'm forever interested in the human element at work, and I got the impression that, given total freedom to review the data, they would have opted to stick with the prospective, randomized trials. I draw this impression from the fact that in the primary ACS article, the observational studies were considered as helpful, while in the companion article from Duke (p. 1629), the observational data "did not substantially reduce uncertainty about the magnitude of benefit."

An interesting side note: one of the meta-analyses included in the ACS/Duke review calculated a 19% relative mortality reduction with screening overall, including women ages 39–74. Remarkably, this came from the High Priest of screening nihilism, Dr. Peter Gøtzsche from Denmark. Was he still reeling from the worldwide condemnation after his 2-study meta-analysis found "no benefit at all to screening mammography"? Did his overzealous anti-screening study from the past prompt a redemptive effort, this time including *seven* clinical trials albeit only a modest mortality reduction of 19%?[5]

I'll leave that to the reader, but keep this in mind, as I'm voting for recalcitrance—in a 2011 editorial in the *Canadian Medical Association Journal,* Dr. Gøtzsche wrote: "The best method we have to reduce the risk of breast cancer is to stop the screening program."[6] This is not taken out of context. Dr. Gøtzsche's entire career is built on the hope of abolishing screening, fueled by his undying belief in the spontaneous regression of tumors as the explanation for overdiagnosis. He builds the case for massive overdiagnosis using numbers and assumptions, while those of us who actually see breast cancer every day have never seen it happen even once, much less to the soaring degree theorized by the cadre of nihilists.

One burning question should be: Did the ACS/Duke review include the Canadian NBSS? Of course it did. Only the World Health Organization has had the temerity to toss it out. For screening minimalists, it's a god-send. It has been so thoroughly anointed by so many that it would have been "heresy" to exclude it. Regardless of propriety, the CNBSS hurts the combined data. It dilutes the benefit of mammography. This does not prevent commentators from saying that this ACS/Duke effort confirms only "modest" benefit and that the 19% mortality reduction calculated by Gøtzsche probably reflects Reality better than the higher benefit calculated by others.

So, given the inclusion of the CNBSS with its "no benefit" dilution, one should also ask, "Was the U.K.'s AGE Trial included, the only semi-modern prospective RCT, designed exclusively for women in their 40s?" Yes, it was included. But only the 10-year follow-up, before a statistically significant reduction was announced in 2015. This is understandable, of course, as medical periodicals are written long before they appear in print.

Then, much to my surprise, I noticed in the closing paragraphs of the Duke article, a last minute online search (within weeks of publication) was made to determine if any new studies were worthy of inclusion. Indeed, 2 updates had been published on RCTs that had already been included in their meta-analysis—the 25-year follow up from the CNBSS, as well as the 17-year follow up from the AGE Trial. It was not felt, however, that anything had changed. True for the CNBSS (no benefit), but the AGE Trial had achieved statistical significance subsequent to the 10-year follow up used in the meta-analysis. Of course, by the time it's blended into the other trials, it's only a drop in the bucket.

But that drop happens to come from the only RCT that used technology anything close to what we do today. Furthermore, it's the only trial ever performed that addressed the predefined age group (40–49) by capturing women *as they were turning 40* in order to document nearly a full decade of impact through *annual* mammographic screening (through age 48). In contrast, the Canadian trial enrolled women "in their 40s" in the CNBSS-1 limb, so the absence of any benefit here is even more remarkable as some participants were nearly 50 when they agreed to participate.

The AGE Trial had a much more difficult task in trying to show a benefit, by including women that, overall, were being screened at a younger age than the CNBSS-1. As we will see in an upcoming chapter, the AGE Trial demonstrated a statistically significant 25% relative reduction in mortality for women in their 40s in the first decade after diagnosis (this effect gradually disappearing after the control group began routine screening according to NHS guidelines). The point of introducing the AGE results here is that this was the most powerful evidence in mammographic history for screening women in their 40s, *starting at 40*, yet the recommendation emerged to start screening at 45 (and the only ACS recommendation to be listed as "Strong").

Again, it's always helpful to recall our X + Y = Z equation. *Biology (X) + Sensitivity (Y) = Screening Effectiveness.* Meta-analyses and combined reviews don't help one bit with the "Y" factor. Mammographic Sensitivity (Y) levels from 30–50 years ago do not seem to invite "adjustments" that are so common in statistical methodology elsewhere. On the other hand, the "X" (Biology/interval) was studied in detail in formulating the new American Cancer Society recommendations. The Breast Cancer Surveillance Consortium, serving as advisors to the ACS, calculated (from a sample of 15,440 breast cancer patients) that the proportion of tumors that were Stage IIB or higher, even those larger than 1.5cm, was greater when screening was performed every 2 years as opposed to annually, though this was true only for *premenopausal* patients.

This information added support to the ACS recommendation to continue annual screening in younger women (again, the screening interval is used to address tumor biology, or "X"), but simultaneously calls into question the starting age of 45. If longer intervals mean larger tumors, *especially in younger women*, why change the starting age to 45 (and on the heels of the fresh results from the AGE Trial)? This only creates a new interval—a 5-year interval, in fact—from 40–44 where tumors are free to do whatever they want. It is fairly easy to see why the ACS left the old recommendations as part of the new, even if they are embedded as a secondary option.

Within hours, the Society of Breast Imaging, in concert with the American College of Radiology, weighed in with their recommendation to stick to the old ACS guidelines. Acknowledging that the effort by the ACS was vastly superior to the isolated approach of the Task Force, the fact remains that less screening translates to more lives lost.

Landmark articles are usually accompanied by editorials in the same issue of the journal, an honor traditionally bestowed on experts in the same arena. Sometimes these commentaries will be supportive, sometimes not.

To accompany the new ACS guidelines, the *JAMA* editors invited Drs. Keating and Pace whom we met earlier with regard to their study of a "proper" informed consent (and for which my letter to *JAMA* addressing seat belts was soundly rejected). Their editorial response offers semi-support, as one would expect given the compromise position of the ACS, moving closer to the Task Force. Yet the authors remain overly consumed by dark clouds of overdiagnosis, and they are disturbed about the excessive harms in younger women. "Yes, tumors are probably larger when you screen at longer intervals in younger women, but that doesn't necessarily translate to a mortality reduction," said the ants talking to a world of incredulous spiders. And, when it comes to the ACS and the Task Force, "both guidelines agree that for average-risk women younger than 45 years, the harms of mammography screening likely outweigh the benefits."

Again, you can use empiricism to calculate harms, and you can use empiricism to calculate benefits (albeit these numbers are easily and widely manipulated), but when it comes to that final judgment call claiming, "harms outweigh benefits," that balancing act is 100% subjective. And in today's bizarre climate where honeybees are disappearing, that subjectivity is wrapped in a cloak of certainty and delivered to the public as scientific fact. To quote Kurtz the ivory trader, or Kurtz the general, "The horror! The horror!"

If I were locked in a cell, given only bread and water, and was told I would not be released until I had written guidelines that served as a *compromise* to bridge the gap between specialty societies and the Task Force, I might well have come up with these 2015 ACS guidelines. However, I'm not sure I would have been clever enough to embed the old guidelines within the new as an option. Still, I would have much preferred waiting until age 70, after most of the storm had passed, before switching from annual to biennial (as opposed to switching during the years of peak incidence of breast cancer!). Of course, my resistance would depend on how long I'd been locked up.

That said, if 45 is the new 40, some lives will inevitably be lost while women wait to turn 45 to begin screening. Of course, lives are lost already because we have so little to offer average-risk women *under* age 40 who will be diagnosed with breast cancer (5% of all breast cancer cases). And now, we add another 7% of eventual victims between the ages of 40 and 44 to be disenfranchised with the new ACS guidelines, and we're up to 12%. But if we adopt Task Force guidelines to start at 50, excluding women 45–49, then recall that nearly 25% of eventual victims are being separated from the option of mammographic screening. This is a startling consequence of the Task Force, and completely ignores the post-mortem Harvard study (euphemistically called a "failure analysis") where, in a previous chapter, we saw the widely disproportionate number of breast cancer deaths in women who had not been screened, especially younger women.[7]

So was 45 chosen as a compromise position before the process even started, then the data made to fit accordingly? I don't know, and I'm not sure if it matters. Certainly, the ACS laid out a detailed case that age 45 is grounded in some objective evidence. The incidence of cancer from 45–49 is closer to the 50–54 group than it is to the 40–44 group (barely), as is the mortality data (barely). Then, in the distribution of "person-years of life lost due to breast cancer," the bar in the graph peaks in the 45–49 group. Importantly, the greatest rate of callbacks and other "harms" occur in the younger age groups, so raising the starting age to 45 has a favorable impact on the harm-to-benefit ratio. The ACS openly admits that they are responding to a *greater emphasis on the harms of mammography* than what was done in the past.

I won't dwell on the ACS dismissal of the clinical breast exam as part of the routine evaluation of average-risk patients. Certainly, in my high risk program I tell patients that my primary goal, through multi-modality imaging and research, is to make the clinical exam obsolete. Though to be exact, these ACS guidelines are addressing the average-risk patient, not the high-risk population. Still, it is bothersome to see yet another part of the traditional physical exam go by the wayside, under the header of evidence-based medicine. Using the reductionist principles so beloved by empiricists, one can completely dismantle the traditional physical exam into nothingness. There is precious little data one way or the other on the benefit of routine clinical breast exam, but are we to buy into the ACS justification that this will give more time for the doctor to discuss screening recommendations? Speaking as a seasoned cynic, if more time is generated for the doctor by excluding the clinical breast exam, it will be used for data entry into the electronic health record, not in the discussion of screening recommendations.

In the *TIME* magazine coverage of the ACS recommendations (November 2, 2015), Dr. Kevin Oeffinger, chair of the ACS guideline committee, is quoted as saying, "The evidence simply no longer supports one-size-fits-all. In medicine we are moving closer and closer to bringing about a personalized approach."

"Personalized screening" sounds wonderful, as do all euphemisms. The problem, once again, is that "average risk" women are at high risk for breast cancer relative to other diseases—12% lifetime. Shifting to lifetime *mortality* risk (3%) may appear to lessen the problem through a different endpoint, but simply being *diagnosed* with breast cancer wreaks special havoc, cured or not, so the 12% reigns, in my view, even though that risk is spread out over a lifetime. Still, when talking about such a common disease, women should be on guard when the term "personalized screening" is bandied about.

Dr. Stephen Feig has already sounded the alarm, pointing out the "personalized screening" in average risk women is actually "restricted screening," a wolf in sheep's clothing. Indeed, these ACS guidelines do not open up screening to a single new patient, rather, they unilaterally diminish screening for women at average risk. If most women were once compliant with the old guidelines, then if all were to switch to the new guidelines, the result will be more breast cancer deaths with the new guidelines (roughly, 1000 per year, a tiny drop in the epidemiologic bucket). This is the problem with "backing off" from current guidelines. Had the U.S. the foresight to start off with less screening from the get-go in the 1970s, it would not be so painful today to switch. Yes, the new ACS guidelines are more in line with the rest of the world, but even Dr. Tabár has admitted that the U.S. approach likely saves more lives than his own Swedish Two-County approach.

Well, it could have been worse. The ACS had the option to jump in the pool of Kool-Aid® with the Task Force. So kudos for proposing a compromise. Yes, at first glance, it adds to the confusion. But if both warring parties will admit the need to quit battling in the public eye, perhaps we would see more compliance overall. After all, 90% compliance with the new ACS guidelines would actually lower the number of breast cancer deaths overall, compared to our moderate compliance currently (as variably defined).

Included in the *JAMA* article on new guidelines, the ACS (p. 1611) expresses its dismay about the "contentious nature of debates surrounding breast cancer screening," offering this instead: "Given the weight of the evidence that mammography screening is associated with a significant reduction in the risk of dying from breast cancer after age 40 years, a more productive discussion would be focused on how to improve the performance of mammographic screening."

First of all, age 40 in the sentence above is not a misprint. Saved lives in the 40–44 group is the Reality, but the harms have been deemed by the ACS and others to outweigh the benefits. Secondly, "improve the performance of mammographic screening" is being accomplished like never before, by innovators who happen to be the pro-screening breast radiologists engaged in this debate, not content with the status quo. Yet the armchair authorities who are screening minimalists, or even nihilists, have contributed absolutely nothing to these imaging improvements while, at the same time, have dragged down the efforts of those radiologists who must spend a considerable portion of their professional lives in self-defense.

Importantly, the American Cancer Society is not done yet. In fact, they were the first organization to introduce the good side of "personalized screening"—that is, *doing more* for women at higher risk when they introduced a special set of guidelines for high-risk screening (using MRI) in 2007. This was a bold step, taken without proven mortality reduction. Other organizations followed, notably the NCCN. Very soon, the 2007 guidelines will be revamped, and we're hoping to see better options for women at intermediate risk. The very high risk patients are covered—annual breast MRI and annual mammography, starting at age 30. But for those somewhere in between, at more modest risk elevations, e.g., a woman having a single first-degree relative with breast cancer diagnosed at 50, women are stranded between very high risk and average risk. Ideally, we should stratify patients into 3 groups as has been previously suggested,[8] coupling risk level to breast density level, then offering screening ultrasound and/or MRI, less aggressively than the very high risk group, yet more than what is offered to the average risk patients.

Unfortunately, the "less is more" doctrine regarding screening for breast cancer has been ill-timed, arriving on the social scene at the same time that we're in a technologic explosion, putting "old-fashioned" mammograms, when used alone, out to pasture. One hundred percent of the data being analyzed and argued for these new guidelines *does not include this new technology*. The 3-D tomosynthesis mammography increases Sensitivity (more benefit) while at the same time improves Specificity (fewer harms)—that is, more cancers detected, fewer call-backs and fewer benign biopsies. This will cause a shift in the notorious harms-to-benefit ratio that has prompted the decrease in screening of late. The balance should therefore tip the scales back to more comprehensive screening, starting at ages younger than 45 and screening at one year intervals, just like the good ol' days. Of course, it will be no problem at all for the screening minimalists to shift the fulcrum of the teeter-totter. Remember, the final step after objectively calculating benefits, then objectively calculating harms, is to pin the tail on the donkey.

# 19

# A Journey to the Pathology Lab
# to View By-Products of Screening

It is quite possible that you, the reader, have already been through the screening jungle where a biopsy revealed something of concern, only to be told "it's not really cancer" even though the official report boldly states "carcinoma." Or perhaps you've received a report that your biopsy was "benign, but had features called atypical hyperplasia." Or maybe you were diagnosed with a complex sclerosing lesion that was described as "nothing important, but we're sending the slides to an expert to make sure it's not cancer."

If so, this chapter is for you. If not, it's still for you. If you are female, the potential is always there that it will happen someday. If you are a male or female health care provider, you will face these issues with your patients at some point if you are in primary care.

Anti-screeners would be quick to point out that these "iffy" pathology reports are by-products of deception, that is, mammography is stirring up trouble where none would have existed otherwise. And there is some truth to this. That said, there seems to be selective amnesia on this issue, given that these same pathologic entities were known prior to the screening era, commonly seen when the norm was surgical excision for benign lumps. When the shift came toward biopsies that were generated by mammographic findings, these same challenges on pathology became more frequent and drew more interest. So, we are really looking at by-products of biopsies, related to screening indirectly.

Recall the saga of pathologist Dr. Robert W. McDivitt who reviewed slides from the BCDDP starting in the 1970s, labeling 506 cases as "minimal breast cancer," raising questions as to how these should be treated. But worse, 66 cancer cases fell short of the "minimal" label, that is, there was no cancer at all. Since most of these 66 had undergone mastectomy already by the time of Dr. McDivitt's expert review, a firestorm erupted prompting back-and-forth arguments from the operating surgeons vs. the lone pathologist. As a result, new interest in breast pathology arose in these areas: (1) defining the benign patterns that mimic cancer, (2) distinguishing atypical hyperplasia from carcinoma in situ, and (3) trying to get a handle on the natural history of these "minimal cancers."

The disheartening study that we reviewed earlier by Elmore et al. in the March 15, 2015, issue of the *JAMA* indicated that we have not come very far since the days of McDivitt. With 115 pathologists attempting to pinpoint biopsy results as benign, atypical, in situ carcinoma, or invasive carcinoma, there was only 75% concordance with the expert panel that had earlier reviewed the same slides (with this panel of 3 experts even disagreeing among themselves in certain cases). Most dramatically, in one case, 40% of the 115 pathologists called a completely benign finding "invasive cancer," as had occurred decades earlier in the BCDDP. Granted, this should be tempered by the fact that practicing pathologists have access to deeper cuts, special stains, the input of their colleagues and expert opinion.

Trying to explain the inherent limitations of breast pathology to non-pathologists is a major challenge—the ambiguity is simply not believable. Static images of dead tissue under the microscope are supposed to translate into viable, animated, dynamic stories where the pathologist can describe past, present and future behavior of the cells now buried between slabs of glass. The limitations go far beyond breast pathology—huge gaps can exist between what is seen under the microscope and what evolves in clinical practice. Fortunately, the gaps get smaller and smaller as advances are realized in cellular and tissue analysis.

Would we have the same problems without mammography? Absolutely, though anti-screeners would like for you to believe otherwise. The problem arises in that screening mammography magnifies the difficulties because it generates greater numbers of these controversial findings, sometimes resulting in overtreatment. So, in this chapter, we are going to walk through some of the common by-products of mammography in order to offer insight on the complexities. Anyone can go online and discover canned answers for each of the following diagnoses, but rarely do these snippets tell the whole story.

Before we can talk about specific entities, however, we have to ask, "Is the diagnosis correct?" And, as we've seen above, it may not be the case. In my practice, heavily devoted to these borderline lesions and minimal cancers, we frequently request slide reviews by recognized breast pathology experts. Yes, there may have been two or more pathologists already look at the biopsy and agree with the diagnosis, but when these doctors are all in the same group practice, there tends to be more agreement than is seen with outside review, a product of human nature.

In contrast, consultative experts have a different starting point, that is, they are comfortable in a quasi-adversarial role, prepared to disagree from the beginning. And they do. That said, as we've seen, even the experts don't always agree. In that situation, it is my job to explain to patients why there is a controversy in the first place, and now, what are the options based on a *range* of possible diagnoses and outcomes. And away we go....

*Fibrocystic change.* The older term "fibrocystic *disease*" had such a broad definition, ranging from clinical manifestations (lumps and pain) to microscopic findings, that it was hard to escape the label. Most women had it, making it hard to call it a disease. By dropping the word "disease" and focusing only on the term as applied to biopsy results, "fibrocystic" still remains an all-inclusive term for benign changes. Such a wide scope prevents "fibrocystic" from being clinically useful if it stands alone. Today, most pathologists make further distinction by dividing "fibrocystic" into (1) non-proliferative changes, (2) proliferative changes (or disease), or (3) proliferative disease with atypia (atypical hyperplasia).

When a core (needle) biopsy is performed, the primary task of the pathologist and the radiologist is to determine if the abnormality in question has been adequately sampled. This exercise depends on the descriptors in the pathology report plus open communication between the two specialists. Often, the radiologic images and microscopic images are compared side-by-side in the conference setting.

If the biopsy is confirmed as "benign" after adequate sampling, all parties involved are happy and relieved, but screening minimalists with retrospective certitude replace the word "benign" with "unnecessary." Yet benign biopsies can sometimes offer helpful information, specifically related to risk stratification. While a tissue sample obtained by needle core is a far cry from thorough cell sampling as performed with a Pap smear, there are certain features that can have clinical implications.

*Non-proliferative changes.* Fibrosis, microcysts, calcium in normal structures, duct ectasia, apocrine metaplasia, etc., do not impart a significantly elevated risk for breast cancer. Yet some of the mathematical models used in breast cancer risk assessment ignore this fact and calculate an elevated risk for any biopsy, regardless of the exact tissue abnormalities present. After 3 or 4 of these biopsies over the course of many years, some women will be erroneously placed in a high risk category where they might be advised to take tamoxifen or raloxifene to reduce risk, or to undergo screening MRI, or on rare occasion, to consider preventive surgery. Yet their breast cancer risk, in reality, is only slightly increased over women in the general population. Since no clinically useful information comes from this category, there is the downside potential of excess risk attributed to the patient.

*Proliferative disease (without atypia).* Moderate, severe or florid hyperplasia, adenosis of various types, radial scars and complex sclerosing lesions impart an increased probability of developing breast cancer, usually a 2-fold risk, though some studies indicate florid hyperplasia and the overlapping term papillomatosis can carry a 3-fold risk. Alone, this degree of risk is usually not enough to warrant interventions, but when combined into a total risk profile, proliferative findings can make the difference as to whether or not a patient should be entered into a high risk protocol.

Given that one million benign breast biopsies are performed each year in the U.S. alone, you would think that we would put these benign findings to work. Unfortunately, when "tissue risk levels" were proposed and popularized by Drs. Page and Dupont in 1985,[1] some pathologists began including the relative risk numbers on their reports. At that time, there were no mathematical models for risk analysis outside the arcane epidemiology literature, and very few clinicians made a distinction between relative and absolute risks. A 2-fold risk seemed high, and it was not uncommon in my practice to see patients referred for preventive mastectomies with proliferative changes as the only risk factor. This troublesome scenario was one of several that prompted my interest in formal risk assessment where the totality of risks and protective factors are considered for each individual, then comparisons made to the general population and the no-known-risk population.

After over-reacting to the tissue risks imparted by proliferative change, pathologists dropped the numbers from their reports, while at the same time, mathematical models appeared on the scene where, this time, proliferative changes were helpful in stratifying risk. This tool is underutilized, as is risk stratification in general. Instead, results in this category are characterized by screening critics as "unnecessary biopsies."

*Proliferative disease with atypia.* Proliferative disease with atypia is commonly called atypical hyperplasia (AH), more specifically, atypical ductal hyperplasia (ADH) or atypical lobular hyperplasia (ALH).

The first decision to be made following this diagnosis on core needle biopsy is to consider a surgical excision of the area, the concern being that there could be carcinoma in situ, or even invasive cancer, living nearby. The likelihood of an upgrade to more serious pathology is stronger with ADH, a 10–20% chance, while ALH upgrade probability is in the 0–5% range, making the latter more controversial as to the need for surgical biopsy.

Beyond this difference, when it comes to the future risk for breast cancer imparted by ADH or ALH, the numbers are so close together than they can be considered together (AH), where the 4-fold relative risk has been documented in several series now, confirming the original risk level assigned by Dupont and Page. However, in sharp distinction to their pioneering work, where AH and family history were synergistic, elevating risk to 9-fold, subsequent series have not duplicated this finding. In fact, relative risks (RRs) seem to hover around a 4-fold risk regardless of family history, an important issue given that the mathematical models in common use today still incorporate an element of synergism that can render risk calculations higher than reality would dictate.

While the Plymouth Rock of quantifying tissue risks came from the work of Page and Dupont at Vanderbilt, the Mayo Clinic has recently contributed the bulk of new information pertaining to risk levels attributable to various benign pathology findings. Dr. Lynn Hartmann has taken the leadership role here, and she is sometimes assisted by William D. Dupont, PhD, the biostatistician at Vanderbilt who helped launch the study of tissue risks with Dr. Page more than 30 years ago.

In the January 1, 2015, issue of the *New England Journal of Medicine*, a special report was published on atypical hyperplasia drawn from the Mayo Clinic benign biopsy registry.[2] In nearly 700 cases of AH, the 4-fold risk was confirmed once again (for either ADH or ALH or both occurring together), while more solid evidence was presented in the form of absolute risks over time. Patients diagnosed with AH had a cumulative incidence of breast cancer approaching 30% at 25 years of follow-up, or roughly 1% per year, exactly what one would calculate with a 4-fold risk that persists over time.

Astutely, the authors point out that current MRI screening guidelines assign ADH and ALH to the "insufficient evidence" category, along with women who calculate to be at a 15–20% lifetime risk for breast cancer. Yet the American Cancer Society cited a risk of "only" 10 to 20% among women with ALH, while not providing any cumulative risk estimates for women with ADH. The Mayo Clinic data offers the best evidence yet for long-term risk imparted by both ALH and ADH. So, at present, we have the untenable, if not preposterous, situation where a woman who has a *21%* lifetime risk for breast cancer based on family history will qualify for MRI screening, while the patient with ADH and a *30%* risk over 25 years does *not* qualify for MRI. And, if a woman is diagnosed with ADH at a young age, let's say 35, this 30% long-term risk applies only through age 60 where cancer incidence is still peaking, so additional risk will follow over her "lifetime." Such a patient's lifetime risk could end up being double that of the patient who qualified for MRI on the basis of family history that yielded a 21% calculation.

The word "premalignancy" has been tossed about for many years in association with atypical hyperplasia, while the same term has been suggested for in situ carcinoma. It's a weak word, for sure, given that it implies the inevitable development of life-threatening cancer. From the 30% risk as noted above, one can see that the majority of women who carry a diagnosis of atypical hyperplasia will *never* develop breast cancer. So "premalignancy" is considered by many as too harsh in that implies an inevitable 100% probability of cancer.

But what a 30% risk for breast cancer *does* imply is this—all women diagnosed with AH should be informed of the pros and cons of pharmacologic risk reduction, using tamoxifen, raloxifene, or one of the aromatase inhibitors. Why? The risk reduction imparted by these agents is greater for women diagnosed with AH than it is for women who "only" have a positive family history.

This should be no surprise, given that AH is an actual tissue abnormality being targeted by the pharmaceutical agent, whereas a patient with a positive family history might have breast epithelial cells that are completely normal. Furthermore, nearly all AH lesions are "ER-positive" (too many estrogen receptors on the cell surface), and when they do evolve to full-blown cancer, those cancers are most likely going to be "ER-positive," the only situation where these pharmacologic agents work to prevent breast cancer. Indeed, the initial results in the first chemoprevention trial sponsored by the NSABP[3] were unexpectedly strong for tissue risks—in those patients who entered the trial on the basis of ADH, there was an 86% risk reduction in the development of breast cancer, very close to what is accomplished by preventive mastectomies. In contrast, the overall risk reduction in the study was about 50%, still impressive, but less than what was seen specifically in the ADH patients. As time passed, this risk reduction for patients with ADH settled down to 75%, but still … this is huge. And, after a 5-year course of tamoxifen, the durability of its effect can be measured for at least 15 years after the drug has been stopped.

The other interventions for patients with ADH or ALH include MRI screening or, in some cases, women will opt for preventive mastectomies with reconstruction. Mastectomy is not a medical directive as there are no threshold risk levels that automatically prompt surgical prevention. Instead, it is patient-driven choice that is usually accompanied by a family history for breast cancer, where the ADH patient has personally observed breast cancer treatment and/or mortality in her family (even though the risk level may be the same with or without the family history).

After excision of ADH (or ALH), it is easy to wonder, "Why is there still a risk for breast cancer if the problem has been removed?" Good question. The bottom line is this: we have limited information on what else is going on microscopically in the remaining breast tissue after a focal area of AH is diagnosed and removed. But we do have a great deal of information on what happens after the diagnosis—the cancers that occur are usually unrelated to the original AH biopsy site, with a nearly equal distribution between the two breasts. (The Mayo Clinic data suggests an ipsilateral preponderance at first, a precursor-type finding, later evolving to an equal distribution.) This pattern is the conceptual origin of the term "tissue risk factor," where the future cancer could occur anywhere, of any histologic type, that is, the same situation as one might see in a patient with a positive family history. While it is assumed that if AH is in one location, it is probably scattered in other locations as well, we don't usually know for sure. Instead, the published series simply count cancers as they emerge clinically, forming the basis of our risk calculations.

That said, another feature of the Mayo Clinic data is the finding that multiple areas of AH will increase risk beyond the usual 4-fold. Two foci of AH translate to a 5.5-fold risk, while three foci generate a 7.6-fold risk for breast cancer. Other microscopic features have been identified that work in the opposite direction—notably, lobular involution, a shrinkage of the microscopic lobular units (where milk is manufactured). Partial involution is the norm, but complete involution can cut AH risk in half, while no involution nearly doubles the AH risk, to a level comparable to having three foci of ADH.

In my practice, devoted to high risk patients where many patients have ADH or ALH, I slip away from the mathematical models, instead, using this precise data from the Mayo Clinic that seems to trump most family histories (notwithstanding pedigrees that point toward a genetic predisposition gene). Simply put, the mathematical models do not require review of the pathology slides where the AH was diagnosed, and this review can change the calculated risk substantially, in either direction.

*Flat epithelial atypia (FEA) or columnar alteration with prominent apical snouts and secretions (CAPSS) with Atypia* (or any other terminology relating to the same family). Despite the fact that "atypia" and "atypical" would seem to carry the same weight wherever used in the taxonomy of breast pathology, FEA or atypical CAPSS lesions do *not* impart the same level of risk as ADH or ALH. They are not the same thing. To confuse the issue further, FEA and CAPPS with atypia admittedly appear to be signposts along the pathway toward the development of breast cancer. Yet they are different in appearance from ADH and ALH, and as of this writing, they do not seem to impart an independent level of risk beyond that delivered by the background pathology. For example, once again drawing from the richly endowed Mayo Clinic data bank, if FEA is associated with background changes of proliferative disease without atypia, the patient's risk is 2-fold (same as proliferative disease alone). If FEA is associated with a background of ADH, then risk is 4-fold (same as ADH alone). Why bother with such trivia? Because FEA and its ilk are not uncommon findings at all, yet when identified in a risk assessment program that is chained to the mathematical models, patients are often tallied as having AH, generating risk levels far in excess of reality. This is double trouble when one considers that the models have the potential to exaggerate the power of AH in the first place. Only the background pathology associated with FEA or atypical CAPSS lesions should be entered into the computer models used for risk assessment.

*Lobular carcinoma in situ (LCIS).* Here's what the majority of online pundits have to say about LCIS: "It's not really cancer … it's only a tissue risk factor … and that risk is only 15% to 20%."

All three claims are either misleading or incorrect. This is an example of a pendulum having swung too far, an overcorrection and overreaction to the days when women with LCIS were sometimes treated with unilateral Halsted radical mastectomy.

Is LCIS cancer? After all, "carcinoma" means cancer. Of course, it depends on your definition. If you limit your definition of cancer to a disease state that, at the moment of diagnosis, has the potential to spread and kill, then no, it's not cancer. Is it pre-cancerous or premalignant?—again, it depends on the definition, but note the fine line here between a "tissue risk" and a premalignant lesion, a.k.a. "precursor." Some experts have proposed benign-sounding names for LCIS in an attempt to influence behavior through language. Instead, I prefer the term, "non-obligated precursor," which is stating that there exists a direct line of passage from LCIS to invasive *lobular* carcinoma where the molecular biology of the LCIS cells and the invasive cells are nearly identical. At the same time, LCIS predicts an increased risk of the ductal type of cancer as well, not a direct precursor, at least not using the light microscope alone. This would more reasonably prompt the "tissue risk factor," though the molecular biology here is complex and the LCIS-to-*ductal* cancer pathway may be circuitous, but still occurring through specific mutations with LCIS acting as the precursor.

Even though I am using the term "precursor," the qualifier "non-obligated" means that LCIS can stall or regress and never become invasive, that is, it is not *obligated* to progress to invasion. And to refine this definition of LCIS further—if, after wide surgical excision, the final diagnosis is *classic* LCIS, then the best descriptive definition to fit its behavior is this: a non-obligated precursor that sometimes has a widespread geographical distribution in both breasts.

This scattering of LCIS was painstakingly mapped from mastectomy specimens in the 1960s by Oklahoma City pathologist, the late Perry Lambird, M.D., while he was still in training at Johns Hopkins.[4] The diagrams were published in the *JAMA* in 1969, seldom referenced today, but strongly supportive of the concept that LCIS, once diagnosed, tends to be distributed widely. My knowledge of these long-lost LCIS maps by Dr. Lambird came from my years in medical school (1971–1975) working in the pathology lab at St. Anthony Hospital in Oklahoma City where Dr. Lambird was one of the attending pathologists. This widespread distribution of LCIS helps to explain why the future cancers after this diagnosis are often unrelated to the original biopsy site. At the same time, the future cancer will appear at the original biopsy site more often than a simple "tissue risk," and will be invasive lobular more often than is seen in the general population, demonstrating "precursor" behavior more than "tissue risk factor."

Some early studies of LCIS confused the issue by including what today would be called ALH, such that the future cancers were distributed 50–50 between the two sides and were far more likely to be ductal than lobular, endorsing the "tissue risk" concept. However, when stricter criteria for LCIS are applied, we see the "non-obligated precursor with widespread distribution" behavior emerge.

So what is the future risk of invasive cancer after a diagnosis of LCIS? In relative terms, it is twice the risk imparted by ALH or ADH alone—that is, 8-fold—and this RR has been known and accepted for many years, though it needs adjustment based on patient age, that is, the underlying baseline risk. This should translate to a 2% per year risk for breast cancer, a level *not* seen in most longitudinal studies of LCIS where 1% per year is more common, once again because ALH is often mixed in with LCIS. The difference between ALH and LCIS under the microscope is a very smooth continuum where even the experts can disagree, and I would submit that a given pathologist might call a lesion ALH one day, and LCIS the next.

For nearly two decades, those of us performing risk assessments have largely relied on tables provided by Bodian et al.,[5] which offer the long-term risk of cancer in patients previously diagnosed with LCIS who opted for nothing further beyond the biopsy. In the Bodian tables, future risk is about 1% per year, more in line with ALH and ADH, prompting many to use the 1% per year figure for all 3 entities. This 1% per year cancer-risk for LCIS, however, has always been suspect, since some of the first observational studies of LCIS generated risks of 1.5% per year, and in one case, 2% per year. This is not splitting hairs—convert these risks to time periods in excess of 10 years, and there's a world of difference.

Now let's dissect the common online advice about LCIS that claims "15–20% risk" for breast cancer. First of all, this statement violates one of the most basic principles when quoting absolute risks—that is, you must include a time frame. It is absurd to ascribe the same "15%" to a 35-year-old with LCIS and an 80-year-old with LCIS. The very definition of risk assessment is the determination of absolute levels of risk *over a defined period of time*, although I'm admittedly quoting my own definition.[6] Still, this principle is violated routinely in discussions of LCIS.

When the MRI screening guidelines for high-risk women were issued by the American Cancer Society in 2007,[7] the risk for LCIS was minimized by quoting a short-term study. As a result, the LCIS patients were placed in the same category as those women with a calculated 15–19% risk (and those with ADH and ALH), where again there was "insufficient evidence" for using MRI. However, if one draws their LCIS outcome data from a study with 20-year follow-up, then the cumulative risk will be 20%. If the follow-up is 30 years, the risk will be

30%. This is not a difficult concept, yet even the experts will toss around risk percentages with no reference to the other half of the definition—that is, over what period of time does that percent probability apply?

In practical terms, a 50-year-old female with a life expectancy of 30 more years, diagnosed with LCIS, is facing a 30% risk for breast cancer, at least, rendering the "15–20%" misleading, especially when coupled to "it's not really cancer, it's only a tissue risk." Those of us in the screening/diagnostic arena are further concerned about the fact that the invasive counterpart to LCIS, invasive lobular carcinoma, often has a diffuse growth pattern that renders it mammographically invisible. This factor provides further justification for the use of screening MRI, understanding that some lobulars can even squeak through MRI undetected.

Some of the confusion about LCIS relative risks (RRs) not matching the absolute risk has come from the fact that RRs decline over time, not necessarily because the risk loses its power, but because the denominator is increasing. Remember that an RR is actually a fraction, numerator over denominator, and as the incidence of breast cancer rises in the general population, if the numerator is linear, then the relative risk actually decreases. So the RR for a woman diagnosed with LCIS at age 70 is only about 3.0. Don't dwell on this if math isn't your thing, the point is that RRs are always tricky, and what we really want to know is directly observed cumulative risks—absolute risks—over time.

To that end, in 2015, the largest collection of directly observed LCIS patients was assembled by Tari King, M.D., and colleagues while she was at Memorial Sloan-Kettering.[8] In this 29-year longitudinal study, with a median follow-up of 6.8 years (range 6 to 368 months), of the 1,004 patients with LCIS who chose surveillance, 150 developed 168 cancers (63% on the same side as the LCIS, 25% on the opposite side, and 12% on both sides). This translated to an absolute risk of 2% per year, more in line with what one would expect with the 8-fold risk of LCIS. As an interesting aside, chemoprevention dramatically reduced the risk of breast cancer in these LCIS patients by 73%, comparable to the risk reduction quoted earlier for tamoxifen and ADH in the long-term follow-up of the NSABP P-01 trial.

Will this 2% per year hold up over time? We don't know, but one thing is for sure—the pervasive "15–20% risk of cancer" is grossly misleading. In this study from King et al., 15% of LCIS patients had already developed breast cancer after a median follow-up of *only 6.8 years*—hardly a lifetime—and that's with 17% of the women taking a round of chemoprevention. The risk was higher still in those LCIS patients undergoing surveillance alone, without chemoprevention. Furthermore, we know that observed risk for LCIS is persistent for at least 30 years, at a minimum of 1% per year, so even if the 2% per year fades over time, we could still be dealing with the possibility that lifetime risks for young women diagnosed with LCIS could reach 50%, the highest risk ever calculated outside of mutations in the breast cancer predisposition genes.

One more comment before leaving LCIS. I have used the term "classic" LCIS to indicate the textbook picture. Additional risk is probably imparted by extreme examples of LCIS while less risk is generated the closer one gets to ALH. Quantitative efforts have indicated additional risk imparted when the LCIS is present on more microscope slides, as was the case in Dr. King's study, while qualitative studies have indicated higher risk for LCIS when there are more cells expanding the acinar units in the lobules ("histologically flagrant examples"), while risk is lower the closer the lesion approaches being ALH.[9] But again, this is "classic" LCIS. There are other types of LCIS as well.

Pleomorphic LCIS is more concerning than classic LCIS, as it is associated with pleomorphic invasive lobular carcinoma, a high-grade, aggressive version of lobular cancer. The classic version of invasive lobular cancer is composed of small, unassuming cells that often look like normal lymphocytes. In contrast, "pleomorphic" lobular denotes larger cells with a disturbing appearance, varying in shape and size, i.e., "high grade." Importantly, it appears that pleomorphic LCIS behaves more like DCIS than LCIS.

Even rarer than pleomorphic LCIS is a pattern where the in situ cells are not necessarily high-grade or pleomorphic, but there is central necrosis and calcifications,[10] these features being inconsistent with classical LCIS. In fact, the features perfectly match one type of DCIS. So why isn't it called DCIS?

Today, a great deal of faith has been placed in a special stain called e-cadherin that distinguishes ductal lesions from lobular lesions (negative staining in the latter). The reliability of this stain is rather remarkable, as one can see adjacent normal breast tissue and how well the stain is working. Yet, in spite of certain lesions appearing to be straightforward DCIS, the negative staining with e-cadherin evokes an official diagnosis of LCIS, the e-cadherin stain trumping the basic appearance. In the years prior to e-cadherin, these lesions would have been diagnosed as DCIS and treated accordingly.

But is this reliance on the trump card, e-cadherin, the right thing to do? Do we abandon all we know about DCIS and re-name the lesion as LCIS? Sometimes, one has to resort to that timeworn, yet still-esteemed scientific principle—"if it looks like a duck and quacks like a duck, then by golly, it probably is a duck." Bottom line: when it comes to both pleomorphic LCIS and DCIS-like LCIS (features of these two entities can be overlapping), patients should be presented with DCIS options, which at a minimum—unlike classic LCIS—should involve an attempt to get clear margins with surgical excision. Additional therapy such as partial breast radiation or whole breast radiation should be discussed as well, pending confirmatory clinical studies. Large areas of involvement where clear margins cannot be obtained may even prompt a recommendation for mastectomy. Data will eventually catch up and recommendations could change, but right now, these lesions are too rare for anyone to draw upon high-quality evidence-based medicine.

*Ductal carcinoma in situ (DCIS).* As with LCIS, the question is "Is it really cancer?" Unlike LCIS, however, where we have considerable long-term data on women who opt for nothing after the biopsy (where residual LCIS is assumed to be likely), evidence for the natural history of DCIS is mostly indirect, given that women with this diagnosis have been traditionally treated for presumed malignancy. Even when analyzing data from cohorts of women with DCIS who opted for nothing more than wide excision, the natural history is not fully revealed, since the surgical removal with clear margins is often curative on its own.

So is it cancer? For starters, DCIS is not a single entity, making it nearly impossible to adopt sweeping generalizations. But pinned to a wall, I would offer this description, "DCIS is a non-obligated precursor like LCIS, but unlike LCIS, the spatial distribution is located primarily at the biopsy site. Furthermore, the degree and range of obligation to transform into invasive cancer varies widely among the different presentations of DCIS."

Let me back up. When a patient is newly diagnosed with either LCIS or DCIS, there is a critical issue that few like to discuss, that is, what is the probability that an invasive cancer is already present in the patient, but *unrelated* to the biopsy site in question, that is, an "elsewhere" invasive cancer *not seen on mammography*. This information is actually available from mastectomy specimens, but is seldom mentioned, dismissed because the probability is so small. Small, that is, as long as you're not in the 3–4% of women who, upon opting for preventive surgery after a diagnosis of LCIS or DCIS, are found to have *invasive* cancer *unrelated to the biopsy site.*

If a woman is being informed about LCIS or DCIS and is told, "don't worry, it's not really cancer," there is a 3–4% chance that the counselor is making an egregious error. Can we identify those women ahead of time, so that the discussion can proceed along the lines of an accurate diagnosis of in situ cancer only?

We certainly can for DCIS. (LCIS is a more difficult challenge in that small areas of invasive lobular may not show up on any form of imaging.) In a unique study at the time, breast radiologist Dr. Rebecca Stough and I addressed this very issue, using pre-operative MRI in 288 consecutive patients newly diagnosed with solitary sites of DCIS,[11] tallying the findings *to the exclusion of the index lesion.* Our only question was "What's going on elsewhere?" In 10 patients (3.5%), we found invasive cancers unrelated to the DCIS biopsy site, with 6 of the 10 being Stage IIA, not tiny little nothings. In 5 patients, the invasive cancers were located in a different quadrant on the same side, so perhaps whole breast radiation would have unwittingly kept these tumors from getting out of control had we not used MRI. However, 2%, that is, 6 patients (one patient had both multicentric invasion and contralateral invasion), had invasive breast cancer on the opposite side, mammographically invisible, with 3 of 6 proving to be Stage IIA, hardly "subclinical," a word used by critics to disparage MRI findings. In this scenario, however, it's the mammographically-discovered DCIS about to be treated with lumpectomy that deserves the moniker of "subclinical."

If a surgeon performs wrong-side surgery anywhere else in the body, then it is straightforward malpractice with a few headlines tossed in for good measure, estimated to occur less than 1 in 100,000 procedures. Yet here, we have a 2% incidence of wrong side surgery being performed *as the standard of care* for DCIS when patients are treated with lumpectomy, but without a pre-op MRI. The clinical significance and deadly potential of the contralateral invasive cancer easily outweighs the importance of the known DCIS, leaving us with a painful thorn in the side—that is, a tiny probability of a major misadventure. Is this 2% (3.5% when including multicentric invasive cancers on the same side), enough to warrant submitting all patients newly diagnosed with DCIS to a pre-op MRI?

Well, what happens without MRI? Within several years, these contralateral cancers emerge, and few give pause to think, "Hmm, I wonder if that was present when I operated before?" Well, it probably was. This is not conjecture. Our study of pre-op MRI in DCIS was spawned by an observational study performed at M.D. Anderson Cancer Center, published in 2008.[12] In this study, 799 patients with DCIS were followed for a short-term (2.9 years median), where 5.6% of patients had a second event, usually invasive cancer and usually in the opposite breast (understanding that some patients underwent unilateral mastectomy, skewing the proportions, but not the absolute numbers). In fact, 3.9% (31/799) of patients developed invasive cancer as the second event within this very short time frame, essentially the same number that we demonstrated up front with pre-op MRI (3.5%).

This relatively high rate of invasive cancer in the short-term did not go unnoticed in the editorial response provided by Drs. Lagios and Silverstein who stated the obvious—with such a short follow-up period, these cancers were likely present at the time of the original surgery, but undetected. Pre-op MRI had not been utilized in this series. And while overall survival was 97%, consistent with a DCIS diagnosis, in contrast, for those patients with a second event, the survival was only 76%. The conclusion from the M.D. Anderson study was succinctly stated: "Second events following DCIS occur primarily in the opposite breast and have a negative impact on survival."

Instead of increasing awareness about the problem of "elsewhere invasion," however, there is unrelenting criticism from breast cancer experts about the inappropriate use of pre-operative MRI in women newly diagnosed with breast cancer. Oddly, the criticism is even more intense for DCIS, where admittedly, the evidence for benefit is slim, that is, *whenever the measured outcomes are limited to the site of the index lesion.* While it is true that MRI is of little benefit when it comes to managing the index lesion in DCIS, that's not the purpose—the purpose is to identify "elsewhere invasion," a scenario that has received almost no recognition in spite of its deadly implications.

These are life-threatening cancers on the opposite side, unknown to either doctor or patient, which will be left untreated without adjunct imaging, either ultrasound or, better yet, MRI. There will be no radiation to the opposite side, there will be no chemotherapy to help with the opposite side, and given the in situ pathology as the only thing "known," there may or may not be endocrine therapy after treating the DCIS (where, even if utilized, is usually not enough to serve as single therapy for invasive cancer). And certainly, the hormonal agents are not enough when the majority of these cancers are Stage IIA, as was the case in our experience. Without pre-operative MRI, in the end, the contralateral life-threatening cancer will be ignored 2% of the time, while the radiologist, pathologist, surgeon, radiation oncologist, and medical oncologist all focus their entire efforts on the multidisciplinary management of the wrong breast.

In 2015, Dr. Steven Narod et al. at the Women's College Research Institute at the University of Toronto published a landmark paper on DCIS,[13] based on Surveillance, Epidemiology, and End Results (SEER) data that allowed the investigation of 108,196 women diagnosed with DCIS from 1988 to 2011. For those with 20 years of follow-up, the breast cancer specific mortality was 3.3%, consistent with other reports, always with the presumption that the 3–4% of patients who die after DCIS have a later bout with invasive cancer. The unsettling finding by Narod et al. was that the majority of the women who died from breast cancer in this large series were never diagnosed with invasive breast cancer. Instead, they went from DCIS to metastatic disease and death. One longstanding explanation is the acknowledgment that DCIS can act like invasive cancer, that is, the malignant cells can squeeze through the basement membrane of the duct and access the patient's blood stream even though not seen on routine pathology. Dr. Narod's conclusion does not offer an exact mechanism, but he makes the point that DCIS should be considered to have the same potential to spread as a small invasive cancer. This certainly flies in the face of those wanting to change the name of DCIS because "it's not really cancer."

Another scenario to explain Dr. Narod's findings might be that women have undiagnosed "elsewhere" invasion, as was seen in our MRI study. Perhaps these patients are adequately treated locally, especially when this invasion is on the same side as the DCIS, managed successfully by radiation and/or endocrine therapy such that there is no in-breast recurrence, but still with systemic spread (our Biologic B that metastasizes prior to early detection). Or, in those women who opt for bilateral mastectomy after a diagnosis of DCIS, the contralateral invasion is missed in the routine sectioning done in the pathology lab. Then, when the diagnosis of metastatic breast cancer follows years later (after successful local management) and death ensues, the scenario remains a mystery as to how this could have occurred with a mere diagnosis of DCIS originally, no evidence for invasion. If this is the case, then these Biologic B tumor outcomes would not ordinarily be altered by earlier detection with MRI. However, their discovery up front with MRI would introduce the use of systemic therapies that could improve survival.

So what do we do about DCIS? When Dr. Mel Silverstein wrote and edited his medical textbook on DCIS[14] in 1997, it was 665 pages long. So imagine the futility of any attempt to condense that information to a few paragraphs. There are so many paradoxes and disagreements about these paradoxes that Dr. Silverstein opted for a perfectly appropriate title for Chapter 2—"Insanity of Ductal Carcinoma in Situ."

What makes DCIS so insane? In short, it's the wide and unpredictable range of biologies (natural histories), the wide range of disease extent, and the fact that biology and extent occur in all possible combinations. Thus, you can have an aggressive high grade DCIS that is small in size, easily managed by breast conservation, while another patient might have a very low grade DCIS that involves all four quadrants of the breast, prompting mastectomy. And you can have every combination in between.

This is why Dr. Silverstein and pathologist Dr. Michael Lagios drafted their Van Nuys Prognostic Index (VNPI) in 1996 that included lesion size, grade, and surgical margins, which then converted numerically to local recurrence rates with various forms of treatment. The primary allure of this approach was in the identification of DCIS patients who will do well after excision alone (no radiation). In 2002, "age at diagnosis" of DCIS was found to be a valid prognosticator as well, so this fourth parameter was added to the VNPI, by then called the University of Southern California/Van Nuys Prognostic Index (or USC/VNPI), recently updated with 5-fold the number of DCIS patients since the algorithm was originally developed.[15]

From this rational approach to patient care, albeit initially drawn from retrospective data, patients who need nothing more than wide excision alone can be safely identified as having very low recurrence rates without radiation. While pathology features using the USC/VNPI have now been collected prospectively for 1,704 patients by Silverstein and Lagios, no large scale randomized treatment trials have been performed, rendering this approach as "lower level" evidence, albeit adopted by higher level thought.

At the same time that the Van Nuys Prognostic Index was introduced and undergoing scrutiny, the dominant position on DCIS management was to treat nearly all DCIS as a single biologic entity, using the same approach as invasive cancer, that is, conservation surgery followed by whole breast radiation. Later, adjuvant tamoxifen became a suggested option. This was the position of the NSABP, drawn from the strength of their B-17 and B-24 prospective, randomized trials for DCIS.

This homogenized approach was accepted by many before the social tsunami of "less is more," so the USC/VNPI was slow to earn acceptance. Recall that Dr. Silverstein spent 12 years defending his position that radiation can be safely deleted in selected patients. The National Comprehensive Cancer Network (NCCN), a trusted source for cancer guidelines, finally accepted a Van Nuys–like approach, as an option for DCIS patients with "lower level evidence," given the absence of prospective, randomized trials. Still, making it into the NCCN guidelines is not an easy feat when one proposes innovative approaches that do not easily lend themselves to prospective RCTs. Dr. Silverstein's persistence paid off, and many patients today can attribute their "easy" treatment of DCIS to his efforts, as well as the work by pathologist Dr. Michael Lagios. Today, other pioneers have taken up the charge of minimal treatment of solitary areas of DCIS, but we should not forget that the seeds of excision alone for DCIS were planted in 1982 when Dr. Lagios first reported his "experimental" group of 20 patients with an average lesion size of 0.8cm who underwent no additional treatment after lumpectomy, long before breast conservation had been accepted for *any* stage of breast cancer.[16]

Ductal carcinoma in situ, or DCIS, does *not* mean "small." Although confined to the inside of the ducts, the ductal system itself permeates the entire breast, and communications from one segment to another have been documented. Thus, this "early" form of non-invasive breast cancer can generate challenges in local therapy far more complex than invasive cancer. In the latter, one is usually dealing with a "lump," but for DCIS, the 3-dimensional tendrils can extend irregularly throughout the breast tissue.

DCIS has many presentations:

High-grade DCIS, palpable and involving an entire quadrant of the breast
High-grade DCIS, non-palpable, but involving 2, 3 or 4 quadrants
High-grade DCIS in a single ductal segment that leads up to the nipple
High-grade DCIS forming a mammographic mass, with discrete margins
High-grade DCIS presenting as a small calcium cluster on mammography, but with far
    greater extent in reality
High-grade DCIS presenting as a small calcium cluster, without extending beyond the
    calcifications

Now go through all the possibilities above, this time using "moderate grade DCIS" instead of "high grade," and again with "low grade DCIS," mixing biology and extent of disease. Then, mix in the molecular biologic assays and/or genetic analyses to all the above, and that's what you have today—the Insanity of DCIS. The possibilities are maddening, for both the patient and her doctor.

So what advice can I offer here for DCIS? Right off the bat, as strange as it might seem when breast conservation is the standard and where limited radiation or no radiation at all are possibilities, there are still some patients who require mastectomy for disease control. Chemotherapy, sometimes used up front to shrink invasive cancer, is oddly unreliable in its ability to eradicate DCIS. In some patients with invasive cancer plus some of the original DCIS, the chemotherapy will kill all traces of invasive cancer, yet the final pathology reveals healthy DCIS cells, living "protected" inside the duct system, unfazed. Endocrine therapy helps some, but the main benefit of tamoxifen and other endocrine agents is the preventive effect for the remaining breast tissue, helping to prevent a new cancer. The point is that some DCIS patients have multi-quadrant disease, or a large area of DCIS, for which all treatments, with the exception of surgery, will fail.

Today, however, given that DCIS is usually image-detected, most patients are candidates for conservation, with the same local options as designed for patients with invasive cancer—lumpectomy plus whole breast radiation. The NSABP, in the past, took the position that subtypes of DCIS are unreliable (in contrast to the Van Nuys approach), as a single patient can have a mixture of architectural types and grades within the same lesion, including the measurement of estrogen-receptor status, negative in some areas, positive in others. Thus, in their

B-24 trial[17] that studied whether or not the anti-hormonal effects of tamoxifen would benefit patients beyond the radiation therapy, the protocol didn't require measurement of estrogen-receptor (ER) status. Candidates were randomized to receive tamoxifen or placebo, after primary treatment with lumpectomy and radiation, without measuring ER status and, for that matter, without concern as to the type or grade of the DCIS.

Later on, tissue blocks from the B-24 were carefully analyzed for ER status, and the use of tamoxifen (or other endocrine agents) became a standard option for local control and prevention, albeit not with the intent to improve survival rates as is the indication in patients with invasive cancer.

Today, we are on the lookout for patients in whom we can safely delete radiation therapy, based on the general principles found in the USC/Van Nuys Prognostic Index. The ideal candidates are older patients with low or moderate grade lesions of small size, with final surgical resection yielding wide margins. Some cautious surgeons are adding genetic analysis of the DCIS (Oncotype DX DCIS® was the first to market) to the standard parameters in order to safely select patients in whom the radiation can be deleted.

I've been intentionally ambiguous on my terminology here in order to keep this discussion concise. But if you are wondering what to do about your recent diagnosis of DCIS, the best advice I can give is this: Ask point blank: "Am I a candidate to leave off the radiation therapy?" If the answer is no, and you still want to pursue this, ask the question again in a second opinion, specifically asking for recurrence rates as calculated by the USC/Van Nuys Prognostic Index. Or "Do I meet requirements to delete radiation as outlined by the NCCN?" Or "Would an Oncotype DX DCIS® score help?" If the answer is still no, then ask if you are a candidate for partial breast irradiation, where only the lumpectomy site is irradiated. Another approach is to deliver the radiation as a single dose during surgery, though the DCIS data is lagging behind the data for invasive cancer with all techniques for limited radiation.

To help resolve the DCIS confusion, clinical trials are being implemented to monitor the natural history. Women are being asked if they are willing to go with "no treatment at all" after biopsy, as is currently done for LCIS. In addition, molecular biology of DCIS and genetic analyses are a hot area of research and will continue to address natural history as well.

As for the problems surrounding semantics, some have recommended selective use of terminology, limiting the word "cancer" to high-grade DCIS. There's a measure of historical irony here in that the original comedocarcinoma discovered on palpation in the late 1800s, today called high grade DCIS, was originally considered as a new type of invasive cancer. The basic concept of in situ disease had not yet been worked out. If we return to these historical roots for our semantics, it's because it is likely that a larger proportion of high-grade DCIS progresses to invasive disease, but more easily demonstrated is the fact that this transition occurs within a shorter time frame than lower grades of DCIS.

Mid-range DCIS, or intermediate grade, could be treated with excision and some form of radiation (or excision alone if margins are good), without worrying too much about the exact semantics of the lesion.

But importantly, the recommendation has been made that low grade DCIS be grouped with its so-called benign counterpart ADH, and then designated as a "borderline lesion," the therapeutic implication being *excision alone*. Thus, the criticism of "overtreatment" of DCIS could be largely put to rest by this classification scheme, given that the only difference between low grade DCIS and ADH might be the presence or absence of a full moon.

The "borderline lesion" idea is not new, with several pathologists in favor of the designation over the years, most notably Dr. Rosai in his oft-quoted 1991 article that demonstrated major discordance among pathologists looking at the same lesions in a rebuke to Dr. David Page who claimed that a sharp distinction could be made.[18] Dr. Page countered with his take on the problem, pointing out that if pathologists rolled up their sleeves and followed clear criteria, ADH and DCIS could be distinguished with remarkable concordance, at least among 6 expert pathologists.[19]

In his breast pathology book,[20] Dr. Page provides 16 sketches of architectural patterns that are distinctive for regular hyperplasia, atypical hyperplasia, and DCIS, enough to make you seasick if you stare at them too long. And the diagrams don't even address cellular detail, just the gross architecture. Yet, even though remarkable concordance was reached by Dr. Page and his expert colleagues who participated in the study, the word "remarkable" is relative, and in this case, applies only to concordance as defined within the discipline of pathology.

From a clinician's standpoint, it remains a concern that perfect agreement of 6 pathologists occurred in only 58% of cases reviewed. At the clinical level, this leaves the counseling surgeon in a fix much of the time, whether he or she knows it or not. Too, these were nationally-recognized expert pathologists who participated in the study. The reality, I believe, is closer to what Dr. Elmore revealed in her 2015 *JAMA* article reviewed previously—that is, the distinction between ADH and low-grade DCIS is difficult and inconsistent. *If treatment were the same for both entities, it wouldn't matter.*

Instead, the difference in treatments can be huge—told she has ADH, a patient might opt for nothing further, while the same patient with the same lesion told she has DCIS might opt for bilateral mastectomies. This problem has been recognized, and largely suppressed, for at least four decades, starting with Dr. McDivitt's pathology review for the BCDDP in the 1970s, then the Rosai article, followed by modern day accounts and editorials calling for new terminology.[21]

If the treatment of choice for a small "borderline breast lesion" were wide excision alone, with or without endocrine therapy (as they are nearly all ER-positive), then radiation could be held for the next time around, should there be a next time. The recurrence rate would be quite small, somewhere in the range of 5% or below over the next 10 years. It's time to call a truce on this controversy, with the terms of the agreement being semantically vague in order to match the pathologically vague "borderline breast lesion."

*Lesions that mimic invasive breast cancer.* Separate from the "borderline lesion" question of low grade DCIS vs. atypical hyperplasia, a more treacherous problem exists, exacerbated by mammographic screening—that is, benign lesions that can appear to be invasive cancer, both on imaging studies and under the microscope. This is a family of abnormalities with a long roster of diagnostic terms used throughout the years, but a common theme is "sclerosis." Sclerosis could be called "fibrosis with malicious intent," that is, the sometimes chaotic, and sometimes orderly, deposition of scar tissue that distorts the anatomy in a way that converts benign breast tissue into having a malignant appearance.

Normal structures of a microscopic breast lobule can multiply (adenosis) and then be separated and distorted by sclerosis, rendering diagnoses such as microglandular adenosis or sclerosing adenosis. Toss in some extra cells (hyperplasia) before squishing them down with sclerosis, and these normal cell clusters can look like invading armies of malignant cells coursing through the breast tissue. Sometimes these changes are diffuse, but sometimes they form mammographic masses that can mimic cancer both in the eyes of the beholding radiologist and the pathologist.

Radial scars are small star-shaped masses that can look very much like invasive cancer on mammography, but are usually straightforward as benign when viewed under the microscope. However, as these radial scars persist and enlarge, they seem to create an adverse environment for normal cells such that a common development is hyperplasia to the point of papillomatosis, or even atypical hyperplasia and DCIS, bringing us back full circle to the controversies noted above. Researchers are having a heyday trying to figure out whether the stroma alter the cells or vice versa. While we don't understand the exact process involved, the chance of complex pathology in this family of lesions appears to be size-related, so it has become customary to refer to radial scars larger than 1.0cm as "complex sclerosing lesions," or CSLs, where we usually recommend excision.

Although some consider the large CSLs to be precancerous, they are associated with a much more serious problem than a future cancer, and more serious than the "simple" harboring of borderline lesions (ADH/low grade DCIS)—that is, some of these CSLs can be nearly perfect mimics of invasive cancer, that is, the entire lesion is thought to be a relatively large invasive cancer when, in fact, it is completely benign. This is the scenario most feared by pathologists and those of us who depend on them, i.e., everyone. Oddly, the greater the magnification of the microscope, the harder it is to identify the CSL as such. Backing away to less magnification allows the pathologist to get a "gut feel" and then, special stains can help with the diagnosis, too.

The challenge is "thinking about" a CSL to begin with. A busy pathologist reviewing hundreds of slides every day, including invasive carcinomas of the breast on a regular basis, can label CSL as invasive cancer if the possibility is not kept at the forefront at all times. Because many pathology departments now require two opinions for breast cancer, and special stains often come to the rescue, the problem has been minimized. Still, extreme examples of counterfeit cancer can occur, with a CSL imitating a malignancy on both mammography and pathology.

From the inherently difficult issues above, it is easy to see how anything that magnifies the problems in pathology is going get targeted. And in this case, the target is mammography. Critics of screening can deliver their shots without ever pulling the trigger, that is, without ever mentioning the word "mammography," simply by addressing these issues of microscopy. The anti-screening cadre and screening minimalists don't even have to leave the pathology lab: "Look how some women are getting overdiagnosed and overtreated, simply because of the lack of expertise and standardization of breast pathology."

This is why the argument for "excision alone" for borderline lesions, selected DCIS, and some small, low grade invasive cancers is so compelling. Remove the overtreatment, and the overdiagnosis problem, at least Type III, becomes a non-issue. The problem is real and has largely persisted throughout these many years of screening mammography. Given the highly improbable existence of Type I overdiagnosis (festering cancers), the inability to do anything about Type II overdiagnosis, i.e., the discovery of Biologic A tumors (length bias masquerading as overdiagnosis), we must admit that Type III is a pressing issue, not for screening mammography directly, but indirectly by traveling through the pathology lab.

# 20

# Risk-Based Screening— It Feels So Right, but Wait...

It makes perfect sense. It's both rational and empirical. It fits snugly within the goal of "personalized medicine." It's the long-sought solution to a long-argued problem about breast cancer screening for women in their 40s. What is it? Risk-based screening. In fact, many women have already made it the pivot point when they decline mammographic screening— "I don't get mammograms because I don't have risk factors."

Here are my concerns:

1. It's a feeble answer to the controversies.
2. Risk stratification has reached most of its potential already.
3. We should be thinking about far superior strategies.

Yes, it feels good to adjust screening recommendations to match the patient's probability of being diagnosed with the disease in question. It's a wonderful example of "personalized medicine," a goal we love to tout in medicine even though it is, in some ways, the antipathy of "evidence-based medicine," which homogenizes guidelines based on analyzing the masses. But when it comes to mammographic screening for breast cancer, there are limitations to risk-based decision-making that you might find surprising.

From my résumé, one would think that I would be gung-ho for risk-based screening. My interest in breast cancer risk assessment pre-dated the Mammography Civil War and pre-dated the Gail Model (the first widely used mathematical model to predict risk). My original interest was generated many years ago in the counseling of patients who had been referred to me for preventive mastectomy. From what little epidemiologic evidence I could find at the time (rather, what publications the departmental librarian, Linda O'Rourke, could find in the pre-internet days), the actual calculated risk for breast cancer was usually *far less* than what women perceived. Thus, my counseling sessions were centered on putting risk in perspective, by comparing to the no-risk patient, and looking at alternatives other than surgery.

In spite of the abundance of articles addressing this or that risk factor for breast cancer, very few clinicians at the time were paying attention to the development of formal risk assessment, a means to combine all known risks and protective factors into a single probability for breast cancer. Little wonder that this progress was esoteric, given that the articles were published almost exclusively in the epidemiology journals. By formal risk assessment, I mean

168

this—offering the patient her *calculated probability for the development of breast cancer over a defined period of time.*

In contrast to this definition of *risk assessment,* most individual counseling at the time, if done at all, relied on two misleading approaches: (1) the use of relative risks, and (2) the use of absolute risks without regard for the length of time for which that risk was calculated.

In the first instance, an example would be "With your mother's history of breast cancer, you're at double the risk for getting cancer as well." But double compared to what? What is the denominator that is to be doubled to calculate actual risk? Or, in the second approach, patients might be given an absolute risk, such as "Since you've had breast cancer on one side, your risk for a cancer on the opposite side is 20%." But what about life expectancy? In its absurd extreme, this oft-quoted 20% was applied to the 30-year-old as well as the 75-year-old. As it turns out, calculating contralateral risk after breast cancer is rather tricky, with the effects of treatment lowering risk while, at the same time, pre-diagnosis levels of risk weighing in as well.

In 1991, at my alma mater, we held a "wall-breaking" ceremony to launch the construction of Oklahoma's first multidisciplinary breast clinic. Swinging the hammer with me was the noted breast pathologist, David L. Page, M.D., of Vanderbilt, who was largely responsible for the risk assessment craze by assigning relative risk numbers to specific findings on benign breast biopsies, beginning in the 1970s and reaching clinical medicine in the 1980s. During his brief trip to Oklahoma City, I made an ill-conceived statement that betrayed my ignorance about "lifetime risks," whereupon Dr. Page snapped, "Lifetime risks are poorly understood and often misused, and surgeons are the worst."

That was the official liftoff of my career in risk assessment. Dr. Page gave me the epidemiologic resources I needed, most notably the tables published by his collaborator, epidemiologist William D. Dupont, PhD, that allowed the conversion of relative risks to absolute risks over a defined period of time. I ended up using these tables in my practice even after release of the Gail model software. On occasion, I still use the tables today for rare risks that are not included in the mathematical models.

In 1993, nearly two years after my gaffe with Dr. Page, I announced one of the first formal risk assessment programs in the U.S. In 1996, on the first day it became available and using a strict protocol in place at that time, we added BRCA genetic testing to the mix of risk stratification tools. Although it may seem strange now, at the time, the American Cancer Society had to give its "seal of approval" to those sites pioneering BRCA testing in the clinic. With so many hoops to jump through, given the complexities of counseling, our program was the initial testing site in Oklahoma City.

The point of all this is that I made the assumption that this revolution in risk stratification was happening all over the country, especially after the clinical introduction of the Gail model and its primary use in selecting patients for risk reduction using tamoxifen. I was wrong. Formal risk assessment was still a rarity, so my "pioneer" status was actually bestowed by default.[1]

Only in 2007 did risk assessment/genetic testing became a raging fire of interest, this being a result of the newly announced American Cancer Society screening guidelines using MRI for women at very high risk for the development of breast cancer. Note that this separate set of guidelines for high-risk women include the recommendation to begin screening *at age 30,* using *both* mammography and breast MRI. In addition to categorical risk factors, such as BRCA gene mutations ("BRCA-positivity"), the guidelines included the calculation of lifetime risks (without regard for the admonition of Dr. Page), using any one of several mathematical models based largely on family history. It was the threshold number of "greater than 20–25% lifetime risk" for screening MRI that prompted breast centers nationwide to formalize a strategy for calculating risk levels in women as they passed through the screening mammography mills. Educational courses, certifications, etc., followed soon thereafter, yet it was not until 2015 that the Commission on Cancer in its accreditation program for cancer programs in the U.S. required that a system of risk assessment/genetics be in place.

In spite of my unwitting entrée into risk expertise, my true interest was not in the numbers themselves. My interest was in the *interventions* available that could alter the numbers, or at least, allow early and reliable diagnosis. To believe that the numbers are the endpoint in risk assessment is a violation of Noah's principle: "There's no benefit to predicting rain unless you build the arc."

The "arc" for breast cancer is amazingly sound, especially when compared to other cancer types where fewer interventions are available. For breast cancer, several interventions have been identified that are quite effective. These include surgical risk reduction; pharmacologic risk reduction; and high-risk surveillance.

*Surgical risk reduction.* While preventive mastectomies are often described as mutilating and barbaric, those patients who have undergone nipple-sparing mastectomies and autologous flap reconstructions will argue otherwise. On occasion, I'll hear from a post-op patient that her primary care physician said, "I don't know what procedure was performed, but it wasn't mastectomies." Some implant reconstructions with silicone gel are not far behind.

Nothing has the power of risk reduction like preventive surgery, although breast cancer risk does not drop to zero. Additionally, there is no calculated risk level that defines the threshold for preventive mastectomy. In spite of the excellent cosmetic outcomes that are possible today, the psycho-sexual connotations render this approach as selective and patient-driven. The duty of the risk assessment program is to provide realistic numbers over defined periods of time, and how those numbers compare to the general population, so that the woman considering this approach can make a more realistic decision.

*Pharmacologic risk reduction.* As of this writing, two drugs are FDA-approved to lower the risk of breast cancer—tamoxifen and raloxifene. Other agents will follow. Here, as opposed to preventive surgery, there is a numerical threshold for pharmacologic risk reduction, based on the entry criteria used in clinical trials. The minimum number for use is "1.67," the focus of a failed publicity campaign that tried to indoctrinate both physicians and patients. This number has all the makings of a *relative risk*, given that so many publicized risks are in this range. But it's *not* a relative risk. Instead, 1.67% is a 5-year absolute risk calculation for the development of breast cancer, using the Gail model. In spite of aggressive efforts to promote the number (and the Gail model), patient acceptance for pharmacologic risk reduction is relatively low. Modifications to 1.67% have been recommended to improve harm-to-benefit ratios in different age groups and whether or not the uterus is still present (given the small risk of uterine cancer with tamoxifen), but the number approach has largely failed to impress clinicians or patients. More than 500,000 women take raloxifene for its other FDA-approved use (osteoporosis), yet for some mysterious reason, precious few take it to reduce the risk of breast cancer.

*High-risk surveillance.* Most of the interest in risk assessment relates to qualifying for breast MRI screening, either through genetic testing or through a risk number calculated using one of the mathematical models. To be honest, as a risk expert, I cringed (along with others) the day these guidelines were announced via conference call. Good news: MRI screening was finally endorsed for high-risk patients. Bad news: "lifetime risks" were the standard.

From my "lifetime risk" censure by Dr. Page in 1991 to present day, I have presented and published the many problems that are generated by using lifetime risks to select patients for two-tiered screening—mammography and MRI. First and foremost is the fact that a "lifetime risk" is more accurately described as *remaining* lifetime risk." Without any skills in math, you can readily see the problem—young women, at lower short-term risk, qualify for MRI screening because they have so many more years to live, while older women at substantial risk do not qualify for MRI, even though they are at the age of peak incidence for developing breast cancer. Without belaboring the point here,[2] a 60-year-old can easily be at 4 tmes the likelihood of a breast cancer being detected on MRI during the next 10 years, as compared to a 30 year-old with the same risk factors over the same 10 years. Yet the 60-year-old can easily fail to qualify for MRI (at least, according to U.S. guidelines; in fact, the Brits figured this out well before us, and patients can qualify for screening breast MRI in the U.K. based on 10-year calculations).

Another variant of the lifetime risk problem is the patient who qualifies for MRI on the basis of, let's say, a 22% lifetime risk for breast cancer, originally calculated at age 45, but after 10 years of MRI screening, just as she enters the years of peak short-term risk, her *remaining* lifetime risk calculation from age 55 to 85 drops to 19%, and she no longer qualifies for MRI. Dr. Page was correct—lifetime risks are a messy thing.

Yet another flaw in the guidelines was the placement of a past history of atypical hyperplasia into the "more research needed" category in spite of the fact that younger patients with this diagnosis might be at higher risk than those women who easily qualify for screening MRI on the basis of family history. This inconsistency within the guidelines is a function of the fact that the international MRI screening trials (that prompted the ACS recommendations) had used only family history and genetic predisposition for patient enrollment. In short, the American Cancer Society was going out on a limb with these recommendations, given the absence of any mortality data, and it was considered best to stick closely to the design of the original (non-randomized) trials. Empiricism to the exclusion of rational thought wins again!

The first question on the conference call announcing the 2007 guidelines was directed to this very issue—how do you reconcile the fact that a 45-year-old woman with atypical hyperplasia on a biopsy exceeds the 20% lifetime threshold qualifying her for MRI, yet is simultaneously excluded from these guidelines? "These are only *guidelines*" was the fragile answer, all of us fully aware that third party payors see guidelines as rules written in stone.

At my facility, we began our MRI screening program several years before any guidelines were available. We realized two issues at play—(1) level of risk, and (2) level of breast density. The former is obvious in our attempt to practice cost-effective medicine using an expensive imaging method like MRI, but we realized that the moment you begin to rely on the mathematical models for specific threshold numbers, there are so many caveats and problems, you end up tripping over yourself to avoid conflicting recommendations.

Even as someone using the models every day in my practice to derive specific numbers, I didn't think it was a good idea to unleash these numbers as parameters to qualify for MRI. My answer was to use "categorical risks," e.g., a "sister with breast cancer prior to age 50" or a "prior diagnosis of atypical hyperplasia," rather than a number. Alternatively, short-term risk calculations are the great equalizers, helping to avoid age-discrimination inherent to lifetime risks. This is one reason why the NSABP used short-term (5-year) calculations for their prevention trials.

In addition to categorical risks, it was our contention that breast density should play a role in the decision for screening MRI, not so much for the inherent risk associated with density, although that certainly plays a role, but for the fact that if we are talking about a two-tiered approach to screening, shouldn't the second tier be used more liberally when the first tier is more likely to fail?

Well, the current guidelines didn't approach the problem in that fashion. Instead, "breast density" was treated as though it were an independent issue (and placed in the "need more research" category). Yet density levels are a feature of every single patient being screened. The first screening tier—mammographic density—should play an integral role in whether or not to add a second tier—either whole-breast ultrasound or MRI. So, originally, we used both density and risk levels in selecting patients for screening MRI until third party payors forced our hand to stick closely to the guidelines.

At the 10-year point of MRI screening, we calculated and published our results on those women whose cancers were discovered on MRI alone[3]—*half* of our MRI-detected cancers would not have been found if we had been following even a liberal interpretation of the guidelines. So, today, those women who would have met our original threshold for MRI screening are no longer being diagnosed at the earliest possible point in time. They have become guideline casualties.

The 2007 guidelines for MRI screening introduced by the American Cancer Society were followed shortly thereafter by similar guidelines from the NCCN (National Comprehensive Cancer Network). Seemingly, everyone wanted a risk assessment/genetic testing program at their breast screening center starting in 2007. By this time, I had dropped breast surgery from my practice and was devoted full-time to high-risk patients and what to do about their risk. Although the new breast MRI screening guidelines had stumbled awkwardly into the world of "risk-based screening," there is a key point to be made—risk assessment was being utilized to do something *more*, something *better*, an improvement in early detection.

It didn't take long for breast cancer risk assessment to get hijacked by the screening minimalists as a tool to do *less*. The first time I heard of a strategy to do less was during the Mammography Civil War. I objected then, as I do now. Unfortunately, this is positioning myself against two august bodies—the American College of Physicians and the American Academy of Family Physicians, both of whom follow recommendations for the 40–49 group as outlined by the U.S. Preventive Services Task Force, the former group in spirit, the latter having officially adopted Task Force recommendations.

This policy of risk-based screening sounds fine on the surface. Who could object to having a discussion with your patient as to pros and cons? But remember that the default position for screening during the decade of the 40s is *not recommended* routinely by the Task Force. Yes, the language of a C-recommendation from the 2016 Task Force has softened, but a C is still a C—and a C is not a covered service in the Affordable Care Act. The recommended *default position is no screening*, with exceptions made for women with risk factors and/or dense breasts. This is, of course, the physician-directed version of the untenable statement I mentioned at the beginning of this chapter: "I don't get mammograms because I don't have risk factors."

So, if we're going to *restrict* screening, under the guise of "risk-based screening" or "personalized screening," let's see how the numbers work out.

Family history is the dominant feature for most patients who are at increased risk for breast cancer. The problem in using this risk to base a decision about screening is that 80% of eventual breast cancer patients newly diagnosed will not have a significant family history. So any system based on this risk *will exclude the vast majority* of women who would benefit from screening. This is why I used the word "untenable" for those who rely on family history.

But let's ignore this shaky foundation and move directly to the numbers where we would hope to see a sharp distinction between at-risk patients and no-risk patients.

A 40-year-old woman visits her family physician to discuss mammographic screening, yes or no, pros and cons. She has a single risk factor in that her mother was diagnosed with breast cancer at age 55. "Well, of course, you should begin mammography," says the physician, "your risk for breast cancer is 2-fold the general population."

So let's go to work. The risk of developing breast cancer in the general U.S. population during the decade of the 40s is 1.5%. (It's 2.5% in the 50s, and 3.5% in the 60s, helping to explain why "Number Needed to Screen" to save one life improves over time.) At 1.5% baseline risk over the next 10 years for a 40 year-old, you can readily see that the odds are greatly in the patient's favor that screening won't help a thing, although this is also true of the "lifetime risk" of 12%. Nevertheless, to calculate our patient's individual risk, given her mother's history, it would seem that we should multiply 2 times 1.5%, generating a probability of 3% that she will be diagnosed with breast cancer during the next 10 years. Not a huge difference. Both numbers seem small when cast in this light.

But now, I'm going to nitpick. Let's go back to the 1.5% baseline. This is *general population risk*, not a no-risk baseline. General population risk includes women with risk factors, and that means those women at extraordinarily high risk due to genetic predispositions. Take away all the women with known risk factors, and the baseline no-risk probability of developing breast cancer is approximately 1% over the 10 year period. This is where the "two-fold risk" of breast cancer is applied when talking about relative risks, not to general population risk. Why? Because the original studies that arrived at a 2-fold risk for breast cancer had to use a control group, and this control group is, by intent, a "no risk" population (at least not having the risk being studied), *not* the general population. In this instance, the original studies to determine risk would have used women without a family history of breast cancer.

So we don't multiply 2 by 1.5% for a 3% breast cancer risk over 10 years. Instead, we multiply the 2-fold risk by 1%, and we have a *2% probability* of breast cancer over 10 years for our patient "at risk" in her 40s, compared to a *1.5% probability* in the general population and a *1.0% probability* in the no-risk population. Are these small differences, *spread out over 10 years*, enough to exclude 80% of the population, based on a lack of risk factors? In fact, one can more easily argue no screening for this group as a whole, rather than selectively apply screening to those who have, or don't have, modest risk elevations.

As for the very high risk patient where the calculated 10-year risks can be 10% or more, yes, it's quite easy to recommend more. But it's very shaky to recommend *less* for women at average risk when there are negligible differences from patients with modest risk factors.

From the public health standpoint, when these small differences are applied to a large population, there can be a substantial improvement in cost-effectiveness screening at the 2%

risk level vs. 1%. But at the same time, 80% of women in this age group would be denied screening, and the vast majority of cancers will occur in this denied group! Yet multiple studies have documented the "beauty" of this risk-based approach—in theory—and it forms the very basis of the discussion primary care physicians are told they should have with their patients in their 40s.

The problems only grow more complex when one considers that the 2-fold risk I chose to illustrate here applies only when the first-degree relative is in the age range of 50 to 60. The relative risk is less for older relatives with breast cancer, while imparted risk is higher when relatives were diagnosed in the premenopausal years. Mathematical models are available to clinicians who want to calculate absolute risk over a defined period of time, but the most familiar and easiest to use, the Gail Model, won't help. It *does not include the ages* of the affected relatives, nor does it include second or third-degree relatives with breast (or ovarian) cancer, which can make a huge difference in calculated risk. Other models help us in these situations, but they are more time-consuming for a busy primary care physician, not to mention trickier to use. Thus, risk assessment programs using multiple models are a standard feature today at breast imaging centers.

The bottom line is obvious: there is very little practical difference in risk for women in their 40s, with and without risk factors, with the exception being those women at *very high* risk of breast cancer. But recall that *these women are already covered with our guidelines*—they qualify for annual mammography *and* annual breast MRI. When it comes to defining risk levels that are so low that we can safely say, "No need to screen," there is not a rational cut-off point. The woman at modestly elevated risk for breast cancer is not substantially different from the woman without those risk factors when considering only the decade of the 40s.

If you remember nothing else about the confusing numbers above, be aware that *all efforts to screen only those women at elevated risk will, by definition, exclude the majority of women who are headed toward breast cancer.* In this light, using risk to deny screening is doomed before you start. It should be a one-way street—yes, risk is very helpful to do *more*, but the moment you use it to do *less*, you've excluded the overwhelming majority who would benefit. Recall the post-mortem Harvard study[4] one more time: *"The majority of breast cancer deaths (71%) occur in unscreened women."* And this was especially true for younger women.

My mathematically-modeled theories aside, has anyone actually looked at the problem of excluding cancer detection in young women through risk-based screening? Of course, though they are ignored by the policy-makers. For example, in December 2015, in response to the growing craze of "personalized medicine" (a.k.a. "precision medicine"), radiologists at 3 sites in California, including UCSF, looked at young women diagnosed with breast cancer *by screening mammography* in their 40s, between the years 1997 to 2012.[5] Of the 136 young women with cancer, a very strong family history was absent in 119 (88%), while extremely dense tissue was absent in 117 (86%). Even looking at a risk-based strategy with an expanded definition of high risk—that is, any first degree relative with breast cancer or extremely dense tissue—*66% of the malignancies would have been missed.* How's that for "precision medicine?" Incredibly, risk-based screening to decide the 40–49 controversy is the dominant "cutting edge" belief of the day.

As often occurs, critics of mammography will drag other types of cancer into the picture for the purpose of analogy, even when there's nothing analogous at all. For instance, one type of cancer that is very much disposed to risk-based screening is lung cancer. In fact, the U.S.

Preventive Services Task Force recommends annual screening for lung cancer with low-dose CT in adults aged 55 to 80 years who have a 30 pack-year smoking history and currently smoke, or have quit smoking, within the past 15 years. I won't waste space here quibbling about limitations of a 30 pack-year history, or exactly 15 years of abstinence from smoking, as if risk disappears overnight. Suffice it to say that this is risk-based screening at its finest (I'm serious).

A little history is in order. Once, it was good practice for all adults to have a yearly chest X-ray, a holdover from the days when tuberculosis was rampant. Although a variety of health issues could be evaluated with a chest X-ray, one of the alleged benefits was thought to be early detection of lung cancer. Turns out, of course, that lung cancer was mostly limited to smokers, not to mention that the routine chest X-ray was not a great way to detect early lung cancer. No mortality reduction from lung cancer could be demonstrated in controlled trials. Enter low-dose CT where successful screening trials were achieved when participants were smokers.

And this is where things start to separate from breast cancer. Recall that only *20%* of eventual breast cancer patients have a positive family history, such that restricting screening to that group alone excludes *80%* who might benefit. Contrast that to lung cancer where *90%* of the eventual cancers occur in smokers such that only *10%* are excluded by this policy. Furthermore, the risk for lung cancer imparted by heavy cigarette smoking is *20-fold* the risk in the general population, whereas the breast cancer risk of a first degree relative having the disease is only *2-fold*. A third point can be made as well—in lung cancer, the low sensitivity chest X-ray failed whereas the high sensitivity CT scan was successful. (Remember this when we discuss the sensitivities of mammography and MRI.)

**Percentage of Cancers Addressed by Focusing on the Most Common Risk:**
Lung Cancer—90%               Breast Cancer—20%

**Power of the Most Common Risk Factor in 2 Types of Cancer:**
Lung Cancer (smoking)—20-fold     Breast Cancer (one 1st degree relative)—2-fold

Risk-based screening certainly has its place, but it falls short in breast cancer when used to justify a no screening policy.

Some might respond with "Okay, if that's the case, we should be working to perfect the science of risk assessment. After all, we have SNPs (single nucleotide polymorphisms, which are best conceived as variations in DNA rather than mutations) and other high fallutin' technologies that can separate who needs to screen and who doesn't."

Forgetting that some of the proposed measures add substantial cost to the goal of cost-cutting, we are still faced with the problem that there's simply not a sharp dividing line like we have in lung cancer—smokers vs. non-smokers. Improvements in risk assessment can predict slight benefits in cancer yields, but still to the exclusion of many eventual breast cancer patients.

For instance, a recent article in the May 2015 issue of the *Journal of the National Cancer Institute*[6] was impressive, first by its listing of *more than 200 authors* who studied 77 SNPs in 33,673 breast cancer cases vs. 33,381 controls. Lifetime risk for breast cancer in the lowest quintile (lowest-scoring 20%) was 5.2%, while those in highest group had a 16.6% lifetime risk. That's actually pretty good separation for SNPs. But still, if you limit screening to the highest quintile, i.e., the top 20%, then you exclude the vast majority of eventual victims. Besides, we already know that women without traditional risk factors are at 7% lifetime risk for the development of breast cancer, not really different from the SNP-based 5.2%.

Combined with the family history of a first-degree relative with breast cancer, the division between top and bottom quintiles using SNPs was more impressive, but the "lowest" risk was still 8.6%, justifying basic mammographic screening as we currently do anyway, while the highest risk was 24.4%, the implication (in my view) being that these patients now qualify for *more* screening, that is, both mammography and MRI. Some epidemiologists will swarm over this data to show us how we can apply it to screening mammography, using large population numbers to make their point, primarily with reference to doing *less*.

But the fact remains that a risk-based approach for "no screening" is a losing proposition in breast cancer unless someone comes up with a test that has profound strength in negative predictive value, that is, the capability to offer assurance that an individual is *not* going to be diagnosed with breast cancer. In the meantime, the baseline risk is simply too high to ignore.

Let's use the lung cancer comparison once again. The distinction here for CT screening is drawn sharply through smoking vs. not smoking. Smokers have roughly a 25% lifetime chance of developing lung cancer, whereas non-smokers have a 1% risk. Not much going on "in between" those numbers. If a SNP test for breast cancer predisposition could draw an equally sharp distinction, allowing us to identify a group of women at only a 1% lifetime risk, then yes, it would prompt us to limit screening in that group. But the current best with SNPs of 5.2% (yet to be validated prospectively) is still too close to our known 7% baseline risk in the no-risk population.

With the exception of SNPs, however, very little research is invested in the goal of negative predictive value. Most are trying to identify women with occult risk factors, that is, women thought to be at average risk who are actually at high risk. The purpose here is to do more, of course, not less. So we have minimalists clamoring for less screening when, in fact, hardly any inroads have been made toward identifying women at an extremely low risk who can skip mammographic screening, if only in the decade of the 40s. Our basic scientists, out to discover occult risks, are sometimes out of synch with our epidemiologists and public health experts who want the exact opposite—the identification of women at very low risk.

It bears repeating—risk stratification is the best method available for selecting patients to do *more*—that is, multi-modality imaging. However, this approach has nearly reached its maximum effectiveness. That is, women at the very highest risk for breast cancer as defined by genetic predispositions (where lifetime risks may be as high as 85%) will still only end up with 3–4% yields on a single breast MRI, gradually decreasing to 2% yield per year as the "steady state" is reached after multiple screens. While these yields are higher than the 0.5% annual yield for general population screening with mammography, they are still marginal when it comes to cost-effective screening when using MRI. A question we will ask later: "Is there any way to generate cancer yields using MRI that are higher than the current maximum?"

Again, in summary, using risk stratification to do *less* automatically excludes the *majority* of women who will develop breast cancer. Excluding patients from screening is not a well-conceived strategy when there is so little difference in yields between the modest risk patient and the "no risk" patient due to the high baseline risk. Unlike lung cancer where there is a reasonably sharp division between the 25% lifetime risk of cancer in smokers from the 1%

risk in non-smokers, there is nothing comparable in breast cancer to pinpoint the safe exclusion of basic mammographic screening.

Hang on. We are only a few chapters away from a proposed answer to the problem of proper patient selection to "rule in" and "rule out" screening—and it has nothing to do with lifetime risk calculations.

# 21

# The Greatest Story Never Told

When the breast conservation trials began in the 1970s, pitting lumpectomy vs. mastectomy, a new standard was forged in surgical science—the application of prospective, randomized controlled trials in determining best practice. The concept of using prospective RCTs had already been applied in other areas of medicine,[1] but it lagged application when it came to surgery. Dr. Bernard Fisher of NSABP fame, whom we've met previously, is credited with introducing surgeons to the world of strict scientific method, and his starting place was in breast cancer.

Prior to that time, surgeons were reporting their results on breast cancer randomly, primarily focused on minor variations in technique. And though it's difficult to imagine today, different surgeons used different staging systems. One surgeon might report results based on the Manchester system, while another would use the Columbia system. The adoption of the current TNM system from the American Joint Committee on Cancer later emerged as a consensus for staging most cancer types today.

Now imagine you are a woman newly diagnosed with breast cancer in 1978, and you hear about a clinical trial where you might get the opportunity to save your breast. It's worth investigating, so you learn that the study has three limbs—mastectomy (the control group), lumpectomy with radiation, and lumpectomy without radiation. Your placement in one of those three groups will be done on a random basis. That is, after you sign on the dotted line, you will draw a number from a hat, so to speak, and it will determine which of the 3 groups you will enter. Not bad. You have a 2 out of 3 chance that you'll get to save your breast in an era when mastectomy was the norm. But what if you get randomized to mastectomy? You will end up getting the identical treatment as if you had simply followed standard of care. The only way to be assured of saving your breast would be to seek out a surgical maverick; otherwise, take your chances in the NSABP B-06 trial (or other smaller trials of that era).

Well, as it turned out, few women signed up. The idea of keeping or losing your breast on the basis of a random draw was simply too much to ask. So the NSABP tweaked protocol a little bit, and performed what they called "pre-randomization" so that women knew the group to which they would be assigned before actually signing that dotted line. This maneuver has been long forgotten by most, and if it were tried today, I suspect epidemiologists would cry "Foul!" Nevertheless, it worked beautifully and enrollment soared.

But that's not why I'm re-tracing history. For those "pre-randomized" to one of the two lumpectomy limbs, there was a caveat—if the surgeon doing your lumpectomy ended up with a positive margin on pathology, that is, tumor cells at the edge of the lumpectomy specimen, according to the protocol you had to return to the operating room for a mastectomy.[2] Indeed, this happened about 10% of the time. So you might think that once the mastectomy was performed, the patient would move over to the mastectomy group. "Foul!" "Pre-randomization" might slip through, but not a gross violation of the "Intent-to-Treat Rule," which states, "Final analysis is performed on the basis of the group to which you are assigned, not on the basis of the treatment actually received." The Intent-to-Treat Rule is integral to the conduct of prospective, randomized controlled trials.

Furthermore, there was an additional caveat for women in the two lumpectomy limbs. If you developed a recurrence in the breast later on, it was also automatic mastectomy. For the group that received radiation, this was not nearly as frequent as the group randomized to no radiation where 39% developed local recurrences (or new cancers) over the course of the next 20 years. Add that 39% who underwent delayed mastectomy to the 10% who underwent mastectomy up front for positive margins, and you have *49% of the women in the lumpectomy alone limb who actually had mastectomies performed*. In the 20-year follow-up of this B-06 study, where there were no survival differences among the 3 groups, the "lumpectomy alone" limb seems like a misnomer, with half the group having undergone mastectomy.

Rest assured, other trials have confirmed the equivalency of breast conservation with mastectomy, my point being a dramatic introduction to the "Intent-to-Treat Rule," something foreign to many of us. In fact, the first I ever heard of it was by listening to Dr. Bernie Fisher discuss the NSABP B-06 in the 1980s.

The application of this rule to screening mammography is less dramatic than losing one's breast, but in fact, has more of an adverse impact on determining the power of screening mammography. After all, in the B-06 study, all received their assigned surgical treatment, though some got more than they bargained for. *Equivalency* of the 3 treatment strategies was the goal. With mammography, however, where we are trying to prove a *difference* between two groups, we have two forces at work—compliance and contamination—and *both* work to hurt the measurable impact of screening.

Compliance refers to those women assigned to get mammograms, but don't do it. Contamination of the control group is the opposite, that is, when women assigned to *no* mammograms proceed on their own to have mammograms performed. Yet both scenarios in prospective RCTs count patients in the group to which they were assigned, *not* what they actually did.

Why would this be considered the standard? And not simply a standard, but a rule so firm as to be unbreakable? Remember, the purpose of randomization is to control for confounding variables. The moment you start excluding people from analysis for non-compliance, your groups theoretically become unequal and bias is introduced. This is not a popular rule, by the way. Investigators readily see the absurdity of having their drug, or treatment plan, bashed when the real problem might have been non-compliance. As a result, some researchers try to worm their way around the rule by designing trials called "*modified* intention-to-treat analysis" but the evidence-based aficionados see right through this ruse and take great delight in condemnation.

Another justification for the rule has to do with "health policy." If you are trying to establish a formal policy, it makes no sense to expend great effort on promoting a drug or a test or a treatment if compliance is low. So, when it comes to screening mammograms, the epidemiologists want to know what the impact is going to be when a certain policy is applied *to a given population*. This is *not* the same as determining the power of screening mammography on compliant patients. Thus, we have two sets of data that we've already encountered in discussing the clinical trials—mortality reduction based on "*invitation* to screen" vs. mortality reduction in those who actually "screened." Or "number needed to *invite* to screen" to save one life (NNI) vs. "number needed to screen" to save one life (NNS).

These numbers are different! In fact, when better outcomes are seen in compliant patients, we have another ounce of evidence that mammograms are working. Imagine this— what would be your conclusion if there was a 15% mortality reduction seen in women *invited* to screen and a 15% mortality reduction for those who *actually* screened, even though compliance was only 50%? You would be hard-pressed to believe that mammograms were responsible for the mortality reduction.

And it's not easy or straightforward to calculate compliance and contamination, by the way. Imagine a 10-year trial of annual mammography where the goal is 10 mammograms total. How do you count compliance if a woman gets 7 mammograms, or 3 mammograms? Or what if she allows a 5-year gap in her 10-year plan, while compliant the other 5 years? How do you count contamination if a woman only gets 2 mammograms as opposed to zero? Worse, how thorough is your data, considering you are trying to register the mammography habits of 50,000 women or more, where you must follow them long after the actual screening is over? What were their mammographic habits afterward? These variables spell trouble in that they allow all sorts of manipulation of the data. It makes your head spin until you drop in a heap and surrender allegiance to the intent-to-treat rule.

When the prospective RCTs are published, compliance data with analysis are included, but this doesn't count when it comes to the final outcome. When the results are published and promoted, you'll never hear anything about the outcomes that considered compliance and contamination unless you obtain the original article and read it for yourself.

Suppose you were in charge of designing the definitive mammographic screening trial. How would you set this up, knowing that it would be nice to include 100,000 women so that your statistics were air tight? Ideally, you would want the actual screening duration to be 10 years or so. Shorter trials are the rule, based on practicality. But the shorter they are, these trials have a disproportionate number of women who enter the study with "prevalence" cancers, that is, cancers detected on the first screen that have been "building up" prior to the mammogram. "Incident cancers" are those detected on subsequent mammograms. Prevalence tumors are larger, and thus, a higher Stage, so that the benefit of long-term screening is not fully appreciated.

The Canadian NBSS, for instance, performed only 5 years of active screening. It takes nearly that long to achieve what some call the "steady state" where you are detecting incident tumors only, where the optimal impact of screening is to be found. Short duration of screening is a rarely discussed weakness in the prospective RCTs. The long-term follow-ups quoted are, in fact, long durations of time *after* the screening study period has ended.

Next, in your study design, you would like to ensure that all women randomized to mammography comply at the 100% level, and those in the no mammography group are not allowed to have a mammogram (unless they develop a palpable lump). Compliance and contamination would be reined in nicely. Then, a drastic maneuver—at the end of the relatively long 10 years of screening, the mammography group must stop, undergoing no further screening for another 10 years, while the control group is not allowed to screen either. Why? To allow correction of lead time and to control for overdiagnosis bias (slimming down the bloated numbers we hear about today).

This design has never happened and it never will. Prospective randomized trials, which work so well when determining if a drug is effective, aren't nearly so pristine when it comes to screening (or, for that matter, radiology or surgery in general) where "blinding" cannot be done. It should be readily apparent that you can't stop women from screening, especially once the "formal screening phase" is over. Bottom line: the study of mammographic screening does not lend itself well to prospective RCTs, no matter how loudly our public health experts scream. To make matters worse, the controversies today surround trials that used Jurassic Mammography. Is it any wonder that Dr. Robert A. Smith of the American Cancer Society made his recent statement that it's time we monitor what's happening in actual screening situations, rather than regurgitating the trials of antiquity? This, of course, would mean excluding nearly all of the evidence used by the Task Force in their calculation of harm-to-benefit ratios.

One more point about our imaginary trial—how do you recruit 100,000 women? This is no small matter, and it's responsible for much of the ongoing battles today between pro-screeners and anti-screeners, still arguing over study design and its impact 30 years later.

The Canadian NBSS opted to use volunteers. Sounds perfectly reasonable. And, in fact, the Canadian study can boast one of the highest compliance rates of any of the trials due to their participants being highly motivated in the first place—100% compliance at the start, drifting down to 86% 5 years later in the NBSS-1 (though contamination in the control group was 24%). It has to be considered, however, that volunteers can be motivated by their personal risk factors as well as concerns they already have about lumps on self-exam. This skews the population from the beginning, and the CNBSS made matters worse by their physical exam performed prior to randomization that resulted in the corrupted control group.

But what if you simply send out *invitations* to participate? This may help avoid a skewed population, but still has a volunteer aspect in those who accept. However, these women are not as highly motivated after receiving "junk mail," and compliance is lower, sometimes dramatically so. Many other nuances exist in this process of patient selection, and since no method is perfect, opponents delight in pointing out the deficiencies of others.

Now let's see how these principles work in an actual clinical trial, a study we've only breezed by at this point, yet it is the most important clinical trial ever performed when it comes to determining the benefit of screening mammography for women in their 40s—the AGE Trial, from the United Kingdom.

One often hears from journalists (and misinformed doctors) how the Canadian NBBS is unique in that it was the only mammography trial where the 40–49 age group was pre-defined. *This is not true.* One also hears how the CNBSS was the largest trial ever performed for women in their 40s. This is not true either. The AGE Trial was devoted entirely to the 40s question, and in fact, enrolled women at the ages of 39–41, screening every year to age 48 (as opposed to the Canadian trial where entry could be anywhere in the 40s, and screening lasted only 5 years). Thus, the AGE Trial is truly a study about screening in the 40s, whereas the CNBSS-1 was about *starting* to screen at some point in the 40s.

As for size, the AGE Trial included twice the number of women in their 40s who received mammograms, that is, more than 50,000 in the AGE Trial compared to 25,000 in their 40s in the mammography limb of the Canadian trial. The control group in AGE was based on a

2:1 ratio, so more than 100,000 control patients brought the exact total to 160,921 patients in the AGE trial compared to 50,430 in the Canadian NBSS-1 for women in their 40s.

The AGE Trial is sometimes referred to as the "only modern trial for screening mammography," and indeed the patient accrual from 1990 to 1997 was still taking place during the Mammography Civil War. Mammograms of the 1990s had advanced greatly since the 1970s and 1980s, but still would be considered inferior to today's mammograms. Another limiting factor in the AGE Trial is that 2-view mammography was performed for baseline at the time of entry, but after that, the remaining screens were *single view studies*, using the best view—the MLO (mediolateral oblique)—the view not included in the CNBSS until the final few years. But the MLO view is still not as good as two-view mammography that includes both MLO and the CC (craniocaudal) views. Approximately 20% of cancers will be seen only on the CC view.

But let me dig the hole so deep that the AGE Trial is bound to fail. Compliance was only 68%, a function of the polite approach of a well-worded *invitation* to screen. At 10 years of follow-up, a preliminary report indicated that the trial had, indeed, failed. In the December 9, 2006, issue of *The Lancet*,[3] the mortality reduction of 17% failed to reach statistical significance.

From our tedious coverage of "statistical significance," we know that this does *not* mean that mammography was not saving lives. It simply failed to conform to our arbitrary designation of "statistical significance," and that with more time, "significance" might be achieved. The results, however, were remarkably pinpoint, dead on, exactly what was perfectly consistent with what was already known. That is, the meta-analysis used by the 2002 Task Force calculated a 15% mortality reduction that did, in fact, reach statistical significance for screening mammography in the 40s. Although the p-value was too anemic to count in its 2006 publication, the AGE Trial essentially duplicated the Task Force calculations when it reported a 17% relative reduction.

Recall that the 2009 Task Force then stated that "new data" had prompted their reversal, but the only thing new on the plus-side was the 2006 results of the AGE Trial data that didn't change a thing in the benefit column. The 17% (insignificant) results blended into the 15% mortality reduction, and guess what—the benefit was still a 15% reduction in mortality, exactly what you would guess without knowing anything about statistics. As we saw earlier, the real reason for the policy reversal had nothing to do with the AGE Trial. It was the Task Force adopting a new method of calculating the harms of mammography, and the decision that those harms outweighed saved lives.

Now let's look at the fine print in the AGE Trial where compliance data was presented. In fact, when considering only those women who actually underwent mammograms, the mortality reduction was 24%, and it missed statistical significance by only a "hair." To be exact, the 95% Confidence Interval (CI) was 0.51–1.01. In order to reach "significance," the upper end of that CI cannot cross the 1.00 line, but look how close it came. Again, the mere fact that compliance data is superior to what was found under the "intent-to-treat" rule is evidence in its own right (lower level, of course) that mammograms are doing exactly what they are designed to do—save lives.

Then the Greatest Story Never Told—in July 2015, the 17-year follow-up was published for the AGE Trial.[4] Screening women in their 40s reached a *statistically significant 25% reduction in mortality* in the initial 10 years after diagnosis, the first time statistical significance had ever been demonstrated prospectively for this age group, and to a degree greater than ever seen in a prospective, randomized trial. *There wasn't a peep from the media.*

This was not the compliance-adjusted figure mentioned above, but the "intent-to-treat" data, such that one could expect an even greater reduction in mortality with compliance. Interestingly, the benefit could not be demonstrated so clearly in the years that followed the 40–49 screens, the most plausible reason being that once the trial was over, women in the U.K.'s National Health Service are ordinarily invited to screen starting at age 50 (currently, in the process of changing to 47), so the control group had begun their routine mammographic screening. This meant no difference between groups in the decade of the 50s. So the 17-year follow-up from the start of AGE, by definition, included the "no difference" years in the 50s, diluting the overall results to a 12% mortality reduction that missed significance by another hair (95% CI: 0.74–1.04). Perhaps this is why journalists didn't want to touch this critical study with a 10-foot pole. They didn't understand the impact of "losing" the control group to mammography. Or perhaps the reason runs deeper than that.

Oh, and by the way, the number of cancers found in the screened group and the control group were virtually the same after the effect of lead time had passed, and the authors made no bones about it—*"overdiagnosis" was almost non-existent.* Or, in their words, "at worst a small amount of overdiagnosis."

Consider now the official renderings of a "good informed consent" being proposed by public health experts where we are admonished to tell patients that they run a 30% risk of overdiagnosis with screening mammography, even with invasive cancer. There's a big difference between 30% and "at worst a small amount." Furthermore, the Task Force would have us tell women in their 40s that harms outweigh benefits. My bias is this: there is potential harm generated by these informed consents in and of themselves, ironically designed to prevent harms.

In the next chapter, we are going to switch gears to Another Story Never Told—the true percentage of cancers detected by screening mammography—that is, Sensitivity.

# 22

# The Myth of Mammography

You've seen the "10 Myths" about anything and everything online, and in print media, but there is one myth you will not see listed, simply because it has been so thoroughly embraced by so many for so long. The myth that refuses to die is the "80–90%" Sensitivity of mammography.

For many years on a regular basis, the American Cancer Society has published a document called *Breast Cancer Facts and Figures* where, in the past, it would state that mammograms detect "80–90%" of cancers. However, the ACS did not provide a reference for this "fact," even though the document overall was highly accurate and heavily referenced. In the most recent edition, however, the statement is no longer present, nor is it replaced by another number. It has been deleted.

I don't believe for a moment that 90%, or even the more modern "80%," has been intended to deceive. "80–90%" Sensitivity is a deeply held conviction by many, if not most, today. This is strongly reinforced at many facilities where the data collection (for accreditation purposes) does not properly capture the normal mammograms performed in the months prior to the cancer diagnosis, generating numbers such as "95% Sensitivity," and with it, self-congratulation.

In the opening chapter, I mentioned the fact that my entrée into breast imaging occurred in the late 1980s when I asked this simple question of a breast-dedicated radiologist in the university setting—"What's the origin of the 90% detection rate for mammography?" (Back then, few would even stoop to 80% as a possibility.) In the years since, I've made it a hobby, of sorts, to navigate the various tributaries that led to a wide expanse of miscalculations.

Let's first clarify our definitions. By "detection rate," I'm talking about Sensitivity, in this case, the percentage of breast cancers detected by mammography. The inverse of Sensitivity is the false-negative rate. So, if mammograms detect 90% of cancers, then the false-negative rate is 10%. If they detect 80%, then 20% is the false-negative rate.

Specificity and its inverse, the false-positive rate, is an independent parameter. That is, it is calculated without regard for Sensitivity. A Specificity of 70% means that there is a 30% false-positive rate. Again, effective screening (saved lives) is a function of two variables: vulnerable *Biology* and *Sensitivity* of the screening tool. X + Y = Z. Specificity doesn't count when it comes to effectiveness. It's not part of our equation. Specificity is important with regard to the pragmatic application of a screening tool, not its effectiveness. Poor Specificity means more false-alarms and thus, higher costs and greater anxiety, but it doesn't impact the number of saved lives.

The two basic parameters used to judge medical testing can then be combined into Accuracy, not to be confused with the lay use of the word. Accuracy is a mathematical formula that combines Sensitivity and Specificity, and it can be quite misleading. A test with 90% Sensitivity but only 40% Specificity will end up with the same *Accuracy* as a test with 40% Sensitivity and 90% Specificity. Yet the difference between utility in those two examples is huge. To make matters worse, Sensitivity and Specificity dwell in a delicate balance. As you improve one, the other will usually suffer. As I mentioned earlier in the book, Sensitivity and Specificity are at war with each other, while Accuracy gives the illusion of peace.

Ignoring formulas, the practical definition of mammographic Sensitivity sounds straightforward—the percentage of breast cancers detected. Unfortunately, the waters get muddy as soon as your feet get wet. Let me be more precise. Sensitivity of screening mammography is the percentage of cancers detected in *asymptomatic* women *over time*. These two qualifiers in italics will make more sense shortly.

As for "asymptomatic," recall the original definition of mammographic screening as proposed by one of the "fathers" of mammography, Dr. Robert Egan who, at the time, was developing the technology at MD Anderson in the 1950s. Dr. Egan emphatically pointed out that the concept of screening should be restricted to women without symptoms (and that includes lumps). Once a lump is present, the mammogram is useful for diagnostic purposes, but if population screening is ever attempted (he was writing when screening was only an idea), it should be obvious that mammography should be judged by its performance in asymptomatic women.

And this is where the confusion begins. The "90%" that was originally quoted for mammographic sensitivity did not spring forth from studies of asymptomatic women. It came from studies that included women with lumps, most notably the massive BCDDP where I already mentioned how, as surgery residents in the 1970s, we referred patients for inclusion in that study *after* we had scheduled them for biopsies of palpable lumps. Indeed, there were more Stage II cancers identified (1,375) in the BCDDP than Stage 0 and Stage I cancers combined (1,306). This was not a study of asymptomatic screening.

However, that did not keep us from making erroneous conclusions after hearing data presented from the BCDDP. Here's a sample from the BCDDP that shows how we were all tricked, intentional or not: In women under 50 in the BCDDP, mammography alone detected 44% of the cancers, while mammography and exam detected another 46%. Thus, in the end, 90% were detected and only 10% of cancers missed by mammography. These words have a magnetic appeal, seeming to confer that mammography has 90% sensitivity, and in fact, it's true for women with palpable lumps. But that's not screening. When women don't have palpable lumps, the tumors are smaller and harder to detect.

In all fairness, it's unreasonable to generate a single number for the Sensitivity of screening mammography (and from here on, I'm talking about asymptomatic women). The range probably extends from 20% to 95% depending on background breast density.

Also, it would be more precise if we had Sensitivity determinations for 0.5cm tumors, 1.0cm tumors, 1.5cm tumors, and so on. The "detection threshold" based on size will play a major role in assessing Sensitivity when we look at modalities other than mammography. Many women newly diagnosed with breast cancer will hear or read (for reasons I don't understand), "Your tumor was likely present 5–7 years before it was detected." First of all, there's quite a bit of wiggle room here, and some cancers are likely present only a matter of months. But ignoring that, the automatic and justifiable response from newly diagnosed women is this: "Then why wasn't it seen on last year's mammogram … or, any of the 5 to 7 mammograms prior to your so-called early diagnosis?"

The answer is "detection threshold." Tumors have to reach a certain size to be detectable. This will play a role when we lower the threshold with other modalities, whereupon it will cast mammography in a worse light than it should. Taken to its extreme, if we were able to detect the very first cancer cell—one cell—all of our measured Sensitivities for mammography, ultrasound, and MRI would plummet to embarrassing depths. Detection threshold, therefore, is an important point, and the most straightforward way of measurement is going to be tumor diameter.

So, now that we're going to restrict the discussion to asymptomatic women, an obvious issue arises (from the days when mammography was the only modality for breast imaging)— "How do you know when you missed a cancer?" After all, if it's mammographically invisible in a screening population without lumps, how do you see invisibility?

The short answer: Follow-up. That is, you count the number of women who develop a palpable cancer subsequent to the negative mammogram. Sounds easy, if it weren't for one annoying variable—time. How long after a negative mammogram are we going to count?

What emerged was a calendar-based approach that, by definition, ignores biology. If cancer was palpated within 12 months of a negative mammogram, it was considered a "miss." So what if a woman jumps the gun and gets her mammograms at 11 months instead of 12, and a cancer is found? Do you count the prior mammogram as a miss? And why 12 months? Why not 15 months? Why not 18 months?

Another way of describing this approach is to count the number of interval cancers, that is, those cancers that pop up on exam between screens. In fact, this is one of the most common ways used today in quoting Sensitivity. When the screening interval is 12 months, we expect an interval cancer rate around 20%. Thus, mammograms capture 80% while "missing" 20%, and this is good enough for most. In fact, many of the best web sites for breast cancer information will quote 80% Sensitivity, usually without a reference since everyone "knows" this to be true. But if a reference is provided for 80%, I can guarantee there's going to be at least one mega-caveat when you interrogate that referenced article.

This approach of using interval cancer rates to generate "80% Sensitivity" could be considered a "practical" reality when it comes to mammographic Sensitivity, but it's not the real reality. Why? Because some interval cancers are rapidly growing tumors that were simply not present on the prior mammogram. Mammograms shouldn't be penalized for cancers that weren't there. So, this "interval cancer" approach, it would seem, casts mammograms in a worse light than deserved. But on the other hand, this approach does not count the cancers that were, indeed, present and *detectable* on the prior mammogram by virtue of size, but did not show up due to surrounding density. As it turns out, this latter probability will prove to be greater than any of us ever imagined.

Using the old, and preferably obsolete, method of 12-month follow-up, what is the current working number for mammographic Sensitivity using modern technology? The best answer comes from the Digital Mammographic Imaging Screening Trial called DMIST,[1] first reported in the *New England Journal of Medicine* in 2005. DMIST included 49,528 women at 33 centers who underwent both film screen and digital mammography. FDA approval for digital had been granted 5 years earlier on the basis of equivalency, that is, digital was at least as good as film screen, but it remained to be seen if digital was actually better.

The DMIST study used 12-month follow-up for its definition of Sensitivity, on the working assumption that a cancer found within a 12 month period was likely to have been present at the time of the prior mammogram, a harsh assumption, for sure. The results demonstrated 70% Sensitivity for digital mammography vs. 66% Sensitivity for film screen, not quite up to the prevailing "80–90%." That said, the primary interest in DMIST was the *relationship* between the two modalities, rather than absolute Sensitivity levels.

But it was a sub-group analysis that came later that raised a few eyebrows. First of all, 10 sub-groups were studied with both modalities (thus, 20 Sensitivity determinations), and not a single group reached the mythical 90% sensitivity. In fact, only 3 of 20 groups were above 80%. The shocker came for film screen mammography in premenopausal women under 50 with dense breasts where Sensitivity was only 27% (recall now how hard it has been to prove a mortality reduction in younger women, esp. since the historical trials *all* used this film screen technology). And while headlines roared about how great digital mammography was for women with dense breasts, the digital Sensitivity for this same group was only 59%, barely more than half.

What about non-dense breasts? Remarkably, the older film screen technology had 69% Sensitivity in the over-65 group with non-dense breasts, compared to only 53% for digital. Few discussants ever mentioned the subgroups where film screen outperformed digital. At the time of adopting digital technology, we knew that the carrot-on-the-stick was going to be future developments, specifically, computer-aided diagnosis and tomosynthesis. But we all focused on the improvement in imaging dense breasts with digital, ignoring the fact that absolute Sensitivity determinations were well below what is often quoted to the public.

But then the sponsoring organization of DMIST, the American College of Radiology, did a strange thing with their Sensitivity calculations. They performed a secondary calculation of Sensitivity based on a *15-month* follow-up definition rather than 12 months. You wouldn't think there would be a great deal of difference between 12 and 15 months. However, as it turned out, digital and film screen mammography had identical Sensitivities overall using the 15-month definition, and both modalities were embarrassingly low—*41% Sensitivity.* Could it be true that mammography misses more cancers than it finds? As we will see, when we base our Sensitivity levels from studies using more than one method of imaging, this 41% will no longer be unthinkable.

If these are the modern numbers, then what were the Sensitivity determinations from the historical screening trials? Wouldn't that be important to know, especially if we are making recommendations today based on a technology in use 40 years ago?

From my decades of sleuthing, whenever an author begins their scientific paper that relates somehow to mammography, they will often begin with something like this: "Mammograms are known to detect 71 to 96% of breast cancers," and of course, they will provide a reference. I've been looking up those references for years, and I'm forever surprised by what's really in print. The example I've used here (71–96%) is one of the more common references in use today. Where did it come from?

In fact, authors are often quoting the *2002* U.S. Preventive Services Task Force article.[2] But like the old game of "Telephone" (a.k.a "Gossip"), as it turns out, the Task Force was merely quoting another article where a retrospective detailed analysis was made regarding Sensitivity in the historic trials.[3] But that source, which came from the Department of Biostatistics at MD Anderson Cancer Center and the Harvard School of Public Health, reveals something that escapes clinicians who don't follow this area closely—there are two sets of numbers for the Sensitivity in those historical trials—in one set, the range is from 71 to 96% as often quoted, but this *only applies to prevalence screens*, that is, the first screen. For all subsequent screens (incidence screens), the numbers take a dive, with Sensitivity ranging from *39% to 66%* when single values were calculated for given studies,[4] that is, roughly 20–30% lower across the board for all screens subsequent to the initial screen.

This *long-term* number is what we really want to know. Otherwise, we're quoting a detection rate applicable to one screen only (the first screen—"71 to 96% Sensitivity"), while the listener is hearing a number that she thinks is applicable for the rest of her life. In reality, the historic trials for the long haul should be quoted as having demonstrated "39% to 66%" Sensitivity (where the distinction between prevalence and incidence was made).

Why would the Sensitivity of prevalence screens be so much higher? The answer is remarkably simple, yet rarely discussed or even considered—Prevalence tumors are larger. Again, prevalence screens are the first screen, representing disease prevalence within a population. The first time someone undergoes screening, there are often several years' worth of cancers "backed up," so not only is the number of detected cancers higher on the first screen, but also, *they are larger.*

This concept of tumors being "backed up" is hard to imagine if you've also heard that tumor "doubling times" for breast cancer are 3–6 months. But remember, those doubling times are calculated using tumor *volume*, not diameter. Geometry can be a stumbling block here, but what we focus on with imaging is tumor *diameter*, not volume. And the relationship is such (forget the formula this time around) that a doubling of volume has only a small impact on diameter. For example, a 1.0cm tumor that doubles in volume will still be less than 1.3cm in diameter, barely noticeable.

Disease prevalence then refers to how many women are walking around at a single point in time with undiagnosed cancers of various sizes, "waiting" to emerge clinically. The number for breast cancer is conjecture, but if we go by the 5–7 year latency period, then the number is well over one million women currently have undiagnosed breast cancer at a subclinical size, perhaps 200,000 with tumors large enough to be detected.

Another key measure is *sojourn time*. This is the time period when a breast cancer first becomes clinically detectable until screening actually takes place. Sojourn times don't help patients make decisions, so I've chosen not to linger on this common term used in the assessment of screening; however, these concepts help explain why prevalence screens are picking up tumors that are "backed up." Furthermore, a single screen doesn't capture all the "backed up" tumors, so epidemiologists point out that it takes several years to reach a true "steady state," where screening is picking up cancers as they emerge. Eventually, "incidence screens" should match, well, disease incidence, thus the name.

Sensitivity is strongly correlated to tumor size, with palpable tumors larger than screen-detected and prevalence tumors larger than incident tumors. So prevalence tumors have higher Sensitivity than incident tumors. In fact, when patients undergo their first asymptomatic mammogram (or their first mammogram after a long skip period) and a cancer is found on X-ray, it is not unusual to perform a careful clinical exam, and in fact, the tumor will be barely palpable. Palpable is largest, Prevalence next, and then Incidence tumors are smallest. It should be no surprise that there are substantial differences in the Sensitivity of each. The surprise is that nearly everyone is quoting the bigger numbers applicable to prevalence screens, or even palpable tumors, pumping the data. Is one mammogram, the first one, what we mean by screening? No. And this is why I put the second qualifier above in italics—the percentage of cancers detected *over time.*

This number-pumping for Sensitivity is the "overselling of mammography," in my view. This is a different definition of "overselling" than the epidemiologists and public health experts use, as we've seen throughout this book. Honestly, I don't think most women care about p-values and NNI vs. NNS in order to save one life. I do think they care a great deal about this question: *"If I get breast cancer, what are the odds that it's going to show up on a mammogram before I can feel it?"* Inherent in this question is the notion that we're talking about a *lifetime* of screening, *not a one-time prevalence screen.*

Now let me slip in a caveat—in truth, we shouldn't be quoting *any* of those historic numbers, or even DMIST, given the latest developments in tomosynthesis, but I'll save the new Sensitivity data for later.

On a personal note, when I first put the contents of this chapter into a Powerpoint presentation in 2002, I was justifying my recommendation for screening patients with breast MRI (prior to any guidelines), the basis of which was the low Sensitivity of mammography, a relatively new concept for most. I would end up giving this presentation at the general assembly session of the American Society of Breast Disease in 2006, one year prior to the introduction of guidelines for MRI screening by the American Cancer Society. My exposé of the remarkably low Sensitivity for *incidence screens* in the historic screening trials would necessarily include the Swedish Trials, including the highly successful Two-County study.

As it turned out, Dr. László Tabár of Swedish Two-County fame was receiving the Pathfinder Award from the American Society of Breast Disease, a lifetime achievement award, given immediately prior to my presentation. As the lights dimmed for my talk, the last face I saw was that of Dr. Tabár who had decided to stay in the audience for the subsequent presentations. All I could think about was my upcoming slide showing "39–66% Sensitivity in the incidence screens," a veritable trashing of mammographic Sensitivity even though it was top-notch quality at the time, largely based on the Swedish studies. Dr. Tabár is not known for reticence, and I fully expected a lashing of my trashing at the end of the talk. To this day, it was my most nervous moment at the podium, ever.

So, after the dramatic tension I've invoked here, what happened? Nothing. No backlash. No criticism of my sources for arriving at the pitiful Sensitivity numbers. After all, those studies had taken place a long time ago (with long intervals that allowed more mammographic misses), and Dr. Tabár has since adopted and promoted new technologies for breast imaging, including breast MRI.

It all began innocently enough. "Where does the 90% come from?" "How do you know when you've missed an invisible cancer on mammography?" From there, I began taking special note of the histology of tumors that did not appear on mammograms in my patients (breast pathology being of particular interest to me). Tumor growth features under the microscope are highly variable and many findings never make it onto pathology reports as they don't impact diagnosis or prognosis. That said, these growth patterns often explain what we see on imaging and why. What I learned from analyzing the "invisible cancers" after they were later discovered was that there is usually an explanation for the invisibility.

In the 1980s, only a few papers had tackled this issue about the pathology of "invisible" cancers, and it had been reported that invasive lobular cancer was not showing up as well as ductal. This should be no surprise. Invasive lobular cancer can invade and travel throughout the breast tissue, with malignant cells in multiple single-file columns, skirting through paths of least resistance, without disturbing the normal anatomy.

But what I found on personally reviewing the microscopy in my patients was that invisible cancers were often ductal cancers, the most common type, something that had not been described in the medical literature. Sometimes, these "ductals" had a lobular growth pattern, but other times, small "tumor nests" would be present rather than a single mass, with these nests peppered throughout a small area of the breast tissue, not anything for the pathologist to get excited about, or even report. Or, most memorably, circa 1990, I came across my first "garden-variety" 1.0cm invasive ductal tumor that was invisible on mammography, even though the background density was low.

Histology in that "routine" tumor revealed (at least in 2-dimensions) that the relatively distinct margins (as opposed to crab-like arms extending into adjacent tissue) were abutted on every side with dense, albeit normal, breast tissue that had identical density to the tumor itself. Background density patterns overall had been newly identified in the medical literature as a problem for Sensitivity, but I realized it wasn't necessarily the overall density pattern that caused the problem—it was the nature of the *density directly touching the tumor*. If the tumor was perfectly encased in comparable benign tissue of equal density, it didn't matter what the overall mammographic density pattern was, the tumor was not going to show up on a mammogram.

This led to my first academic paper,[5] an effort that dealt with the histology of false-negative mammograms. With small numbers and no p-values, such an effort would never be published in today's world. However, given our ignorance at the time as to why some tumors failed to show up on mammography, this article was later cited in the 50th anniversary issue of the *American Journal of Surgery* as one of the key papers in oncology over the past half-century. For me, it would be my first step off the path of surgery toward the world of early diagnosis.

To render this scenario even more troubling—that is, *localized density* surrounding the tumor as distinct from *generalized density*—a paper was published in 2005 indicating that breast cancer was more likely to originate in the patches of white on mammography.[6] If this is true, we're talking double trouble. Not only can cancer be embedded in localized areas of white, these very areas could be giving rise to a disproportionate number of cancers. Is anyone safe? Of course. Patients with complete fatty replacement on mammograms, that is, 100% black on X-ray, don't have much to worry about. There's no place cancer can hide (as long as it's on the X-ray plate), and Sensitivity here is 95%. Unfortunately, the group with no significant density amounts to only 10% of the screening population. The remaining 90% have at least some degree of white on their X-ray, in a continuum to the point where there's nearly a complete "white-out" in some patients.

It didn't take long after we launched our breast MRI screening program in 2003, under the direction of breast radiologist Dr. Rebecca Stough, to see in 3-dimensions what I had only seen in 2-dimensions under the microscope (see photograph).

But as it pertains to our topic here—mammographic Sensitivity—consider this: Without MRI, when the tumor indicated in the photograph appears on next year's mammogram, it will be tallied as yet another example of mammographic success and early detection. *It won't be counted as a miss.* No one would have known it was detectable a year earlier. Thus, our

Sensitivity determinations, be they based on the inverse of interval cancers, or 12-month follow-up, are not counting the *detectable* cancers that are invisible. Our Sensitivity numbers are grossly inflated. Ignorance is bliss. And invisible, yet detectable, cancers are a perfect example that bliss is over-rated.

My 1980s question still holds true— How do you know when you've missed cancers if they are invisible on mammography? The answer will come, not through the inverse of interval cancers and not through these weak methods of measuring Sensitivity such as 12-month follow-up; instead, the answer will come through the introduction of *multi-modality imaging*—that is, cross-checking for missed cancers using different imaging methods in the same patients. This approach renders 12-month follow-up and other calendar-based definitions as pointless.

The pioneers of mammography knew that cancers were slipping through. That's why thermography was originally part of the BCDDP. After this heat-seeking technology was tossed from the protocol, however, a small cadre of researchers started to take a look at breast ultrasound. In its original form, the only benefit of ultrasound was to distinguish a cyst from a solid mass. Then, in the early 1990s, the technology improved to the point one could tell benign from malignant.

Along with this improvement came the realization that *whole breast* screening ultrasound delivers its peak performance

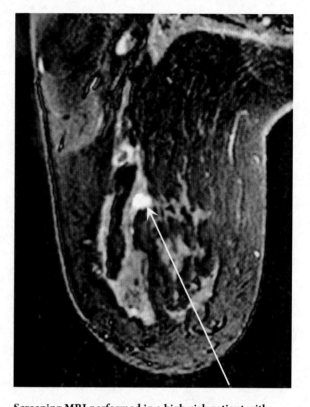

Screening MRI performed in a high-risk patient with negative mammograms and negative ultrasound. The arrow is pointing to an "enhancing" (white) mass that proved to be a 1.0cm invasive ductal carcinoma, Grade 2, negative nodes. The irregularly shaped light gray areas are normal breast tissue, and the cancer is completely embedded in this area of density and is therefore invisible on mammography. The darker gray that makes up most of the area is predominantly adipose tissue (fat), and if the cancer had developed in one of the darker gray areas, it would have been easily visible on mammography. However, given its embedded location, this tumor would not have been discovered until the next screen, at least one year away, or by palpation prior to the next screen. Although this photograph is only one "slice" measuring less than a millimeter, a 3-D look at the entire tumor revealed none of its margins to be interfacing with fat, explaining why it was mammographically invisible.

in mammographically dense tissue. The denser the better. And when studies of women with normal mammograms followed by whole breast ultrasound uncovered almost as many cancers as mammography, the "80–90%" ice began to crack. And, by the time I review breast MRI results, we'll be half-sunk into the chilly waters.

# 23

# Do These Genes Make Me Look Dense?

Shortly before the new year of 2004, an educator from Connecticut underwent her annual screening mammography, as she had been doing for years. As before, the results were "All clear." Six weeks later, she was diagnosed with Stage IIIC breast cancer. She was stunned to learn, for the first time, that she had very dense breast tissue on mammography, the feeble explanation as to why her cancer had been invisible (probably detectable several years earlier with other modalities).

Nancy M. Cappello, PhD, has since joined the list of solo game-changers, that is, non-celebrities who have risen from anonymity to turn their misfortune into far-reaching upheavals that have permanently altered how we manage breast cancer. In the footsteps of Rose Kusher (ending the one-step biopsy/frozen section/mastectomy approach), Betty Rollin (*First You Cry*, the book and movie that introduced many to the emotional impact of mastectomy), Susan Komen and her sister Nancy Brinker (initially, the promotion of screening mammography, then breast cancer research in general), Nancy Cappello set fire to sweeping reforms as to how women are informed about their breast density.

As of this writing, nearly half of the 50 states have passed legislation requiring radiologists to inform patients when mammograms are dense (white on X-ray) and to describe additional imaging modalities that might help, most notably ultrasound. Federal legislation is being considered as well. Through the Are You Dense? organization (RUdense.org) that Dr. Cappello founded, Connecticut became the first state to require that high density information be given to patients, then she has encouraged all states to do the same. Additionally, Connecticut became the first state to pass legislation requiring third party payors to cover ultrasound screening for women with dense breast tissue.

What added fuel to Dr. Cappello's conflagration was the discovery that the medical profession knew about the problem of breast density all along, but did precious little to inform the public.

I sympathize without excuse. I do have mixed emotions about legislated physician practice, but the bundle of provocative and worrisome data about density had been dropped into a deep well, it seems. As an aside, it has always been a curious phenomenon that some information new to the scene is processed quickly and new standards adopted "overnight," while other innovations or ideas are ignored even though well-grounded. After decades of medical literature warning about the danger of breast density, it was like the boy who cried "Wolf," with readers becoming numb to the published data, if they paid attention at all.

And for those historians of breast density who have already groaned at the pun, it was Dr. John N. *Wolfe* who first drew attention to mammographic density patterns, publishing his classification system of N1, P1, P2 and DY that decorated the bottom of mammography reports starting in 1976.[1] I received my first mammogram report with the Wolfe pattern noted in 1980, my first year in practice. The reaction was straightforward at that time—so what? There were no alternative methods for imaging (or treatment for that matter), and the focus then was *not* on mammographically invisible cancers. Dr. Wolfe proposed his system entirely on the basis of *imparted risk* for breast cancer, yet there were no interventions available at the time short of preventive mastectomy. In fact, Dr. Wolfe was so convinced that women with the DY pattern were headed for breast cancer (45% lifetime risk by his calculations) that he felt they should seriously consider preventive mastectomies. And with the introduction of breast implants at about this same time, "subcutaneous mastectomies with implants" were already being performed for reasons far less impressive than Wolfe DY patterns.

But then, we entered a silent period, where at the clinical level, Wolfe patterns were gradually dismissed, sometimes as old-fashioned "folly." Certain investigators, though, were using different classifications schemes, but still coming up with the same conclusion—denser breasts translated to greater risk. Still, the focus was on imparted risk. It was only later that clinicians began to appreciate that breast density was double jeopardy. Not only was density imparting elevated risk, but also it was responsible for hidden cancers missed by the very mammography that defined density in the first place.

After Dr. Wolfe, only a handful of researchers devoted their efforts to exploring the origins and implications of mammographic density. As one of those pioneers, Dr. Norman Boyd (Ontario Cancer Institute) stated in the *Journal of the National Cancer Institute News*, March 17, 2010: "While the field is now … well funded and populated, till the mid–1990s you could fit all of us into a phone booth."

What is most peculiar in re-tracing my steps during this era is that no one was arguing anything different. It wasn't controversial, rather, it was esoteric. The risk data for density was consistent no matter how the density levels were described—the highest density breasts had roughly a 4- to 6-fold relative risk for breast cancer when compared to the lowest density breasts. Yet, lagging behind, only a handful of studies prior to 1990 showed the danger of density when it came to early detection and invisibility. The vast majority of clinicians believed the "90% Sensitivity" for mammography, independent of density levels.

A reminder about 4- to 6-fold relative risk. Recall from the Number Games that *relative* risks (RRs) are fractions with a numerator and a denominator. When the word hit the street about the 4–6 fold risk, many patients and their doctors were unnerved by these numbers. The problem with this particular RR is that the number applies to the highest density (10–15% of the population) compared to the lowest density, the latter also present in only 10–15% of the population (hardly the average woman). In epidemiology-speak, the "referent" was this low density group, not the average woman. Indeed, even the "average" density patient is at 2-fold risk for breast cancer when compared to predominantly fatty breasts.

How can someone be "average risk" and "2-fold risk" at the same time? By switching out the denominators. That's why they are called *relative* risks. The RR will change if you alter either numerator or denominator. If we compare women with extremely dense tissue to the *average patient* (not the low density group) we get a more acceptable RR of 2.0. This degree of risk is more in line with having a first-degree relative diagnosed with breast cancer at age 45, whereas an RR of 4.0 would be like having two first-degree relatives diagnosed with breast cancer at 45.

And while the risk might not seem quite as powerful when stated in those terms, it may well be the most pervasive risk in existence, given the commonality of dense tissue. More women have above-average breast density than those with a positive family history. The term for this is *population attributable risk*, and mammographic density ranks as #1 in this category, if we don't count age and female gender.

While nearly all the focus was on the imparted risk of mammographic density, pioneering radiologists interested in ultrasound saw immediate application for screening women with dense breasts. Radiologist Dr. Thomas Kolb, then at Columbia University in New York City, was certainly at the forefront and became an activist for screening ultrasound. Within a decade, at least 10 large studies, totaling 60,000 patients, had been published,[2] all showing similar results—the number of additional cancers discovered after negative mammograms and negative clinical exam ranged from 2.71 per 1,000 to 4.61 per 1,000. Roughly speaking, this is a *relative* 50% (or greater) improvement over mammograms alone.

The evidence for MRI screening began trickling in about this same time as well, so at my facility, we created a "Breast Density" brochure in the early 2000s, describing the double jeopardy of density as well as the recommendation to consider multi-modality imaging with either ultrasound or MRI. At the time we initiated this program, there were no screening guidelines for multi-modality imaging at all, so we developed a scoring system that combined risk and density for patient selection, giving equal weight to both. After all, if one is going to recommend a second tier of imaging, then it should be based on the probability that the first tier is going to fail,[3] and the most powerful predictor for first tier failure, by far, is breast density.

While the primary interest in breast density seemed fixated on the associated cancer risk rather than the hidden cancer rate, even the risk agenda failed to generate momentum. To this day, only a few mathematical models incorporate density levels into formal risk calculations. This, after scores of articles have confirmed the relationship of density and risk.

A decade ago, in my presentations about multi-modality screening, primarily MRI, I would offer the overwhelming evidence that mammographic density is a risk factor, then call it "The Rodney Dangerfield of Risk Factors." It doesn't get any respect. Fortunately, times have changed.

In 2009, a study published in the *Journal of the National Cancer Institute*[4] described a meta-analysis of 47 studies of breast density related to breast cancer risk, involving 28,521 cancer patients and 3 different ways to categorize density levels—all 3 methods showed the same thing—a 4-fold risk for breast cancer when the top category is compared to the bottom category, and approximately a 2-fold risk when compared to the average patient. Once we add the possibility of invisible (or "missed") cancers on top of the risk problem, the Rodney Dangerfield reference was really an understatement. All that has changed now, with the heightened awareness of density, not via 47 studies combined into one meta-analysis, but through one woman trying to reach 50 states.

The double jeopardy concept seems to trip up even the experts. We have already seen how the 2007 guidelines for screening MRI from the American Cancer Society treated breast density as an isolated risk factor, rather than the greatest predictor of a tier one (mammographic) failure. Fortunately, the recommendation for adding ultrasound to screen high-density women was adopted by the Society of Breast Imaging. But sad to say, experts are no longer the voice of authority. The Society of Breast Imaging guidelines have gone largely unheeded. The powerful and consistent evidence for adjunct ultrasound screening in women with dense tissue will have to wait for those who know very little about ultrasound, but are masters of statistics.

As we saw earlier, the 2016 U.S. Preventive Services Task Force has weighed in and rendered an "I" grade for whole breast ultrasound for women with dense tissue—that is, "insufficient evidence." And they didn't restrict themselves to ultrasound, extending their "I" to breast MRI, 3-D tomosynthesis, or any other modality being promoted to screen women with mammographically dense tissue. Their "wet blanket" assessment for all multi-modality imaging means they are endorsing only one methodology, mammography, the *least reliable* detection method of all when tissue is extremely dense.

This is evidence-based medicine at its scariest—mammography is the only acceptable imaging method because it is the only modality that has a demonstrated mortality reduction through prospective, randomized trials. Forget that the reason mammography struggles to do better is the high breast density in those very same trials. All evidence other than the prospective RCTs is shredded and burned. The Task Force will always be irrelevant with this approach, as the technology leaves them in the dust. In 2009, they gave the cold shoulder treatment with an "I" for digital mammography as well, so after every facility in the U.S. switched to digital, the Task Force tucked their tail and simply didn't bring up the issue of digital in 2016, moving ahead with their next set of "I's."

No one has attempted an ultrasound screening trial where the endpoint is mortality reduction, given all the problems we've seen already with mammography, not the least of which is obsolete technology by the time the requisite follow-up is complete. Instead, we have relied on prospective trials (non-randomized) where participants undergo multi-modality imaging, and then cancer yields are recorded for each method individually—mammography, ultrasound and MRI—and in combination. Improved cancer yields are indirectly reflective of a mortality reduction, though purists will be quick to point out that we can't rule out the impact of the Big Four biases.

We have very good offerings for imaging beyond mammography available now, underutilized, though with much improved outcomes based on cancer yields:

**Mammographic density and no other risk factors = whole breast ultrasound**
**Mammographic density plus additional risks = ultrasound or MRI
(perhaps alternating, or perhaps biennial MRI alone)**
**Women at very high risk, regardless of density = MRI**

Nancy Cappello saw the problem shortly after her own diagnosis. Breast density is double jeopardy. It is a risk factor, and it is a predictor of mammographic failure.

Several questions often arise with regard to breast density. First, "How did I get it?" And second, "What can I do about it?"

Baseline breast density is a product of your genes, though environmental influences do cause alterations. Interestingly, some of these alterations are associated with a similar change in breast cancer risk, raising the question as to whether or not density can be used as a surrogate measure for risk-reducing strategies. Each pregnancy lowers breast density a bit, and breast-feeding does as well, both known to be protective factors when occurring in the younger age groups.

Postmenopausal hormone replacement therapy, especially estrogen and progesterone, can result in an increase in mammographic density. And the use of SERMs (Selective Estrogen Receptor Modulators—tamoxifen or raloxifene) can lower breast density, perhaps reflecting when they are also preventing breast cancer.

Taking "statins" to prevent cardiovascular events and death is widely accepted, even though, as with any preventive health measure, it is only the minority who benefit. Yet the surrogates—blood lipid levels—have become endpoints unto themselves. "We've successfully treated your hyperlipidemia" ignores the fact that the goal is something else entirely—that is, reducing the probability of cardiovascular events and death.

The lack of such a surrogate may be one of the reasons why so few women accept a recommendation to take one of the SERMS, which are FDA-approved to reduce the risk of breast cancer. Fairly good evidence suggests that the same women who have a lowering of their breast density pattern while on SERM therapy are the same ones benefitting most from the drug. Perhaps someday, breast density will become an official surrogate, and pharmacologic risk reduction will enjoy greater popularity.

Other factors don't fit so well into the density picture. Body fat (BMI = body mass index) is a confounding variable that doesn't always match up with breast density risk, with higher BMI being associated with higher cancer risk in postmenopausal women even though it is also correlated to lower density. In fact, for many years, it slowed down acceptance of breast density as a risk factor. Ethnicity doesn't always match either. Asian women, in general, have a much higher density level than African American women, yet the breast cancer risks are higher for African Americans.

A common misconception is that "young women have dense tissue, while older women do not," thus explaining the superior efficacy of mammography in older women. While these differences may be true in general, exceptions are quite common. Some women who start screening in their 30s will have low density mammograms, and we see 80-year-olds with mammograms so dense we can't see a thing. Some women gradually become less dense after menopause, others do not, especially if they take estrogen-plus-progesterone hormone replacement therapy. And there is no sharp and rapid loss of density at menopause. In fact, if you look at density in the 40s as a whole and compare it to density in the 50s, there is very little difference.

The point is that breast density is a highly individual situation. I've included an assessment of density in my risk assessment program for more than 20 years. My reasoning for this was based on the double jeopardy issue, and I've made it a practice not only to adjust risk levels accordingly, but also to individualize an estimate of Sensitivity should breast cancer occur, a distinct number from density as a risk factor. Example: "Your risk for breast cancer, including your near-100% density level, is going to be such-and-such lifetime, such-and-such for the next 10 years, and if cancer occurs, the odds are less than 50% that we will see your cancer using mammograms alone."

Now, one quibble with the Are You Dense? educational efforts. As often happens in medicine, we are confronted by continuums for which we must create artificial (and subjective) classification schemes. Are You Dense? has opted to use the dichotomy approach—two groups, dense and non-dense, with 50% density as the dividing line, an approach used in some clinical trials as well. The problem here is that the 50% point is where subjectivity is at its worst.

Picture a bell curve, which is what we nearly have in breast density, from 0 to 100%, with most women bunched in the middle. Then, you draw a line straight down from the peak of that curve, and you have the majority of women bunched at the dividing line. Not only do radiologists routinely differ in their density assignments at this point in the dividing line, but also studies have shown that the same radiologist will assign a different density level from year-to-year in the same patient, even when the density level is unchanged.

This is no one's fault—it's simply the nature of subjectivity applied in a quantitative fashion to a phenomenon that has a strong qualitative feature as well. In other words, it's not merely how much density is present, but what is the nature of that density—small patches of white? Large patches of white? Diffuse haziness? Net-like strings of white? Net-like strings of white interconnecting small white patches with a diffusely hazy background? It goes on and on. The qualitative differences are huge, and Sensitivity will vary with the confounding variable of tumor growth pattern if cancer occurs.

Once breast density became an accepted risk factor and predictor of mammographic failure, an entire industry arose in order to quantify it in a meaningful fashion, using software that spits out exact percentages of density, a number that can be translated to both "risk levels" and "sensitivity levels." The resilient Dr. Kopans, surfacing again on this issue, has spent considerable effort trying to educate the world about the subjectivity of breast density, pointing out the extreme complexity that underscores all attempts to simplify the problem, that is, the qualitative issues are every bit as important as the quantitative. Indeed, the software programs attempting to objectify subjectivity generate divergent outcomes from one company to another.

For the past 20 years, the American College of Radiology has required that interpreters of mammography describe the degree of breast density, dividing into 4 categories. The definition for each category has changed slightly over time, but what used to be Levels 1–4 are now called Levels A-D, originally based on quartiles of density: 0–25%, 25–50%, 50–75%, 75%-100%, though now with qualitative modifiers. In years past, radiologists were directed to dictate "in cypher" using a formal lexicon. For instance, "scattered fibroglandular densities" was code for a Level 2 (now called Level B) mammogram, or 25–50%. Primary care physicians grew immune to the redundant terminology, but you can imagine Nancy Cappello's shock to discover that this density information rarely made it to the patient. Today, the American College of Radiology insists that Level A through D be included as part of the official report, and directives also include a method for patient awareness of same.

In my practice, as I am reviewing the mammograms for double jeopardy, I attempt to incorporate the quality of density as well as the quantity, the latter having already been addressed by the radiologist with A, B, C and D levels. In my mind's eye, I picture a small invasive cancer, about 1.0 to 1.5cm, and I move that imaginary cancer around both the MLO views and the CC views while asking myself a simple question: Is there anywhere this (imaginary) cancer could hide? Invasive lobular carcinoma can prove problematic to this approach, as the diffuse growth pattern in some lobulars allows them to hide anywhere they want. This approach is still subjective, but it's not a false dichotomy. Generally speaking, the overall percentage of white reflects the imparted risk level, while the qualitative pattern of the white allows me to predict the probability that a small cancer will be detected (Sensitivity).

Importantly, this "roving" 1.0 to 1.5cm (imaginary) tumor approach is based on the premise from the previous chapter that overall density pattern is only an indirect predictor of invisible cancers—the real problem is the density immediately adjacent to the tumor that could completely encase the cancer. When you consider the possibility that the origin of cancer might be primarily within the white patches, it can render some uncomfortable conclusions about mammography as used alone, as well as the shaky premise of density as a dichotomy.

Another word about DCIS, usually presenting in the form of a calcium cluster, that is, tiny white dots in a grouping on X-ray. Calcium appears on mammography better than ultrasound or even MRI, so mammography has held the top spot in the hierarchy of screening. But now that DCIS is dropping in popularity as a worthy goal, ultrasound has gained momentum in that a higher percentage of ultrasound-discovered cancers are small invasive cancers, rather than DCIS. To be specific, mammography-discovered cancers will be DCIS about 25–40% of the time, while ultrasound-discoveries are DCIS only 10–20% of the time. So some observers (certainly not the Task Force) claim superiority of ultrasound over mammography in the very high density groups, given one or the other. This introduces the speculative, but attractive, notion of screening with whole breast ultrasound alone in selected patients.

Certainly, mammograms alone in this highest density group (greater than 75%) have failed to deliver. I once encountered a breast center that had a disclaimer at the bottom of all of its reports: "4% to 8% of breast cancers are not visible on mammography." I did not make any friends when I openly stated that the only way such a statement could be true in a patient with extreme breast density was to add a zero to both numbers—that is "40% to 80% of breast cancers are not visible." People thought I was kidding, or at least exaggerating. I was not. Years later, when DMIST demonstrated the sub-group of young women with dense breasts, with only 27% Sensitivity using film screen technology (a 73% miss rate), I was vindicated, although still not popular.

With the great advantage of lower cost and greater patient comfort when compared to breast MRI, whole breast screening ultrasound has some distinct advantages. The drawback is Specificity, with more benign biopsies than occur with mammography or MRI. Most studies show that an ultrasound-generated biopsy will be malignant only 5–10% of the time (compared to 20% for mammography and 30–40% for MRI). These extra biopsies negate much of the up front cost advantage, while simultaneously adding to patient anxiety.

Furthermore, there is a bigger difference in technique and interpretations with ultrasound than mammography, very much related to experience and skill. To that end, a new development (albeit in research status for 40 years) is "automated whole breast ultrasound," which gives a standardized picture of the entire breast that should be very desirable for the screening setting. While handheld ultrasound will likely be maintained for diagnostic problems, automated whole breast ultrasound should be a great addition to the screening tools available for women with dense mammograms, but without other risk factors.

Although single-center studies and multi-center studies have revealed that screening ultrasound increases cancer yields by 3–4 per 1,000 above the 5–7 cancers found by mammography, I'm only going to review one of the most important studies—ACRIN 6666.[5] The American College of Radiology Imaging Network designed a trial to study ultrasound as a complement to mammography in high-risk, high density patients. Notice that participants had to have both—traditional risk factors in addition to the inherent risk of breast density. Although there is not a control group (no imaging at all) in a study like this addressing cancer yields, care was taken to account for as many variables as possible. For instance, patients were randomized as to which study was performed first (mammography or ultrasound), and the radiologists were blinded as to the results of one study when interpreting the other.

Kudos to the trial designers who addressed every possible criticism that I can dream up concerning current multi-modality guidelines. First, the study designers realized the age-discrimination inherent when lifetime risks are used as a sole criterion. The 60-year-old patient with risk factors, and at peak short-term incidence of breast cancer, often won't qualify for MRI because of fewer remaining years in her lifetime. So the ACRIN 6666 team came up with short-term risk calculations, as well as standard long-term calculations.

Then, designers also realized the "qualitative" problem of density, allowing certain patients to qualify for the trial if there were large patches of white even though overall density was less than 50%. Indeed, one-fourth of participants would be called "non-dense" if only "percent density" had been the guide.

And then, one of the most subtle, but perceptive, entry requirements allowed an adjustment in traditional risk requirements based on density level, that is, the extremely dense patient did not need as many traditional risk factors to qualify, and conversely, the lower density patients needed higher calculated risk. I can't say it made any difference in the outcome, but I will offer personal testimony to this—these entry requirements were so sophisticated in design that they could be used for all forms of multi-modality imaging. Enough praise to Dr. Wendie Berg and her team, moving on to results.

From 2004 to 2006, 2,662 women (with both density and traditional risks) at 21 sites underwent 3 rounds of double screening with mammograms and bilateral whole breast ultrasound, at 0, 12 and 24 months. From the boatloads of data generated, let me summarize.

Thirty-three cancers were detected by mammography alone, 32 detected by ultrasound alone, and 26 were seen on both mammography and U.S. Clearly, the modalities are detecting different aspects of cancer, as less than a third of the cancers were seen on both modalities. This suggests a powerful complementary role to ultrasound. In fact, ultrasound appears equal to mammography in this population, if picking one or the other.

A breakdown of tumor size shows that mammography-detected tumors had a mean size of 1.15cm whereas U.S.–detected tumors had a mean of 1.0cm. The comparison in size indicates that U.S. is finding cancers slightly smaller (earlier?) than mammography, but more importantly, it is capturing the cancers that ought to be large enough to be seen on mammography, but were missed, presumably due to density. Yet there is an important difference: 75% of the cancers were invasive by ultrasound, while only 52% were invasive by mammography. Because these ultrasound-discovered invasive cancers were small and usually node-negative (4% with positive nodes, compared to 33% node positivity for mammograms alone), ultrasound could again be declared the winner in head-to-head competition. That said, ACRIN 6666 was not looking for an either-or "winner" when it comes to these two modalities. The study was assessing the role of complementary imaging to mammography.

Beyond digital mammography, ultrasound generated 5.3 cancers/1,000 the first year and 3.7 per 1000 in each of the second and third screens. What about Sensitivity, documenting the benefit from a different angle? Discounting the first screen (as a prevalence screen), the next two incidence screens revealed a Sensitivity of 76% ... combined! That's right. Both mammography and ultrasound together missed 24% of cancers. Sensitivity of mammography alone was 52%. Granted, this is not your average patient population, but "risk levels" have no influence on Sensitivity levels. Density, on the other hand, is the primary determinant of Sensitivity.

But that's not where the story ends. ACRIN 6666 designed a sub-study, where women could undergo a single breast MRI at the conclusion of the 3 screens with mammography and ultrasound. Only 612 women of the 2,662 moved ahead with this aspect of the trial, so a separate set of statistics was created for this group. An additional 9 cancers were discovered on the single MRI (8 of 9 were invasive cancers with an average diameter of 0.85 cm, all patients node negative).

Converted to our 1,000 standard, this was an additional cancer yield of *14.7* per 1,000. Had all 2,662 women participated, an extrapolation would indicate that *39 additional cancers* would have been detected, in a group that had been cleared as "good to go and cancer-free" with 3 sets of negative mammograms and 3 sets of negative ultrasounds.

The smaller tumor size with MRI is a little more impressive than the difference between ultrasound and X-ray, now comparing 0.85cm with MRI to the 1.15cm of mammography. So MRI has lowered the threshold of detection, which automatically hurts the other two forms of imaging when it comes to Sensitivity. To the point, when Sensitivity for mammography and ultrasound are now recalculated while including the MRI-detected cancers, then the *Sensitivity for mammography and ultrasound combined was only 44%.* A 56% miss rate using clinical exam, mammography and ultrasound together, three times, over the course of 24 months!

These study results are both sobering and confusing, if those two descriptors can fit in the same sentence. As a result, the 2012 headlines surrounding this landmark study were mixed, as if the investigators interviewed were baffled by their own data, leaving the journalists bewildered, yet eager as ever to report.

Consequently, some headlines pronounced ACRIN 6666 a clear victory for screening ultrasound, while others proclaimed the superiority of breast MRI. But one headline was never used and never considered for this patient population: "Mammograms alone are good enough."

Wendie Berg, M.D., PhD, breast radiologist, was the study chair and principal investigator for ACRIN 6666. In January 2014, two years after the trial results had been released, Dr. Berg underwent a digital mammogram with 3-D tomosynthesis, which showed Level C density (50–75%), but no cancer. Because she had a positive family history, she decided to proceed with adjunct breast imaging, and in April 2015, she publicly announced that a 0.9cm invasive carcinoma had been discovered—using breast MRI. A new activist group was formed—DENSE (Density Education National Survivors' Effort).[6]

# 24

# The Emperor of All Modalities

The well-known actress was seated next to her medical oncologist, facing Oprah. She had recently undergone bilateral mastectomies for a small cancer that had been discovered on breast MRI in 2008, invisible on mammography. Although a lumpectomy candidate, she was not excited about the prospect of radiation that usually follows removal of the tumor. Instead, she chose bilateral mastectomies for the preventive component of that surgery because she had tested positive for one of the BRCA genes. Thus, even if cured of this first cancer, she was facing a high risk for new breast cancers in the coming years. Of special note, the actress had been so astonished that MRI had discovered her cancer after failed mammography that she had already announced her intent to establish a foundation to help women pay for their breast MRIs.

The medical oncologist, however, had a different focus. She wanted to talk about genetic testing, and how this had been the key to successful disease control. But Oprah seemed more fascinated with the MRI discovery, and finally blurted something like "Well, should we all be getting MRIs?"

It was a moment for the ages. Breast MRI had become clinically available early in the 2000s, lagging well behind the rest of the human body after MRI's clinical introduction circa 1980. The momentum was slow at first, but after the 2007 guidelines from the American Cancer Society for high-risk screening with breast MRI, we entered a new era of multi-modality screening. Yet the word about the imaging revolution was slow to travel, the cost of MRI was high, and the third-party payors were deeply troubled. But now, on *The Oprah Winfrey Show*,[1] breast MRI would be introduced to an audience of women greater in number than the combined outreach power of every breast cancer specialist in the country. Finally, the word would be broadcast at this pivotal moment in time.

Then came the shocking words from the oncologist: "Oh, no, no. MRI misses too many cancers, mammograms are still better," or something like that. My mind went blank; otherwise, I would quote the oncologist more accurately. Nonetheless, the oncologist lowered the boom with a dismissive statement that throttled Oprah, while the actress was blank-faced (not a particularly strong plug for her new MRI foundation). After dousing the fire of the best technology in medical history to define breast cancer independent of breast density, the oncologist then gushed about the exciting new role of genetic testing (we'd already been testing for 12 years at that point).

Again, Noah's Principle: "There's no point in predicting rain unless you build the arc."

201

The medical oncologist was all about forecasting the weather, forgetting the intervention, forgetting the thing that made the difference, forgetting that it does no good to find a BRCA-gene–positive patient unless you can do something about it. And I can't think of an area in breast medicine where the ability to alter outcomes is greater than screening with MRI. And don't be fooled by the critics of MRI who squawk about its "poor Specificity of 37%," quoting a paper from the Dark Ages of MRI. Today, once the baseline MRI has been established, the false-positive rate with screening MRI is no different than screening mammography at centers of excellence.

With a nod to the marvelous book by Dr. Siddhartha Mukherjee, the *Emperor of All Maladies*, I've adjusted the last word of his title to describe MRI—that is to say, breast MRI is king, or queen, what have you, it's the Emperor. Nothing can detect breast cancer with greater Sensitivity than MRI. Granted, positron emission mammography (PEM) and molecular breast imaging (MBI) come close, and when one considers fewer false-positives, the case can be made that these modalities deserve top billing as additional Emperors. That said, both are nuclear medicine studies that include the injection of a radionuclide that delivers a small amount of radiation body-wide, clinically unimportant in a single study. Both approaches are generally considered a good alternative to pre-op staging with MRI in newly diagnosed cancer patients, though we're not sure yet about long-term screening (not that we fully understand the impact of gadolinium exposure 30–40 times over a lifetime either). In recent years, I've served on panels with Carrie B. Hruska, PhD., and Deborah J. Rhodes, M.D., both of whom are on the development team at the Mayo Clinic where MBI is being introduced. Indeed, we could deliver each other's presentations by simply filling in the blanks with MBI or MRI.

Breast MRI does its thing, not so much through the thin "cuts" where remarkable details are provided in 1mm slices, but through the intravenous injection of gadolinium "dye," a metallic element that rests comfortably as number 64 on the Periodic Tables that hang in high school chemistry classes worldwide. Without the contrast agent, it may surprise you to learn that cancers can still hide when embedded in dense tissue on the MRI, even in 1mm slices. Breast cancer generates its own blood supply, called angiogenesis, and these vessels are not normal, so the "dye" makes cancer "enhance" on MRI, a bright white area, brighter than the background breast tissue.

Don't look for prospective, randomized controlled trials with mortality as the endpoint when it comes to screening with MRI. We do have preliminary mortality data in the BRCA-positive population that shows exactly what you would expect—saved lives—but nothing near the ballpark that would satisfy an evidence-based think tank. As always, when comparing two or more imaging methods, we have prospective trials for *cancer yields*, a surrogate for mortality reduction. But without control groups, we can only hold court in a lower venue. As we've seen from the beginning of this book, the Four Horsemen are always lurking.

In these prospective cancer yield studies, all participants undergo all modalities being evaluated. In the early days of MRI, 7 international trials[2] were performed in Canada, the Netherlands, Germany, Italy, Austria, U.K., and USA. All 7 included mammography, while 4 of 7 studied ultrasound as well. The superior Sensitivity of MRI was so profound that, in 2007, the American Cancer Society adopted its guidelines without the benefit of a proven mortality reduction. The conclusion was straightforward for most of us—if you have a modality that is finding double or triple the number of cancers, you can't wait 20 years for someone to do the definitive prospective RCTs. You must act now.

So what were the Sensitivities of MRI? The range might surprise you, starting with the worst—71%, 77%, 77%, 86%, 89%, 91%, and 100%. These studies were in the developmental phase of MRI, and some countries focused on "dynamic MRI," which had lower Sensitivity and higher Specificity than what we use today ("high spatial resolution MRI"). High spatial resolution is high Sensitivity, lower Specificity, but by combining the technologies, it has been shown that both Sensitivity and Specificity are in the 90% range with modern MRI.[3]

But there are other reasons why the MRI Sensitivity was on the low side. Mammograms detect lower grades of DCIS that don't have much in the way of angiogenesis. Thus, they don't show up well on MRI. This may not be a bad thing. As it turns out, X-ray and MRI are visualizing different things when it comes to DCIS. Angiogenesis in invasive cancer is associated with a more aggressive biology, so it may turn out that MRI is only identifying the biologically important DCIS. But in these trials where small areas of DCIS were detected by X-ray calcifications, it would sometimes count as an MRI miss.

There's a strange thing about DCIS Sensitivity—it depends on which modality came first as the referent. If you take all the mammographic-detected DCIS, then perform an MRI, the latter won't perform very well. But if you take all the MRI-detected DCIS, then perform mammography, it will be the X-ray that flunks. Basically, two modalities are detecting two different, overlapping groups of DCIS, and it will be our job in the future to sort this out as to whether or not MRI-detected DCIS is more important.

Back to the subject of Sensitivity where I haven't yet given you the performance data for mammography or ultrasound. First of all, there wasn't a single study where mammograms detected more than half the cancers, the range being from 33% to 50%. In 2007, a combined analysis of 5 of the 7 studies[4] tallied 81% Sensitivity for MRI, 43% Sensitivity for ultrasound, and *40% Sensitivity for mammography.*

No one likes to quote mammography as having only a 40% Sensitivity, but it's routinely done when discussing these alternative imaging methods. Sometimes, the coverage is schizophrenic. A popular news magazine (I won't mention names this *TIME*) once featured the breast MRI revolution, revealing numbers that indicated mammography had only a 40% Sensitivity (correct). Yet the sidebar that accompanied the article described mammography with its "90%" Sensitivity. It's mind-boggling how we continue to cling to the Myth. How is it done? And 40% and 90% in the same breath?

One way to live with cognitive dissonance is to claim that the results showing profoundly low mammographic Sensitivity are not reflective of the general population, given that these were imaging studies in high-risk women But while higher density means higher risk, the reverse is not necessarily true. In fact, high risk patients have the same bell curve of density. This plays out most dramatically in the only MRI screening trial (Canada) that was limited to women with a proven BRCA gene mutation. As it turned out in that study, Sensitivities were no different for women over 50 than under 50, and in a shocking addendum, there was only 33% Sensitivity for mammography in patients in the lowest quartile of density (Level A), and the same 33% for Level B.[5] So much for density being the only determinant as to when MRI can help. As the photos in their article reveal, even a benign-looking "wisp" of tissue, the only white on the X-ray, can turn out to be malignant.

The other way in which poor Sensitivity for mammography can be dismissed is by claiming that MRI is only lowering the threshold of detection. We've talked about this before. If a new technology is able to find breast cancer at 0.2cm instead of the 0.8–1.0cm average of MRI, then it's going to make MRI look bad. There's a second volley of rhetoric that accompanies this stance, expressed like this: "And furthermore, we don't need to find cancer earlier with MRI. Detecting cancer at 1.0cm with mammography is fine, where the cure rates exceed 90–95%." I agree. But that's not what MRI is doing, at least not entirely.

Recall the MRI picture I showed in a previous chapter—that patient did not experience "earl*ier*" detection. That was a 1.0cm tumor, the size that is *supposed* to be visible by mammography. I agree we don't need to focus on detection of tumors much smaller than 1.0cm, but we clearly need to find the 1.0cm tumors currently being missed by mammography. In other words, we need more *reliable* detection, rather than earlier detection. We know (that is, we believe) that mammography saves lives through detection of tumors in the 1.0–1.5 size range, so we need to find the remainder of those same-sized tumors. Thus, our goal is not to find cancers *earlier*, nearly as much as it is to find those cancers large enough to be seen on mammography, but missed.

Let me return to "sojourn time" even though a mystical science surrounds its calculation. In brief, the sojourn time extends from that point when an asymptomatic cancer first becomes detectable until it becomes clinically apparent, the implication being the window of opportunity for screening. The earlier that reliable screening is performed, the shorter the sojourn time (and incidentally, the longer the lead time). Although I have chosen in this book to describe the two key elements of effective screening as *biology* and *sensitivity*, some prefer "sojourn time" over biology, which is another way of saying the same thing. I chose "biology" in order to avoid the calendar as much as possible.

Sojourn times are iffy, in that cancers have widely different growth rates, but that hasn't stopped sophisticated analyses used to arrive at *mean* sojourn times. I've used more concrete terms, e.g., "threshold of detection," to remind the reader that breast cancer is present for some unknown duration of time prior to being detectable, then sits silently in the breast (during its sojourn) for another duration of time prior to actual detection.

That said, I have no way of precisely adjusting the 40% Sensitivity for mammography upward, to account for the impact of the slightly lower threshold of detection with MRI. But I do know the pathology data that comes from MRI screening, and not all studies show smaller tumor sizes with MRI-discovered cancers. One of those studies is our own[6] where, updating our results since that publication, the average tumor size of MRI-detected cancers is 1.17cm (skewed higher by some invasive lobulars) and the median size is 0.9cm, essentially the same size as tumors found on mammography. This implies that the MRI effect is mostly through capturing tumors *missed by mammography*, rather than by lowering the threshold of detection, or "earlier" detection, or if you must, altering sojourn times.

From multiple indirect sources, giving mammography the benefit of the doubt, I add 10 points' worth of Sensitivity to the 40%, to account for the slightly lower threshold of MRI detection. My construct gives me a nice round number of 50% to deal with, and I've never found any evidence to suggest I should budge on my belief that mammography has a 50% Sensitivity when all ages and densities are considered. Before, we never knew how many cancers were hiding on normal mammograms. True Sensitivity was only a guess, based on weak definitions. Multi-modality imaging has changed everything.

Remember, though, I stated earlier that a single number for mammographic Sensitivity is an unfair question to begin with, given the remarkable range as a result of density, from 20% in the patient with a complete white-out (near 100% density), all the way up to 95% Sensitivity in the patient where the entire mammogram is black. More recently, I've heard podium presentations by breast radiologists acknowledge, "Mammograms detect 80% of cancers overall, but only 50% in premenopausal women or women with dense breasts."

My 50% conclusion is only an approximation when talking about the average patient, keeping in mind that the 40% Sensitivity drawn from the 7 MRI screening trials was in patients where density was slightly skewed higher due to younger women in those trials, while ACRIN 6666 participants had both high risk and high density. Anything I quote for the general population is an educated guess, but I can assure you that, overall, Sensitivity does not reach 80% if multi-modality comparisons are the standard. Without multi-modality cross-checks, Sensitivity *appears* to be 80% because people are only counting the interval cancers that pop up in between annual screens as the "miss" rate. Additional women, with their 1.0cm tumors embedded in white densities, will be detected the next year on screening, and are never counted as a miss. Yet they were *detectable* a year earlier—that is, the sojourn clock started ticking. Unfortunately, the tumors were located in the wrong place at the wrong time.

To summarize, breast MRI has two effects that generate surprisingly low Sensitivity determinations for mammography: (1) Sojourn time is extended by MRI, given that detectability is redefined as "earlier," and (2) Even without threshold of detection being altered, MRI detects those cancers that were large enough for mammographic detection, but were embedded in areas of dense tissue. Restated, with both #1 and #2 in play, mammographic Sensitivity is 40%, but if we look at tumor sizes generated by mammograms vs. MRI, it appears that #2 is the bigger issue.

Why do I persist in making this distinction? Again, some radiologists have been dismissive of the 40% by claiming the entire effect of MRI is through #1, lowering the threshold of detection. I maintain that #2 is more commonly the culprit, giving more credence to the lower values for mammographic Sensitivity.

From multiple angles, evidence supports my contention of 50% Sensitivity for mammography. In 2003, in an effort to help defend radiologists who were spending more time in court than a physician typically desires, a study by mammography experts[7] was performed to make a simple point—most of the time (58%, in fact), a retrospective look on the mammogram in the year prior will show a subtle abnormality where the cancer later appeared on the next year's mammogram. Note that these cancers did not pop up in between screens. They were diagnosed by mammography, *all* considered "early diagnosis," yet 58% of the time, there was a tip-off that something had changed a year earlier.

The point of this study was that radiologists can't be held responsible for subtle changes (easy to see in retrospect by juries and plaintiff's attorneys), that are not enough to warrant a call-back. If such subtleties were deemed as worrisome, then radiologists would be calling back many more patients, and the false-positive rate would skyrocket. Yet, had MRI been performed on these patients, I venture the guess that nearly all 58% would have had their cancers detected in the year prior (90% of the 58% to be exact, or 52%). If more than half of cancers can thus be detected a year earlier, this is more indirect support for a 50% Sensitivity for mammography *in the general population.*

More solid proof would need to come directly through an MRI screening study performed in the general population at average risk. Given the high-cost of breast MRI, given its intravenous injection of gadolinium, and given the cumbersome nature of the procedure, I stated for many years that it would never happen, that is, we would never see MRI screening results from a general population study. *But if it ever did*, the prediction was easy—if mammograms are detecting only half of detectable cancers, then an MRI screen (after a negative mammogram) would have the same yield as occurs in general population screening with mammograms. That is, mammograms would detect the first half, then MRI would do clean-up and detect the second half.

In predicting exact numbers for the general population, the range of cancer yields usually falls between 3 and 5 per 1,000, the higher end of that range occurring when there are more prevalence screens included and/or patients with large gaps in between screens. The lower end of that range is when incidence screens predominate in a compliant population.

If we select 5 per 1,000 as the average cancer yield for mammography, and if this represents only half of detectable cancers (50% Sensitivity for mammography), then a study of MRI screening in women with negative mammograms would yield another 5 cancers per 1,000. Mammograms detect the first half, then MRI detects the second half that were missed by mammography.

After a decade of stating "a general population study of MRI screening will never happen," I was surprised to learn of a general population study of screening MRI that was performed by noted breast MRI expert, Dr. Christiane Kuhl, and her group from Aachen, Germany.[8] Dr. Kuhl's associate, Dr. Schrading, announced the results at the 2013 San Antonio Breast Cancer Symposium.

Mammographic Sensitivity cannot be measured directly from the 1,725 women who enrolled in the study because, by definition, 100% of the women had negative mammography performed prior to entry. Not only that, but 100% had negative clinical exams and 89% had negative whole breast screening ultrasound. This was a population of women thoroughly cleared as cancer-free. Yet, in this "average risk" population, 18 cancers were identified on breast MRI. The yield was 11 per 1,000, or 1.1%. Using my 50% Sensitivity premise, I would have predicted 5 per 1,000 cancer discoveries with MRI, or 0.5%, so now my theoretical 50% Sensitivity for mammography in the general population appears to have been too optimistic.

As for the DCIS: invasive ratio, wherein critics like to charge that MRI is "too sensitive," detecting "harmless" cancers like DCIS, there were 7 DCIS and 11 invasive cancers in the study of general population MRI screening from Germany, but importantly, 5 of 7 DCIS, and 6 of 11 invasive cancers were high-grade, thus considered more biologically significant. Were the invasive cancers only tiny things, subclinical and still cured if discovered 1–2 years from now? Well, the average tumor size was 1.1cm, *identical to mammographic detection threshold*. Again, we are not finding cancers *earlier* with MRI nearly as much as we are simply finding the cancers *missed* by mammography, the ones we know where lives can be saved.

"But you're only making overdiagnosis worse!" "You're finding harmless, low grade tumors, while it's the interval cancers that kill." Review of pathology, however, doesn't jive with this criticism. In general, MRI-discovered pathology is a close match to mammographically-discovered pathology. Some, but not all, studies show a slight shift toward DCIS in MRI-detected cancers. And some, but not all, show a slightly smaller size when detected by MRI. Most, however, show a remarkably lower incidence of lymph node involvement. If average tumor size is held steady at 1.0cm, but lymph node involvement is less, this can also be explained by length time bias—that is, "you are only finding tumors that are less aggressive."

In the aforementioned study of MRI screening at our facility, we encountered a remarkably low incidence of lymph node involvement with MRI-discovered cancers. While mammographically-detected cancers have a 25–30% chance of positive nodes, at the time of our publication, we had only a single patient with a single micrometastasis in a single node after 10 years of screening (4%). Post-publication, we had another patient with a single positive node, after 50 cancers had been discovered through MRI, 80% of these cancers being invasive.

While length bias will always be at work in this situation, there are several other explanations for the low positive-node rate. First, recall that slight differences in tumor diameter translate into much larger differences in actual tumor "volume." So, if MRI is detecting invasive cancers at a mean size of 0.8cm, as opposed to mammography's 1.0cm, the former volume per MRI is actually *half* that of the 1.0cm tumor. This would mean that *earlier* diagnosis does make a difference, something I've heretofore downplayed.

Another explanation has to do with the *range* of tumor sizes detected through screening MRI, which is much tighter than with mammography. Mammographic screening has more outliers with larger tumors having more nodes positive. In contrast, few MRI-discovered cancers exceed 2.0cm.

But perhaps the most intriguing data that minimizes the impact of length time bias in MRI screening has to do with our old nemesis, the interval cancer, those allegedly "aggressive" tumors that pop up in between screening intervals. Critics have been pointing out for years that these are the killers, while we keep detecting the namby-pamby cancers through screening.

As we saw earlier, many have questioned the traditional teaching about interval cancers, and modern studies now reveal these cancers to be a mixture—maybe a third of them are classic, aggressive tumors that arose quickly and grew quickly, for which screening doesn't help. But the surprise finding has been how "ordinary" most of these interval cancers are. Yes, length bias is always at work, but oddly, interval cancers nearly disappear once you begin multi-modality screening with MRI. This is consistent with the proposition that most "interval cancers" are not unique at all, rather, they were simply invisible on the prior mammogram, embedded in dense adjacent tissue.

In the general population undergoing routine screening with mammography, interval cancers number around 20–25% of the total. However, in the high-risk populations, the interval cancer numbers are higher, more in the 30–40% range, or even higher in the BRCA-positive population.

Now, here's what happened to the interval cancer rate when MRI was added to mammography in the international screening trials—0, 2.3%, 3.5%, 4.5%, 5.7%, and 9.8%. Had these high risk women been screened with mammography alone, the 30–40% interval cancers would have been called "more biologically aggressive, and the very reason why screening doesn't work." In fact, the sharp decline in interval cancers strongly supports the notion that most interval cancers are not "aggressive," but are merely invisible on the prior mammogram. Thus, length bias may not be as powerful as once thought.

To be sure, one outlier has been identified concerning interval cancers. A 2010 update from the Netherlands MRISC Screening Study revealed 10/31 (32.3%) invasive cancers in the BRCA-1 population that occurred during the screening interval, using both MRI and mammography. This was isolated to BRCA-1 patients only, given that BRCA-2-positive patients and other high risk women still had very low interval cancer rates of 6.3% or less. To adjust for this finding in BRCA-1 patients, many breast centers now stagger the two imaging studies at 6 month intervals, so that the 12-month interval is cut in half. Whether this was a fluke due to relatively small number of cancers, we don't know. But as a reference point, the

Canadian MRI screening trial (not the CNBSS) that included screening ultrasound as well as mammography and MRI was composed entirely of women with BRCA mutations, yet of the 22 cancers discovered, only one was an interval cancer.

Returning to the study from Germany by Dr. Christiane Kuhl, using MRI to screen average risk women with negative mammograms, an update of the 2013 presentation was delivered at the 2015 ASCO Breast Cancer Symposium. The outcomes continued to amaze, prompting Dr. Kuhl to state in an interview in *The ASCO Post* on October 25, 2015: "In other words, mammography fails to detect up to half of all breast cancers." But of all the compelling data she presented, perhaps the most game-changing statistic was this: there were *no interval cancers* encountered in the study of over 2,000 women, even among those where the interval between MRIs was three years.

Distinct from the many commentaries in my files that have addressed the U.S. Preventive Services Task Force, I have a personal objection that I have yet to see in print. Perhaps no one else objects. Perhaps no one else obsesses over Sensitivity. Perhaps given the widespread belief in exaggerated Sensitivity for mammography, no one noticed. But in their 2009 report that rendered an "insufficient evidence," or "I" for MRI screening, the statement was made that mammography has a Sensitivity of "77% to 95%," while MRI Sensitivity ranges from "71% to 100%." In the Health Care Reform Bill of 2010, 500 million dollars were appropriated for "comparative effectiveness research." Now, study how those two modalities were compared by the Task Force—the Sensitivity ranges are essentially the same, in spite of the fact that MRI finds double, or even triple, the number of cancers in head-to-head comparisons with mammography. The two sets of numbers cannot co-exist without extraordinary stretching of the facts.

Of course, a trick has been played with the numbers. But my concern is that neither side of the warring parties—epidemiologists or breast radiologists—will budge on these incompatible ranges of Sensitivity for the two modalities. Let's take a closer look—where did the Task Force of 2009 get its "77% to 95%" Sensitivity range for mammography? Well, the reference they provide is themselves, that is, the 2002 version of the Task Force. But if you go to that reference, you will find that they are merely quoting an earlier study,[9] discussed in a previous chapter. Fine, so far, given that the "gossip trail" is common in medicine where one reference only leads to an earlier reference, and on and on. But here's the problem. The 2009 Task Force, like many authors, quoted only the *prevalence* numbers provided by the 2002 Task Force, that is, the calculated Sensitivities from the historical trials for the *first screen only*. The 20–30% drop in Sensitivity for all subsequent screens, provided by the 2002 Task Force, is nowhere to be found in 2009.

Now let's turn to the "71% to 100%" Sensitivity for MRI, which I've addressed previously in explaining the lower end of that range. Furthermore, rather than pure prevalence screens allowing the higher numbers for Sensitivity as was quoted for mammography, we have a mixture of prevalence and incidence screens with MRI, dragging the number lower. Additionally, the low end of that range for MRI Sensitivity (71%) no longer existed by 2009 when it was quoted. Instead, 90% Sensitivity for MRI is the accepted number, while mammographic Sensitivity, I maintain, is 50% (ignoring the very wide range that is dependent on density). If you double the Sensitivity, then you double the number of cancers detected. The MRI screening trials did exactly that, and more. It's a pretty simple concept, uncontestable, yet the Task Force opted to quote nearly identical Sensitivity ranges, and at the same time, the radiologic community didn't argue the numbers either.

First, we must admit there's a problem. We must admit that mammographic Sensitivity needs help before we can advance. But in this unique situation, neither side will come clean. Some breast radiologists have moved beyond the grumbling that comes with enlightenment and have admitted in print that the Sensitivity numbers are not as good as once thought, a casualty of multi-modality imaging; however, they'll also point out that this awareness could not have emerged at a worse time than now, when mammography is under such attack already. Silence ensues.

Then, on the other side, the Task Force and its ilk fully realize the obvious conclusion if 50% Sensitivity for mammography is accepted as the new Reality—it means radiologists will go hog wild with multi-modality imaging, which will only make length bias, overdiagnosis and the other harms of screening worse. And all this, without a shred of (acceptable) evidence!

What 50% Sensitivity means is this: (1) there is much more room for improvement than generally believed, and (2) given our duo of "Biology + Sensitivity" for effective screening, it means that breast cancer is far more vulnerable to early detection than we ever dreamed. It means that the modest mortality reductions from the historic trials are calculated with a screening tool that detected only half of the cancers. X + Y = Z. If mammography is saving lives with one hand tied around its back, detecting only half of detectable cancers, then imagine the impact on the mortality rate if we were to find the other half!

# 25

# The Bright Side of the Dark Side of the Force

Along the road to Reality, non-randomized trials tend to generate *false-positives*. Prospective, randomized, controlled trials (RCTs) are the next step on the path, but can generate *false-negatives* in spite of clear trends, simply through lack of statistical power. Meta-analyses then blend comparable RCTs in order to gain statistical strength and shed the *false-negatives*. And when the meta-analyses don't agree, "systematic reviews" of multiple meta-analyses are at the top of the evidence-based ladder. It should be no surprise by now that different outcomes can be achieved with different systematic reviews by different experts and/or think tanks.

In the mammography screening trials, investigators enrolled huge numbers, anticipating that relatively few would die of breast cancer during the study. It's not enough to *detect* breast cancer in a screening trial—the endpoint is the death tally. By the time we get to breast cancer mortality in the historic trials, statistical power is often lacking, especially in the under 50 group. That's why it took the meta-analyses to convince the majority (not everyone) that mammography saves lives.

The bickering still in progress relates not only to the cost and harms of screening mammography, but also to the magnitude of the screening benefit. Remarkably, the debate has raged over a tiny fraction of the total evidence, that is, the prospective RCTs that are, in many ways, irrelevant today. Let's review the unique features of the 9 international trials that should give us pause when we hear claims that modern "systematic reviews" give us the most accurate benefit for screening—a mere 20% relative reduction in mortality when all ages are considered.

*First generation mammography.* With the exception of the AGE trial, the remaining 8 studies had completed the screening phase of the trial *before* mammography quality measures were introduced, and all studies were performed with original film screen technology. Then, the only trial that didn't even trend toward a benefit was the Canadian NBSS where quality was so poor that only 32% of the cancers in the mammography limb were actually discovered by mammography.

*Single views and long intervals.* Hamstringing the potential benefit of mammography were single view studies (missing 20% of cancers), and screening intervals as long as 33 months.

*Poor study design.* By today's standards for prospective RCTs, all studies fall short.

*Confirmation that deaths were breast-cancer specific.* Cause of death is not always clear from medical records or death certificates, prompting different methodologies in the trials; ideally, these should be "blinded" reviews where the examiner does not know whether the patient was screened or not. Nevertheless, there is a significant margin of error inherent in this process.

*Differing time frames for counting deaths.* Some trials focused on the mortality of cancers diagnosed during the screening phase, while others counted patients diagnosed after the study period had ended.

*Inclusion of palpable cancers.* By definition, screening means patients are asymptomatic, so the inclusion of women with lumps into screening trials is a major confounding variable. Clinical exams performed *after* the start of a trial are one thing, but palpable lumps known to be present at the time of entry are a major problem when it comes to measuring the impact of mammography. The Canadian NBSS took it a step further, first by identifying the lumps prior to randomization, then placing them disproportionately into the mammography limb.

*Poor compliance (women in the mammography limb not getting mammograms) and contamination (women in the control arm getting mammograms anyway) based on the Intent-to-Treat Rule.* Women are counted according to their originally assigned group, not by what they actually did. Both compliance and contamination *worsen* over the course of the trial. While the Intent-to-Treat Rule is a standard requirement for prospective RCTs, its impact on the mammography trials is 100% unidirectional, that is, it works to *diminish* the measureable impact of mammography. Nothing about the Intent-to-Treat Rule balances results in the other direction.

*Erratic screening after the study phase.* Women in the no-mammography arm initiate their own screening strategy after the trial, while some women in the mammography arm stop screening, and women in both groups screen erratically after the study phase.

And finally, the *poor sensitivity* of the tool being studied—mammography—with Sensitivity being a remarkably low 39–66% for incidence screens in the historic trials subsequent to the initial prevalence screen. Granted, the long intervals in the historic trials allowed more time for cancers to emerge in between screens and thus be counted as a "miss." Yet, once the modern definition of mammographic Sensitivity emerged through multi-modality imaging, it turned out that the 39–66% range of Sensitivity was probably accurate.

My point: Given the long list above, it is nothing short of a miracle that mammography was able to impact mortality at all!

Why are public health experts so fixated on a mere "20% relative mortality reduction" when the deck is so thoroughly stacked against mammograms?

For starters, toss out the CNBSS and recalculate data from those trials that measured only the impact of mammography. This is not an oddball concept at all. The World Health Organization did it. And the previously referenced definitive 2001 study of mammographic Sensitivity and sojourn times from MD Anderson and Harvard (Shen and Zelen in the *Journal of Clinical Oncology*) had this to say: "*the Canadian studies were not designed to evaluate mammography compared with no mammography.*" So why do most meta-analyses and all systematic reviews include the CNBSS? Short answer to a long problem—politics and personalities.

Next, we've already seen how the "compliance" data within the RCTs fits nicely with the observational studies, with a *greater* magnitude of benefit. It should be no surprise that when you compare women who actually had mammograms to those who didn't, the benefit is going to be greater than when compliance drops to as low as 65% over time.

There are many ways to use rational thought when addressing these trials, but the ant-like slaves to pure empiricism aren't going to budge on a single grain of dirt as they build their hills.

Excluding the "modern" AGE Trial (screening completed by 1997), recall that the historical trials began in 1963, peaking in the late 70s and early 80s, with the final screen in the Gothenburg trial in 1991. Yet the mesmerizing magic of the words "prospective, randomized, controlled," has anointed these primitive studies to the point that multiple transgressions are dismissed with a shrug of the shoulders and the comment "But it's all we have." The problem is clear—the procedure being so hotly debated today is not even being performed anymore. We're two generations of technology removed from these trials (film screen, then digital, and now tomosynthesis), so calculated benefits of "20% mortality reduction," or even the more favorable analyses that generate a "30% mortality reduction," are from yesteryear.

For those considering *all* the evidence, the impact of screening mammography appears to be greater than what was seen in the historical trials.

And this brings us back to the opening chapters where I presented the $X + Y = Z$ formula, and noted we would be returning to that concept again and again, allowing perspective to develop along the way. So, for the last time, here it is again:

**Biology ($X$ = vulnerability to early detection) + Sensitivity ($Y = 90\%$) = Screening Benefit ($Z$)**

Now, if the Screening Benefit ($Z = 20–30\%$ mortality reduction) is fixed, and you then *adjust Sensitivity down to 50% from the perceived 80–90%*, as I've spent this whole book doing, the vulnerability of the biology to early detection must be greater than what we have believed in the past.

**Biology + Sensitivity (90%) = Screening Benefit**
**Biology** + Sensitivity (50%) = Screening Benefit

"Biology" does not lend itself as well to numbers as does Sensitivity and Mortality Reductions, but stated alternatively, Goldilocks biology must be far more common, or more powerful, than we originally considered. If so, we should be doing *more, not less*, to ensure that we detect as many early-stage cancers as possible.

It's a concept of staggering simplicity, yet the bone-crushing grip on "80–90%" Sensitivity for mammography keeps progress in check. Drop that truism down the drain, replacing it with mammography that detects only *half* of detectable cancers, and again, *mammography is saving lives with one hand tied around its back*.

Stated again, two implications are closely related, but conceptually a shade apart, the most obvious being (1) that there's plenty of room to improve on Sensitivity, shooting for a true 90% or greater, plus (2) given greater biologic vulnerability to early detection than previously considered (more Goldilocks tumors), *any modality* that can increase cancer yields (Sensitivity), should result in more saved lives. Number 1 is fact, while number 2 is theory (but a good one).

Yet, at this critical juncture, where imaging research and developments are generating vast improvements in Sensitivity with several modalities, we have a social tsunami with surf-riding anti-screeners telling us to slow down, or even to stop screening entirely. From the perspective of those of us on the front lines involved in early detection, we see many outside our arena—researchers, physicians, patients—switching to the Dark Side of the Force.

Gloom and doom, yes. But actually, there is a Bright Side.

While Think Tanks are scouring archaeological ruins for data, breast imaging research remains in juggernaut mode, with radiation physicists, computer scientists, and radiologists forging ahead with developments as if the Mammography Civil War and the 2009 Task Force never happened. It's enough to make a cost-containment expert sick. Whereas mammograms were fairly static for many years, today, multiple imaging options and benefits are changing so rapidly that Think Tanks don't have time to think.

Tomosynthesis ("3-D") is the greatest technology leap in the history of mammography, doing exactly what critics of screening claim that we need—improving Sensitivity, but more importantly in the eyes of many, improving Specificity (fewer false-positives). Yet what did the 2016 Task Force say about it? "Insufficient evidence." Screening ultrasound improves cancer detection rates, mostly invasive disease, in multiple studies by 3–4 per 1,000, slightly more effective than the addition of 3-D tomosynthesis. The Task Force response: "Insufficient evidence." Breast MRI screening in the general population? A whopping 11 additional cancers per 1,000. The Task Force? "Insufficient evidence." There is a fine line between sharp discernment and global skepticism, the former requiring a host of talents, while the latter requires nothing special at all.

Consider these words from the 2016 Task Force addressing 3-D mammography—"Available data also suggest that tomosynthesis increases the cancer detection rate compared with 2-D digital mammography alone. However current study designs do not answer the question of whether all of the additional cancers detected would have become clinically significant (i.e., the degree of overdiagnosis), or whether there is an incremental clinical benefit to detecting these cancers earlier than with 'standard' 2-D digital mammography."

A valid concern, but global skepticism is easy. It's much harder to consider the data I've presented in this book and make the highly probable prediction that if we increase the Sensitivity of the screening tool (Y), we will improve upon screening effectiveness (Z), considering what we know about the vulnerability of breast cancer (X).

So what would Think Tanks such as the Task Force like to see? The all-inclusive answer is: prospective, randomized trials with mortality reduction as an endpoint. But recalling the challenges in demonstrating mortality reductions when the historic control groups were randomized to *no imaging at all*, imagine what it would take, in size and cost, to measure incremental improvements, such as tomosynthesis over digital, when the control group would be screened. It's not merely improbable ... it's going to be impossible to answer these questions with prospective RCTs for each new technologic advance. And rather than study all available data and offer rational solutions, the Think Tanks will forever be obstructive to the many advances that are underway. "Insufficient evidence" is a cop-out, but that's the only thing the Task Force can offer, forever in the chains of their own choosing.

We've already seen what "insufficient evidence" meant for digital mammography in the 2009 Task Force report. What good did that do anyone? The Task Force was left in the dust, hoping that people like me wouldn't recall that they were never able to pass judgment, and that in 2016, they simply acted as though digital was the standard. Geeez. Now tomosynthesis is the new kid on the block and by the time the next Task Force convenes on this topic, tomosynthesis will already be the standard while the Task Force renders "insufficient evidence" for the next technologic advance.

Quoting the Shen and Zelen (MD Anderson and Harvard) article again, their opening statement in the Discussion section states: "It is important to evaluate early detection trials as soon as possible without waiting for long-term mortality results. For this purpose, screening sensitivity can be used as an early indicator to assess the screening efficacy." (And that's coming from biostatistics and epidemiologic experts, so my apologies if I have stereotyped this group—it was for literary effect.)

Yes, the data is early for tomosynthesis, but that's where those who use it every day have the advantage. We see the cancers present on 3-D, but not 2-D. We monitor the frequency, we get to see the biopsy results, and we get to see the final pathology and stage. In addition to our own experience, we see the "cancer yield" literature indicating that Sensitivity is going higher with tomosynthesis, maybe by as much as 40% in relative terms, 20% in absolute terms (my prediction: from 50% to 70% overall Sensitivity).

Will different imaging modalities pick up different biologies? Yes, to a degree. We've already seen a higher ratio of invasion-to–DCIS with ultrasound than we see with mammography. And guess what—the vast majority of cancers missed on 2-D but found on 3-D tomosynthesis are invasive! This technologic advance is not adding to the DCIS "problem," but is doing exactly what we want—improving the Sensitivity of biologically more significant disease.

The next decade will bring forth a great deal of information about the pathology and molecular biology of those breast cancers discovered by different imaging modalities. And from that information, we will need to make inferences for many imaging combinations that will *never* be addressed through prospective, randomized trials.

What about our high-density patients and our high-risk patients? In 2009, the Task Force issued an "insufficient" for both digital mammography and MRI. In 2016, they limited their recommendations to women at average risk, but again, issued an "insufficient evidence" for MRI, ultrasound, tomosynthesis, "or other modalities in women identified to have dense breasts on an otherwise negative screening mammogram."

Now, let's go back to ACRIN 6666 for women with high density and modest risk—how many cancers were detected by mammography alone for the sub-group that also underwent a single MRI? The answer: 31%. That's the endorsed modality—mammograms alone—by the United States Preventive Services Task Force, for women with dense breasts plus modest risks. So what is the biology of the remaining tumors, the ones left behind after mammography? Are the remaining 69% of undetected breast cancers to be called "overdiagnosis" if we use ultrasound or MRI to find them? That's the presumption of the Task Force—overdiagnosis until proven otherwise.

Now it may be clear why I spent so much time at the beginning of this book describing how anatomic stage in breast cancer, as opposed to prostate cancer, is uniquely positioned for anatomic screening to work. That is, the discovery of earlier stage disease *ought* to reduce the number of breast cancer deaths. Yes, there are other explanations for the beneficial outcomes seen in the screening trials, but they are not the default position. It should not be "overdiagnosis until proven otherwise," as is the stance from the Task Force and other Think Tanks. Lives are being lost while we argue these points, now for a half-century. The default position, without any data whatsoever, should be that the discovery of earlier stage disease through screening *ought* to reduce the mortality rate of breast cancer. What has been so remarkable about this entire controversy is that the data does, in fact, support the default position.

In lieu of prospective, randomized trials for each and every technologic advancement (that will be outdated before the trial is over), we need to accept the fact that Sensitivity in the form of "cancer yields" in comparative imaging studies must be treated as a *reasonable* surrogate for mortality reduction. If not, then Think Tanks are going to remain in their stance of global skepticism, comfortable watching women die unnecessarily in the name of "good science," while crowing endlessly about "insufficient evidence."

With breast MRI, ultrasound and tomosynthesis all at work in various combinations, it is very difficult for a breast cancer to get beyond Stage I at the time of discovery. Yet, a mega-chorus of third-party payors, screening minimalists and screening nihilists are doing every-thing possible to restrict or eradicate the use of these modalities, by calling forth "length bias" and "overdiagnosis" at every available opportunity. It makes you want to cry.

Do you recall the question about radiation-induced breast cancer due to mammography in a previous chapter? These theoretical calculations are admittedly difficult, and impossible to prove. However, from the Biologic Effects of Ionizing Radiation report,[1] the risk of a fatal radiation-induced breast cancer for a woman 40–49 years old is approximately one in 100,000 for a bilateral two-view digital mammogram. And this minuscule risk decreases as women age. But here's what the Task Force came up with—27 breast cancers induced out of 100,000 mammograms, with 5 breast cancer deaths.

We have *zero* empirical evidence to support this claim that comes from many supposi-tions and premises that feed on each other. Critics have alleged fundamental errors by the Task Force in estimating radiation dose, for instance, incorrectly combining the mean glan-dular doses ascribed to each breast, thus doubling their dose estimates.[2] Furthermore, when it came to the new technology of tomosynthesis, the Task Force quoted a doubling of the radiation dose again, true for the first-to-market equipment (still within FDA guidelines), but *not true* by the time the 2016 Task Force drew up their 2015 draft—by then, General Elec-tric had already introduced its technology with radiation exposure unchanged from 2-D dig-ital, other companies to follow.

(As a point of interest, although it may be considered quirky by some, there is actually a school of thought, called "radiation hormesis," that proposes that a small amount of radiation is slightly beneficial. The phenomenon can be demonstrated in the lab, but has never made the leap to human studies.)

The range of *guesswork* on this issue is miles wide, but why would the Task Force pick one of the highest imaginable numbers and offer it as dogma? Why didn't they draw from their old familiar "insufficient evidence"? Instead, they toss out scare tactic numbers without a shred of "high quality evidence" when it comes to this potential harm from mammography. But let us detect more cancers with tomosynthesis, ultrasound, and breast MRI, and "Oh my, no, all these additional cancers could simply be overdiagnoses, and we can't risk that!" (Adding their insult to our injury, neither ultrasound nor MRI add *any* radiation exposure to the screening process.)

By now, the theme is clear—anything that smacks of harm is inflated, while the benefits of screening are arrested, questioned and tortured.

Over the years of dodging the anti-screening bombs lobbed at us pro-screeners, I've morphed from curious bystander to cynical bystander to cynical activist. Gradually and qui-etly, I converted from surgeon to quasi-radiologist (a term preferable to charges that I'm a pseudo-radiologist). My focus is *theory* of imaging, not actual interpretations. The first step in this journey was mentioned in the opening chapter, with my simple question, "Where does the 90% Sensitivity number come from?" But the second step took place at Dallas in the early 1990s, at one of the few breast conferences held back then.

At the time, outside of radiology meetings, there was a single radiologist, Dr. Steven Harms, headlining the multidisciplinary breast cancer conferences with his work on breast MRI. Then at Baylor, he later moved to the University of Arkansas where much of his patented MRI approach was developed. His presentations covering his progress were both myriad and worldwide. Dr. Harms trained under one of the co-developers of magnetic resonance imaging, 2003 Nobel laureate Paul Lauterbur, and in the 1990s, most practicing radiologists conceded that no one understood the underlying physics of breast MRI better than Dr. Harms. In 1998, he was awarded the "Komen Foundation Scientist of the Year."

In those pre–Powerpoint days, the cutting edge of audio-visuals, favored heavily by radiologists, was the awesome two-projector technique with 35mm slides, allowing simultaneous comparison of two sets of images. In demonstrating his invention, RODEO® MRI³ Dr. Harms would present two images for each patient—the mammograms on one projector, with a simultaneous display of the MRI on the other. The audience could appreciate cancers as beacons, lighting up the screen on the MRI side, and with a completely normal mammogram on the other screen. Over and over and over.

To myself, I said: "So that's why so many of my patients presenting for breast cancer surgery are showing up with their newly diagnosed cancer and their negative mammograms."

Breast MRI would be a revolution whenever it came available, or so I thought. But even then, it was obviously impractical to screen the general population with breast MRI. How could we use this extremely Sensitive imaging tool, so as not to bankrupt the entire health care delivery system? Cost was not a strong agenda in that era, but common sense dictated that patient selection was going to be the chief problem with implementing breast MRI.

At this same time, I was in the academic setting where I had organized a weekly breast cancer research meeting for all interested parties on campus. Once a year, I would also trek across the street to the Oklahoma Medical Research Foundation (OMRF) to give a presentation to the entire body of scientists at that facility to review what was happening clinically in breast cancer prediction, prevention and early diagnosis (my personal triad of interest). The purpose of my talk was to recruit interested parties to our weekly meeting for collaborations. One of those attendees was Paul McKay, PhD, a senior scientist who had been one of my professors in medical school.

Shortly after my return from the Dallas conference, my head still spinning from the MRI presentation by Dr. Harms, Dr. McKay walked into our meeting and showed me a publication written by a scientist, Dr. Chaya Moroz from Israel, working at the Beilinson Medical Center and Tel Aviv University Medical School. The scientific paper proposed a blood test that could possibly detect the presence of breast cancer.⁴ This was back in the pre–PubMed days when literature searches were very tedious. In fact, the article had been published (and gone unnoticed) about 15 years before Dr. McKay discovered it and brought it to our meeting. "Any reason that a blood test could help in breast cancer?" he asked me.

At the time, research on available "tumor markers" (CEA, CA15–3, CA27.29) was mixed, with only modest predictive value for detecting recurrent or metastatic disease, so the idea of detecting an early breast cancer, while still localized in the breast, was not on anyone's agenda. Why would we need it? After all, we already had mammography, and in this antebellum period, the belief was strongly entrenched in its 90% Sensitivity.

But in my mind, the linkage of breast MRI and a blood test became a permanent fixation, later obsession. If used to complement mammography, then if a patient's blood test proved to be positive, but mammograms negative, this would be the indication to proceed with an MRI. The blood test didn't have to be perfect, just good enough to make MRI cost-effective. That linkage has persisted, unchanged, to present day, more than 20 years later.

Breast cancer had barely been tagged with pink ribbons at the time, but I had a squadron of fund-raisers who wanted to see improvements in how things were done. With 50–50 funding from this small army and from OMRF, we brought Dr. Moroz from Israel to Oklahoma City for a visit and lectures, while I offered her a locale to base a clinical trial for her proposed blood-based screening tool—at Oklahoma's first multidisciplinary breast center, under construction. She spent several days in OKC lecturing, and we poured over potential study designs for many hours. This led to seven years of colorful experiences and unwavering hope, but in the end, we didn't test a single patient.

In the meantime, however, breast MRI crept closer and closer to clinical use, and by 2002, it was commercially available. I had recently moved to my current location at Mercy Hospital-OKC, with the proviso that my "blood test" agenda would be supported through equipment and personnel, anticipating Patient #1 in a research study someday. The second half of that research agenda mandated the adoption of breast MRI, a goal that was greatly facilitated when breast radiologist, Rebecca G. Stough, M.D., agreed to spearhead a breast MRI program. Through her dedication to high quality MRI, we adopted the RODEO® MRI format and generated truckloads of data that will take years to get in print.

Most notably, Dr. Stough recognized the challenging learning curve for breast MRI, seeing patterns in the breast tissue she had never seen before, thus prompting her to read the first 1,000 breast MRIs personally, before teaching her colleagues. And, for that first year after introducing breast MRI, we suspended our multidisciplinary conference in favor of a MRI-pathology correlation conference so that we could compare MR images to biopsy results, in order to accelerate our learning curve. We believe it paid off, with fewer false-positives and no evidence of overtreatment as is often reported with MRI. But still, cost-effectiveness was a challenge.

The internet allowed monitoring of research activity around the world, unimaginable in years past. And I began to scour the corners of Earth, looking for researchers who might be interested in blood samples that were accompanied by an extensive database *that included MRI results.* This assurance of true-negative control samples, as defined by a negative MRI, was unique. I'm not aware that a similar bank of blood samples existed anywhere else at the time.

With Institutional Review Board approval, we have drawn blood samples from more than 2,000 volunteer patients in Oklahoma. In addition, these samples are then divided into small aliquots and frozen at minus-80 degrees for the long-term. Thus, a single donor might generate up to 15 or more specimens that can be distributed around the world, which is exactly what we did.

More than 10,000 samples have been distributed as of this writing, so a single patient might have had her samples sent to biotechnology companies in the U.S., university cancer centers, and research centers in Norway, England and Italy. Out of 30 or more verbal and written interactions with various research sites around the world, we sent our samples to 9 sites over the years,[5] with two sites advancing to the point of a clinical trial. The first formal trial sponsored by a U.S. biotech company failed in 2006. However, in 2015, a multi-site clinical trial sponsored by Provista Diagnostics (Scottsdale/New York) included more than 1,000 patients in 15 locations,[6] and results appear promising, with good Sensitivity and Specificity that is maintained across all levels of breast density.[7]

When there is very little grant money available for a maverick agenda—that is to say a "high failure rate," the crowd is slow to follow. However, blood-based studies (now being called "liquid biopsy") have gradually gained momentum over the past decade. Still, most researchers are focused on the detection of systemic disease and the potential for intervention before metastases appear clinically. For example, CTCs (circulating tumor cells) are the hot item here. Precious few researchers, however, are aiming at early detection, due to the fact that screening is inherently low yield and costly, and so is the research to improve it.

The Provista test is based on *high-sensitivity/low specificity* protein biomarkers linked to *high specificity/low sensitivity* tumor-associated autoantibodies in a proprietary algorithm. The recent multi-site trial sponsored by Provista Diagnostics was designed so that success would give a new option to radiologists trying to decide whether or not to perform a biopsy. But using it to screen and select patients for MRI is another matter entirely,[8] where current yields for cancer found on MRI are in the range of 2–3%. Can we improve upon that? With sponsorship by the company, we have initiated a "proof of concept" screening trial at my facility, Mercy Breast Center in Oklahoma City, where we are performing the test on women who are already scheduled for breast MRI based on high risk status. After several years of screening, we will re-calculate what the results would have been had we had relied on the blood test to make the decision about performing MRI.

I call this "home run" research, that is, it's either over the fence or a probable out. The ability to convert low yield, high cost breast MRI into a cost-effective, high-yield test would be practice-changing, if not revolutionary. And, with tongue-in-cheek, I'm reminded of Malcolm Gladwell's "10,000-Hour Rule," from his book *Outliers*,[9] recalling that we recently shipped specimen number 10,001 at roughly one person-hour of work per sample.

We should not be relying on long-term risk calculations to select patients for extra screening studies. Long-term risks are poor surrogates for the probability of an occult cancer being present on a negative mammogram at a single moment in time. At a minimum, we should be relying on short-term risk calculations. But at a maximum, we should be developing inexpensive complements to mammography that tell us what's going on *in the present*, at the very moment of the negative mammogram. And for countries that don't have mammography screening infrastructure, a screening blood test could be used as the primary screening method, allowing diagnostic imaging, beginning with mammography, to take place only if the blood test is positive.

In the U.S. and countries with strong radiologic resources, a positive blood test in a patient with negative mammograms would "rule in" MRI for patients not currently qualifying for MRI due to the lack of risk factors. These non-qualifiers make up the bulk of eventual breast cancer patients. However, at the same time, a blood test could "rule out" MRI for high-risk patients who are currently getting the study yearly, given that 96–97% of these women are going to have a completely negative MRI when looking at each imaging study individually. Both "rule in" and "rule out" make for higher yields, while addressing the challenge that *all* women are at substantial risk for breast cancer.

Mathematical modeling allows one to predict the "cancer yields" accomplished with varying degrees of Accuracy (Sensitivity and Specificity) for a blood test. And now we have the MRI screening data in a "normal risk" population, based on the report from Dr. Christiane Kuhl's group in Germany, so we no longer have to theorize baseline MRI yields. Plug in 90% Sensitivity and 90% Specificity for the blood test, and quite simply, you revolutionize the world of breast cancer screening.

But what remains compelling is the fact that you can improve the status quo even with Accuracy well below what many would consider acceptable. A blood test with only 80% Sensitivity and 80% Specificity would generate 4% cancer yields in the "average risk" population, a slightly higher yield than patients who currently qualify for MRI screening due to a mutation in one of the BRCA genes, where published yields are 3.0% to 3.6%. Even this low MRI yield using a blood test as the indication is higher than what will be achieved in longer term studies of MRI in gene-positive patients after the "steady state" is reached with incidence screens. That is, even the BRCA-positive patients are going to drift down to 2% yields with each annual screen, lower still for women having less risk.

But using a blood test is a game-changer—there would be no more prevalence vs. incidence issues. The MRI is done only if the blood test is positive. A blood test doesn't care about anything other than what's in the breast at a single moment in time.

A blood test is not the only way to achieve this "in the moment" concept of performing cost-effective MRI to find mammographically occult cancer.

In July 2014, I was reading the latest issue of *The Breast Journal*, drawn to an article describing a clever way of using computerized image analysis to review *normal* mammograms.[10] The intent was to identify women at very high short-term risk, based on a comparison of density patterns from one side to the other, with the potential to make the same comparison from one year to the next.

To clarify, radiologists already use "computer-aided detection," or CAD, when interpreting mammograms and MRI, but these are systems that serve as a second radiologist, identifying things that can be seen with the human eye. But this new approach, developed by Dr. Bin Zheng and Dr. Hong Liu and their team, described using this "ultraCAD" (my term) on normal mammograms, not for diagnosis of cancer, per se, but identifying high *short term* risk. As it turned out in their preliminary work, a 9-fold short-term risk elevation could be identified, a very powerful predictor of occult cancer.

My thoughts raced, of course, to performing immediate breast MRI if such a pattern should occur. I also considered the scientific paper I described earlier, written by mammography experts, where 58% of newly diagnosed cancer patients have "something" going on at the cancer site one year earlier. Perhaps this "ultraCAD" was identifying the same subtle features, too minimal to call abnormal, but enough to indicate the first changes associated with cancer.

"Who were these guys?" I wondered. Returning to the article header, I was most surprised to discover that their laboratory was located on the Norman campus of my alma mater, the University of Oklahoma. The senior scientist of the group, Dr. Hong Liu, had played a role in the development of digital mammography and had been recruited to OU almost the same month and year that I left. Dr. Zheng had then been recruited as well from the University of Pittsburgh, eager to join forces with Dr. Liu. It was clear to me that this "ultraCAD" system needed clinical confirmation, yes or no—now.

I contacted them at their Advanced Cancer Imaging Lab, then we met on several occasions with our respective teams and decided to collaborate on a small study while applying for a grant from the National Cancer Institute. One year later, July 2015, Drs. Zheng, Liu and I were awarded a $2.5 million R-01 grant from the National Cancer Institute as Principal Investigators, with Mercy breast imaging specialists, Drs. Rebecca Stough and Melanie Pearce as the consulting radiologists.[11] Over 6,000 retrospective cases from Mercy Breast Center will be studied over 5 years, while the key confirmatory group will be an additional 4,000 patients in a prospective trial. We believe 200–400 women from this trial will qualify for an MRI, based on computer analysis of their normal mammograms, and we will see if we can generate yields better than what is accomplished through risk-based screening.

Note the ultimate purpose here is the same as a screening blood test, and the two could even be complementary. But the sequence for proposed use is the same—normal mammogram, but a positive "ultraCAD," would prompt MRI. And, like a blood test, it would open this avenue of MRI to all women, not the current risk-based screening that limits MRI exclusively to those with risk factors.

Research agendas like the two examples above are springing up all over, and the future is going to be a wildly different experience than what we have today. Yet we'll never get off the ground if the nihilists and minimalists get their way, and we end up believing "less is more" in a "kinder gentler world" where we "do no harm."

We can find half of the detectable cancers with screening mammograms alone (yes, 3-D tomosynthesis is taking that number higher), but what if we found the other half through a cost-effective approach to MRI, or ultrasound, or molecular imaging, or *contrast-enhanced* tomosynthesis? If current screening with digital mammography is reducing mortality by 30–40% (my supposition based on Reality rather than the "official" 20% mortality reduction), then would finding the other half, that is, the mammographically occult cancers, reduce mortality by another 30–40%? Is it conceivable that, for those women compliant with aggressive screening using the research tools described above, we could generate a 60–80% reduction in mortality? I say yes. Importantly and maddeningly, *the technology already exists*. It's simply a matter of improving how we select patients for multi-modality imaging.

Yet the mantra today is to *do less*? It makes you want to cry.

By now, the reason for this book should be apparent. The *do less* mantra is exactly opposite of what needs to be done. This is a social tsunami that kills.

*Dark Side* critics point out that the currently accepted "20% mortality reduction" is a relative term, and that the absolute numbers are even less impressive, especially when considering the number of women who have to be screened and all the associated harms.

But look at the *Bright Side*—20% is, in all probability, a serious underestimate of benefit, given modern technology and what we know about women who are actually screened, rather than using numbers that apply to women who receive an invitation to screen. Even my 30–40% mortality reduction could be an underestimate if women are in strong compliance with yearly 3-D tomosynthesis screening.

Still, *Dark Side* critics would say, if you're starting off with only a 3% chance of dying from breast cancer, the best you're doing with current screening is to bring this down to 2%, a mere 1% improvement. Even if the mortality reduction could be doubled, you'd only be lowering the risk of dying from breast cancer by 2% for the individual woman, from 3% to 1%.

But look at the *Bright Side*—a 40% mortality reduction would be saving the lives of 16,000 women a year in the U.S. alone if all are compliant. 8,000 if half are compliant. And if you double that benefit to an 80% reduction, then double those numbers for lives saved. The death toll from breast cancer would plummet. And by the way, when did those of you in public health become so concerned about the individual patient? Shouldn't you be the ones who describe these massive population benefits that I am quoting?

*Dark Side*—Costs and harms will skyrocket with very little benefit if you add multi-modality imaging.

But look at the *Bright Side*—if you have a cost-effective selection process that tells you precisely when to go beyond mammography, costs and harms shrink while benefits rise.

*Dark Side*—But your somewhat outrageous prediction of a 60–80% reduction in mortality is based on tools to assist mammography—blood tests and computer programs—that don't even exist.

But look at the *Bright Side*—the auxiliary imaging tools *do* exist—be it MRI or one of the other options, the point being we don't need any "breakthroughs" in breast imaging when it comes to detecting breast cancer. We need only to develop low-cost methods of proper patient selection for these proven imaging methods. Risk-based screening ignores the majority of eventual cancer patients before you even get started. I envision the day when we can identify, from the general population, those women who need a back-up imaging study because their cancer is hidden on mammography.

*Dark Side*—And who made you Keeper of the Crystal Ball?

# 26

# The Crystal Ball Is Fair to Partly Cloudy

I don't know what people see in them, crystal balls that is. Nevertheless, I ventured a prediction at the beginning of this book that screening for the early detection of breast cancer would remain *foundational* beyond the current generation of doctors, perhaps for the next 50 years.

Why ever stop? Because the research on systemic therapies that sounds like science fiction today will eventually become reality, and breast cancer will be curable, or controllable, no matter what the stage at time of discovery. Be it a pill, a shot, a series of vaccinations, or targeted therapies based on the molecular biology of tumor cells, the mortality from breast cancer will eventually plummet. Only those refusing medical care will form a small cadre of needless victims.

Once screening becomes obsolete, students of medical history will visit the museums and gasp at the sight of a medieval torture device, the mammogram machine, once used to smash sensitive body parts. And to think—"they actually did this on *normal* people with no cancer, a thousand or so, just to save one life. Can you imagine? Why, it's absolutely barbaric."

When that day finally arrives, when established breast cancer can be corralled, early diagnosis will no longer matter. But as I've stated several times already, some clinicians are acting as though we've already landed on Mars. Some forward thinkers have transported themselves "back to the future" and are tripping over their dreams. Unfortunately, many of the miracles that are bubbling and brewing in today's laboratories are decades away from clinical utility. And, given the many types of breast cancer at the DNA level, it will likely require an entire garland of miracles strung between biologies to eradicate metastatic disease completely, and with it, the need to screen for early diagnosis.

Screening minimalists will sometimes say, "We can gradually back off from screening as these systemic therapies improve," but that has a creepy feel to it if you think about it. Translated: "It's okay to let your cancer stay in the breast for another year or two, we'll cure it later on down the road after we can feel it. That is, if it's susceptible to our current systemic therapies." We're not there yet. It will happen, but not yet.

Sure, we have isolated miracles already for some patients with advanced cancers, most notably for HER2-positive disease where biotherapies can sometimes make even Stage III cancer melt away. It's an amazing thing to witness. That said, the spectacular results are primarily in the 20% of breast cancer patients whose tumors are HER2-positive, though research

222

is intense for "triple-negative" cancers and other breast cancer biologies as well. Of course, endocrine therapy can melt away a fair number of tumors as well, but we are inclined to take this for granted as new horizons appear for ER-negative disease. Someday, the phenomenon of melting tumors will work for nearly everyone.

Immunotherapy is on a roll. Cancer vaccines, monoclonal antibodies, checkpoint inhibitors are on fire in the lab, with new products already spreading into the clinical arena with FDA approval. Composite therapies, or conjugates, have also been approved by the FDA, such as a "superHerceptin" (T-DM1) where a cytotoxic agent (a.k.a. poison) is attached to the Herceptin® molecule, so that the cancer cell gets a double-whammy, with chemotherapy delivered to the individual tumor cell by the "B-52" Herceptin® that, at the same time, has landed on the cell surface to do its own damage.

Now, imagine the same "conjugate" approach, but apply it to radiation therapy rather than chemotherapy. In 2013, a first-in-class anticancer agent was FDA-approved that emits alpha particles at the cellular level in prostate cancer that has metastasized to bone. Alpha particles (2 protons fused to 2 neutrons) land a knock-out punch at very short distances, with this first-in-class agent selectively nesting in bone. Now, of course, research is running wild in the attempt to link alpha-emitting particles to monoclonal antibodies, forming conjugates that will deliver radiation therapy to individual tumor cells anywhere in the body, while energizing the immune response to cancer at the same time.

This is only a step away from combining imaging and therapy. Picture this—every 3 to 5 years, women have a routine "breast scan" that reveals the presence of cancer cells and kills them at the same time. If there are no cancer cells, then the contrast-killer has nowhere to latch on, so it's excreted from the body without effect. We will finally have achieved what some erroneously believe that mammograms do today, that is, actively prevent or treat cancer. Today's science fiction is tomorrow's prescriptive non-fiction.

And, yes, costs are running wild in these futuristic scenarios where even today's baby steps are sending third-party payors into fits of pain and protest. Yet, when the day of 100% disease control arrives, bye-bye screening. Treatment trumps screening when the former works all the time, or nearly so. In the meantime, for the foreseeable future (if the future can be foreseen), breast imaging is also bursting at the seams with new developments.

Tomosynthesis is here, finally, and it appears to be fulfilling the expectations that have been predicted for the past decade, with cancers invisible on 2-D brought to life when the 3-D switch is thrown. But this is only half the story with tomosynthesis. If you administer a contrast agent prior to the mammogram, the images start to resemble a breast MRI.

Dr. Kopans was presenting the first contrast-enhanced tomosynthesis pictures at breast cancer conferences many years ago, and I once heard him claim in a friendly chide to breast MRI guru Dr. Harms who was on the same stage: "I'm 10 years behind you, Steve, and I'm catching up." Today, the predictable studies are in progress, that is, head-to-head comparisons between breast MRI and contrast-enhanced tomosynthesis. Somehow, the battered and bruised Dr. Kopans has persisted in these monumental improvements in mammography in spite of the relentless hounds at his heels. What irony that those hounds are so intensely focused on first generation technology that is long gone, while Dr. Kopans has been one of the most important figures in the development of second and now third generations.

At the same time, breast MRI is undergoing an overhaul, and "abbreviated MRI," a 5- to 10-minute study for screening, has been introduced by Christiane Kuhl, M.D., at RWTH

Aachen University in Germany. We met Dr. Kuhl in a previous chapter when her group announced MRI screening results in the "normal risk" population. With MRI becoming shorter and less expensive, while at the same time, contrast-enhanced mammography comes of age, we might end up with an either/or situation when it comes to accuracy and cost. Or one of the two might dominate. Either way, it'll be a win.

The early data on tomosynthesis raised an immediate question—If 3-D tomos are cutting through the density (Greek: tomo = "cut") to find breast cancer, is the addition of ultrasound to mammography as advantageous as we previously thought? A very good question, though cancer yields above and beyond mammography in the ultrasound studies seem slightly better on a consistent basis than the addition of tomo (the latter having the distinct advantage of being a single study rather than two modalities). Still, the trials are underway—digital mammography + whole breast ultrasound *vs.* tomosynthesis alone. We also have trials comparing 3-D tomosynthesis plus ultrasound vs. breast MRI. And "molecular imaging" vs. breast MRI.[1] You name the combination, and someone is looking at it somewhere.

These final 50 years in breast imaging (maybe 100) are going to be exciting times before the final poof of a universal cure blows it all away. If you have a child entering medical school today who is interested in a career in breast medicine, I would recommend breast radiology *or* oncology. However, that child's children will be better off with a career in breast *oncology* where biotherapies will eventually replace cytotoxic chemotherapies, and screening will gradually become of secondary importance before fading away entirely. What about breast *surgery*? This, too, shall pass. (Although paradoxically, DCIS could end up being the last lesion standing for the surgeon.)

"But even if screening disappears, we'll always need radiologic imaging for diagnostic purposes," you might say. Well, maybe not 50–100 years from now. Consider this scenario: the patient feels a lump, the doctor puts a small needle into it, the cytologist confirms malignancy, then an analysis is performed to determine the molecular backbone of the tumor. A personalized potion is delivered, and it's back to work on Monday. Today's throat culture for strep could be tomorrow's cancer culture.

Before this takes place, however, breast imaging is going to enjoy its Golden Age, with vast improvements in accuracy, to the dismay of anti-screeners who will be shouting "length bias and overdiagnosis" at the top of their lungs, while breast cancer mortality rates creep downward. Screening will assume a *more* important role in the near future, not only due to technology and multi-modality imaging, but also due to improvements in patient selection— that is, "Who needs which modality and when?" Yes, there will be modest improvements in risk stratification based on traditional risk factors, genetic testing, and perhaps even the use of single nucleotide polymorphisms (SNPs), but the bulk of progress when it comes to multi-modality screening will come through identifying women who harbor cancers that are mammographically invisible *in real time*, not a "maybe, at some point in the future."

These advances in imaging are coming so quickly that it's absurd to think we can demonstrate mortality reductions for each and every modality, as well as every combination. We must start trusting *cancer yields* (Sensitivity) in radiology trials as surrogates for a mortality reduction, exactly as the American Cancer Society did in 2007 when it fired the first salvo of guidelines for screening high-risk women with breast MRI.

Certain experts never tire in reminding us of the impropriety of that move by the ACS given no proven mortality reduction with MRI; but in fact, it was far more than a new set of guidelines—it was a symbolic measure that said, "Lives will be lost unnecessarily if we don't adopt *obvious* imaging improvements." Is this a departure from evidence-based medicine? I don't think so. It may be a departure from strict empiricism which, as we have seen, has a bad habit of dismissing evidence rather than its stated goal of simply ranking the evidence.

If we are going to stick ourselves in the cement of pure empiricism, then we cannot endorse any mammographic technology used after 1997 when the last mammogram picture was snapped in a prospective RCT. That would include digital mammography, which was introduced a few years later. The only mortality reductions confirmed with prospective RCTs took place through *old-fashioned film screen mammography*. Anything beyond that is a departure from good science, or so we are told by the pure empiricist.

So what did the Task Force do when they raised their periscope and saw nothing but a sea of digital mammogram machines, after having proclaimed "insufficient evidence" for their adoption? They straightened their backs, regained their composure, then boldly shifted their "insufficient evidence" moniker away from digital mammography (without ever endorsing it) and stuck it on 3-D tomosynthesis. Then they lowered their periscope, presumably for another 6 to 8 years.

So let's recap our *cancer yields* for the various approaches to screening, under the presumptive notion that improving yields is a reasonable surrogate for breast cancer-specific mortality reductions, a.k.a. "saved lives":

General population screening with mammography—5 cancers per 1,000 (if a mix of prevalence and incidence screens)

Add tomosynthesis—1–3 (additional cancers) per 1,000

Add ultrasound to the general population with negative 2-D mammograms—2–4 per 1,000

Add ultrasound to high-risk/high density population with negative 2-D mammograms—4–5 per 1,000

Add MRI after negative mammos and negative ultrasound in the general population—11 per 1,000

Add MRI after negative mammos and negative ultrasound in the high-risk population—22–36 per 1,000

Note that, in percentage terms, the range for yields extends from 0.5% in screening the general population with digital mammography to 2.2–3.6% using MRI after negative conventional imaging. I believe cancer yields of 10%, that is, 100 per 1,000 screened, using MRI *in the general population* may be within our reach. Whether it's blood testing, ultra-CAD or something else entirely, we can do much better if we focus on those patients whose established cancers are invisible on mammography rather than the probability that something *might* happen at *some point* in the future.

Yes, many attempts will be made to refine risk-based screening in the future, but the cancer yields with MRI have already "maxed out" at under 4%. That's the best we can do, even though that's limiting breast MRI to only those women at the very highest genetic risk, while excluding the vast majority of eventual breast cancer patients who would benefit with auxiliary imaging. We'll never get above 4% using a risk-based strategy. In fact, the 2.2–3.6% quoted above includes a fair number of prevalence screens, so the long-term yields in this patient population are going to reach the steady state at only 2% with annual MRI screening.

Alternatively, if we focus on occult cancer probabilities instead of future risk probabilities, we can apply our current imaging technology to the general population where most of the breast cancers are preparing to unfold. We should work toward higher yields than risk-based screening allows while, at the same time, introducing the option of multi-modality imaging to all women, rather than a small minority. There is a fundamental philosophic difference in the two approaches—mammographically occult cancer vs. future risk—and apparently, it's not intuitive given the overwhelming dedication to the latter.

The various imaging approaches work for everyone, and for the same reasons. Don't be duped into believing that, somehow, auxiliary imaging only works on women with risk factors. The Sensitivity formula *does not include* risk levels. An imaging modality with 90% Sensitivity works at all levels of risk (though levels of density can matter). The sole purpose of risk stratification for imaging strategies is to improve cancer yields to the point of cost-effectiveness. But when the majority of women who develop breast cancer do not have a positive family history, the very premise of risk-based screening is flawed through exclusion of the majority.

With today's multi-modality technologies, a sneaky breast cancer has a very difficult time trying to hide. Previously, it could remain wrapped in the white zones of mammography knowing it could evade detection. But too many weapons can root it out now. It's only a matter of raising the level of suspicion as to when a cancer is trying to hide, then shining the light on it by using a second form of breast imaging.

My vision of high yield, cost-effective, multi-modality screening can be extended well beyond what I've mentioned above. For instance, what if a blood test could be modified to detect only those cancers that are amenable to early detection? Or what if the blood test could guide eventual therapy? What I've described so far are efforts to find all types of breast cancer, but the potential to target only those tumors with Goldilocks biology would be even better.

I've heard researchers on my same wave length call for a blood test that would detect "only the most aggressive" forms of breast cancer and thus prompt multi-modality imaging; but a word of caution here—these most aggressive tumors might be our old "Biologic B" cancers, where so-called early detection is already too late. Here, we would need to improve systemic therapies above and beyond early detection.[2] It's a fine point, but an important distinction.

Breast cancer biology is currently categorized into sub-groups through DNA microarray analysis, but when these tumors are still "undiagnosed," we don't have the luxury of picking and choosing which ones we want to detect, at least not yet. We go for all of them. And, when all undiagnosed breast cancers are considered as an amorphous cloud of misty biologies, only those with Goldilocks biology will allow a mortality reduction through early detection.

The good news is that we already have the detection technology in place. We don't need to invent anything. The bad news is that we're not very good at selecting the right patients at the right time for whom the technology should be used. And worse, we're nearly at a dead end when it comes to risk-based screening, though the mesmerizing pull of this approach leaves many believing that this is our only alternative. It's *not* our only alternative and, in fact, the occult cancer approach is superior in every way, shape and form, with one little caveat— it's still under development. Succeeding with the occult cancer approach is, however, more real than smoky visions sealed inside a crystal ball.

Unfortunately, at this critical juncture where we can move forward and burst into a new world of cost-effective multi-modality imaging, we have red lights everywhere telling us to stop, back off, slow down, screen less, or not at all—journal editors, science writers, think tanks, the Swiss medical board, dilettantes espousing their opinions based on ancient clinical trials using obsolete technology. They deify and glorify "no benefit" clinical trials that should have been banished to the underworld long ago … it makes you want to cry.

"Stop screening entirely." "70,000 overdiagnosed women a year." "Harms outweigh the benefits." "The most scientifically pure study ever performed shows no benefit to mammography." "Permanent psychologic damage after a benign biopsy." "Using ultrasound or MRI is only going to make overdiagnosis worse."

Red lights everywhere. And it's not limited to those individuals or groups I've repeatedly mentioned in this book. There is a vocal nucleus of women, supported by a cadre of anti-screening experts serving as their gurus, who see mammography as a male-created devilment, the key component of a cancer militia in league with self-serving cancer causes, obsessed with the archaic notion of screening when the future is in curing the disease, *not* photographing it.

These activists' day will come all right, that is, no more mammographic screening, but their vision is premature. And rather than acknowledge screening *and* curing as complementary efforts, these activists are sometimes overtly antagonistic toward screening. Why? I don't know. Perhaps it's the historic "overselling." Perhaps it's the same awareness about the true Sensitivity of traditional mammography that I've covered in this book, only with a fatalistic reaction rather than the Bright Side of the Dark Side. Perhaps many are actual victims of failed mammography. Still, the universal condemnation of screening is premature, and a vote for anti-screening rhetoric is a vote for more breast cancer deaths.

Red lights everywhere. Bias runs rampant.

As for my bias, it's born from multiple sources. From my interest in breast imaging and breast pathology, it's born from reviewing thousands of mammograms and MRIs, comparing images to microscopic patterns on biopsy, as well as the biology and natural history as predicted by final pathology. From the Mammography Civil War, bias is born by my study of screening epidemiology. From my strong interest in risk assessment and genetic testing, it's born through the realization that this approach has both benefits and limits. From simple statistical modeling of alternative approaches to screening, it's born by the realization that we can do so much better than the status quo. In the end, bias is born from an interest in all things associated with early diagnosis—radiology, pathology, natural history, epidemiology, biostatistics, risk stratification, genetics, and screening research. What single specialty incorporates all these things? There isn't one. So what do you call a physician who specializes in all aspects, and only those aspects, of breast cancer that are associated with early diagnosis? The answer: weary.

I've coordinated a weekly multidisciplinary breast conference since 1989, each meeting accompanied by a subject for discussion before moving into patient management. Of course, as the presenter, I am the primary beneficiary of these educational efforts. Many of the conference topics have formed the basis of this book. In fact, my colleagues, if they read this volume, are bound to say, "Well, all he did was put a binder on his weekly conference notes then call it a book. I've heard this stuff for years." And they would be largely correct.

I confess all this, only so the reader will know that I realize that, like every other human, I operate from a position of bias. This might be *confirm*ational bias at times, wherein one readily accepts arguments that help confirm pre-existing bias. Or it might be *conform*ational bias, where one distorts the sensory input to fit pre-existing notions. My only defense is that I have consistently read the fine print of the opposing viewpoints, and that is why I can be such an irritant to the minimalists.

Self-awareness of bias is not an easy task. Very likely, it's impossible to its fullest extent, lest one become paralyzed like the comic character Calvin has warned. Still, one can work at it. I previously mentioned Dr. Richard Feynman, the Nobel laureate, whose career in theoretical physics is lost on most of us, but who is remembered more widely for his wisdom in defining scientific truth and methodology. With countless quotes to his credit, I'll paraphrase the one I draw from most often: When you run a successful experiment and the results prompt your heart to flutter, first stop and think—Is there any other possible explanation for this success, *besides* my hypothesis?

Scientific method is a social construct. We drew up the rules. If we define good science too tightly, we exclude many of the greatest discoveries of all time. If we define it too loosely, then pseudoscience fits the bill on a regular basis. It's a construct. And within this construct, it's impossible to prove anything as "absolutely true" when it comes to a detached Reality. We thrive in the world of falsifiability.

In our discussion here that favors mammographic screening, I have not been defending a counterintuitive position. Early diagnosis *ought* to improve outcomes. Yet, somehow, we pro-screeners have been put on the defensive, having to come to the rescue of common sense. The woman on the street will tell you about the importance of early diagnosis, yet in the battle over screening, we are fighting for your lives to maintain this simple truth. *Proving* it as absolute truth, however, can't be done when we operate under the dominant construct for science that states you can only falsify theories to a certain degree of probability. In practice, if a hypothesis is not falsifiable, it's a waste of time.

As a result of our construct, we talk in terms that use confusing double negatives. So a p-value of 0.05 means there's only a 5% chance that we would get a result, or a more extreme result, given that the null hypothesis is true (no difference between groups). Yet the seductive and deceptive converse is not valid—we *cannot* say that there's a 95% chance that our theory is true. And then, of all things, the standard-bearer of significance in science, $p \leq 0.05$, is an arbitrary number. What a construct we've built for ourselves!

So, in the spirit of double negatives and syntax that may be fair to partly cloudy, let me close with this—Everything you've read in this book may be false, but I doubt it. With 95% probability, at least 80% of it is not untrue. After all, 80% of statistics are made up.

# Chapter Notes

## Chapter 1

1. American Cancer Society, Surveillance and Health Services Research, 2013, ACS Facts and Figures, Page 1, 2013–14.

2. Kinsinger L, Harris R, Karnitschnig J. Interest in decision-making about breast cancer screening in younger women. *J Gen Intern Med* 1998; 13(Suppl):98. Abstract.

3. Wingo PA, Tong T, Bolden S. Cancer statistics, 1995. *CA Cancer J Clin* 1995; 45:8–30.

The decrease from 46,000 to 40,000 breast cancer deaths is further reflected when mortality is population-adjusted. Around 1989, the mortality of breast cancer began to decline from 30 per 100,000 to current levels of 21.9 per 100,000. This 27% reduction in mortality occurred in tandem with the implementation of widespread screening as well as the institution of adjuvant systemic therapy. Most experts attribute an equal contribution from both screening and systemic therapies (above and beyond the benefit of local control through surgery and/or radiation).

## Chapter 2

1. Wilhelm Roentgen made the decision *not* to apply for a patent after his discovery of X-rays. He believed that a tool so revolutionary in the fields of science and medicine should be made available to all without restriction. After he won the (first) Nobel Prize in Physics in 1901, he donated his prize money to his university. After this remarkable display of altruism, Roentgen came to the end of his life nearly bankrupt.

2. As still happens today with every opportunity to exploit science, it didn't take long for someone to mass produce the Revigator™, a radioactive water crock designed for home use, made of radium-containing ore, such that water could sit overnight and, "by morning, drink the radium water to cure whatever ails you." Concerned that charlatans were selling water crocks with no radon production at all, the AMA set standards to make sure that *at least* 2 microcuries of radon were being generated in each liter of water over a 24-hour period. Ironically, the devices were driven from the market, not because they were radioactive, but because they did not produce *enough* radiation to meet AMA standards.

3. As Adolf Hitler came to power, Dr. Salomon was discharged from the University of Berlin and was subsequently sent to the concentration camp at Sachsenhausen. In 1939, through the persistence of his wife, a former opera star, he was released, whereupon they moved to the Netherlands and remained in hiding until the end of World War II. He began life anew in Amsterdam, and in 1971, donated 1,300 paintings to the Jewish Historical Museum in Amsterdam, the artist being his accomplished daughter, Charlotte Salomon, who had been killed in the gas chambers at Auschwitz.

4. William Steward Halsted is considered the father of modern American surgery, introducing many innovations, including the current residency system and a wide variety of surgical principles and techniques. A larger-than-life figure, Halsted once saved the life of his sister who was bleeding to death post-partum. Not only did he perform one of the first blood transfusions in the U.S., using his own blood to give to his sister, he then operated on her to stop the hemorrhage. Self-experimentation was considered the most noble of all pursuits in medical science, and in his enthusiasm to develop the new local anesthetic called cocaine, he became addicted. The treatment of choice for cocaine addiction at the time was the use of heroin or morphine. From that experience, Halsted developed a lifelong addiction to these drugs, such that many of his greatest accomplishments occurred while fully addicted. Together with the infamy associated with his "radical mastectomy," his legacy is unjustly scarred.

5. Bernard Fisher, M.D. (1918– ), has won every major award in cancer medicine, with the exception of the Nobel Prize. At that key moment in history when acceptance of breast conservation was fresh (early 1990s), it became apparent to the NSABP that one of its largest contributors of patients to clinical trials, Dr. Roger Poisson in Canada, had been falsifying data for years that allowed 99 patients to enter the trials who really didn't qualify (the motivation?—more perks come with more patients enrolled). Dr. Fisher and the NSABP were accused of hiding this information during their recalculation of data, prompting a federal investigation that trumped up violations against the sometimes "pugnacious" Dr. Fisher and damaging the great work done at 500 participating centers of the NSABP. The "witch hunt" gained momentum, and when the NSABP required

more time to recalculate than was offered, the National Cancer Institute and the University of Pittsburgh removed Dr. Fisher as head of the NSABP. Fisher countered with a defamation lawsuit that was settled in his favor, including an apology from his alma mater, the University of Pittsburgh, plus reinstatement as Chairman of the NSABP. When the dust settled, Dr. Poisson's patients had not altered the final outcome one way or the other. Yet Dr. Fisher's reputation was sullied, and many believe this explains why the Nobel committee has failed to recognize his singular, courageous contribution to the management of breast cancer. History has already recognized him as the single greatest force that brought an end to the Halsted radical mastectomy.

## Chapter 3

1. An Italian study of breast conservation, a prospective, randomized trial, made it into print before Fisher's landmark NSABP B-06 trial reported its 5-year results in 1985. Led by surgeon Umberto Veronesi, the 1981 report in the *New England Journal of Medicine* described equal survival in two groups of women—349 underwent Halsted radical mastectomy, while 352 underwent "quadrantectomy," axillary node dissection, with radiation to the remaining breast. Dr. Fisher referenced this study often, pointing out that it was *not* grounded in basic science research, nor was it theorizing any underlying paradigm shift regarding the biology of breast cancer. Indeed, Fisher claimed the Italians were fully grounded in Halstedian biology at the time of their study, evidenced by the "quadrantectomy," removing much more tissue than the lump itself, as well as the fact that most patients had tumors located in the upper outer quadrant near the axilla, such that an en bloc resection could be performed as a single specimen, in essence, a mini-mastectomy, still using Halstedian principles. To support this contention, it is a curious fact that, prior to instituting the Italian quadrantectomy trial, Dr. Veronesi was publishing his experience with an "extended mastectomy," a procedure more Halstedian than Halsted himself.

2. Hellman S. Karnofsky Memorial Lecture. Natural history of small breast cancers. *J Clin Oncol* 1994; 12: 2229–2234.

3. Heywang-Kobrunner SH, Hacker A, Sedlacek S. "Advantages and disadvantages of mammography screening." Breast Care 2011: 6:199–207.

4. The difference between Grade and Stage is often confusing, but the former deals with biology, while the latter deals with anatomic extent of disease. Grade, in fact, is the oldest measure of biology, dating back to the first assessments of cancer under the microscope where some cells were quite abnormal (Grade 3) whereas other malignant cells were barely abnormal (Grade 1). Many systems were proposed for different types of cancer; and, even within a single type of cancer, there are different grading systems. For breast cancer, Grade 1 is best, Grade 3 worst, but other "tumor markers" and "genetic profiles" define the biology today such that Grade is now secondary. A strong prognosticator of eventual outcomes is Stage, or the anatomic extent of the tumor. For breast cancer, this is Stage 0 (in situ carcinoma), Stage I (tumors under 2.0cm and negative nodes), Stage II (tumors over 2.0cm and less than 5.0cm and/or up to 3 pos-

itive nodes), Stage III (4 or more positive nodes, or other locally advanced findings), and Stage IV (metastatic to other parts of the body). Additional findings provide more specific sub-groups of A, B, C, e.g., a tumor over 2.0cm, but negative nodes is Stage IIA. As relates to the discussion in this book of "Biology and Size," this is closely related to "Grade and Stage," respectively. One of the controversies today is whether or not sophisticated tumor analyses can finally trump the staging system. Grade alone wasn't powerful enough to do so, but we are on the cusp of switching from anatomic staging to biologic staging.

5. When the NSABP B-06 announced its results showing equivalency of the three groups—lumpectomy alone, lumpectomy with radiation, and mastectomy—the distant disease-free survival curves were often presented as overlapping. However, when the original, detailed graphs are reviewed, there were differences trending, and separate curves are clearly identified—lumpectomy and radiation having the best survival, mastectomy in the middle, and lumpectomy alone with the worst survival. Each of the two conservation groups *were compared only to mastectomy*, with no statistically significant survival differences. However, the two conservation groups (lumpectomy plus radiation vs. lumpectomy alone) *were not compared to each other*, where a difference was strongly suspect, until the survival curves finally began to merge after 20 years of follow-up. Had this comparison been made in the initial analyses, with lumpectomy and radiation having a statistically better survival than lumpectomy alone, the results would not have been supportive of Fisher Theory, given that local variations in treatment are predicted to have little impact on outcomes based on predestined biology in the face of the host response. As the years passed, with larger number of patients participating in multiple trials of breast conservation, a small, but statistically significant, improvement in survival was demonstrated with the addition of radiation to lumpectomy. Although this does not, in and of itself, "disprove" Fisher Theory, it does require us to resurrect those key words that Dr. Fisher used in his writings—unlikely and substantial. Fisher wrote: "Variations in the manner of local control are *unlikely* to have a *substantial* impact on survival."

## Chapter 4

1. Huggins' 1966 Nobel Prize was shared 50–50 with Peyton Rous, M.D. (1879–1970) from Rockefeller University in New York City. In 1910, Rous had discovered the first cancer-causing virus (now called the Rous sarcoma virus). As a pathologist, he diagnosed a lump on a hen's breast as sarcoma (soft tissue malignancy), then began passing extracts made from the tumor into other chickens that also developed malignancies. Interestingly, each newly passed tumor proved to be more aggressive than the last, supporting the concept of "progression," i.e., malignant tumors becoming even more malignant. Viruses were poorly understood at the time, as was the origin of cancer. Years later, viruses emerged as one of the leading suspects for the cause of cancer, some believing viruses were responsible for all cancers. Thus, the Nobel Prize won by Rous came 56 years after his discovery. Although enthusiasm for the "viral theory of

cancer," waned, explaining only a small group of cancers, the Rous sarcoma virus was later tied to the src gene, which formed the early foundation for current theories about cancer causation. The two winners of the 1966 Nobel Prize were not collaborators, instead, working at two different locations on two different projects.

2. Theodor Kocher (1909), Allvar Gullstrand (1911), Alexis Carrel (1912), Robert Barany (1914), Frederick Banting (1923), Walter Hess (1949), Werner Forssmann (1956), Charles Huggins (1966), Joseph Murray (1990).

3. After receiving his medical degree at St. John's University in Shanghai, Ling Yuan Dao came to the United States in the early 1950s, with the intent to do some postgraduate work and return to China. The rise of Mao Zedong prompted Ling Yuan to stay in the U.S. where he assumed the first name Thomas. Dr. Tom Dao (1921–2009) went on to become one of the early pioneers in breast cancer treatment, endorsing and promoting breast conservation as well as his original contributions in the Huggins lab.

4. The PLCO trial (Prostate, Lung, Colorectal, Ovarian), sponsored by the National Cancer Institute, recruited 76,000 men from 1993 to 2001 and randomly assigned them to digital exam (first 4 years) and PSA (all 6 years) vs. usual care. Although screening yielded a 12% higher incidence of cancers, both groups had the same mortality rate, strongly suggesting that overdiagnosis bias was active in the trial. In their 2012 update, published in the *Journal of the National Cancer Institute*, there was still no evidence of a mortality reduction in the screened group after 13 years of follow-up. In contrast, the European Randomized Study of Screening for Prostate Cancer (ERSPC) indicated a mortality reduction for men screened with PSA. The two trials had different designs, but in both, the randomization process was considered good, and intense study is now underway trying to figure out why the two trials yielded different outcomes. The ERSPC was a massive study, enrolling 162,388 men randomized to two groups, PSA vs. "usual." The initial 9-year follow-up revealed a mortality reduction of 15% that was not statistically significant, though many have missed the fact that, by 11 years, the benefit did reach statistical significance and the relative mortality reduction was increasing over time. Importantly, when the screening tool is working, compliant patients in the screened group will have a greater benefit than the screened group as a whole where a fair number of participants are non-compliant. In the ERSPC trial, the mortality reduction for compliant PSA screeners was 27%, as compared to only 21% when the entire group was considered, the latter figure being the accepted standard when following the "intent to treat" rule of prospective, randomized controlled trials. A re-analysis of PLCO is underway as well, given the charge that PSA was commonly performed in the no–PSA control group, perhaps as often, or more so, than in the PSA study group.

5. Haas GP, Delongchamps N, Brawley WO, Ching WY, de La Roza, G. The worldwide epidemiology of prostate cancer: perspectives from autopsy studies. *Can J Urol* 2008; 15:3866–3871.

6. Thompson IM, Goodman PJ, Tangen CM, et al. The influence of finasteride on the development of prostate cancer. *N Engl J Med* 2003; 349:215–224.

7. Welch HG, Black WC. Using autopsy series to es-

timate the disease "reservoir" for ductal carcinoma in situ of the breast: how much more breast cancer can we find? *Ann Intern Med* 1997; 127:1023–1028.

8. Bleyer A, Welch HG. Effect of three decades of screening mammography on breast-cancer incidence. *N Engl J Med* 2012; 367:1998–2005.

## Chapter 5

1. Jatoi I, Miller AB. Breast cancer screening in elderly women: primum non nocere. *JAMA* 2015; 150:1107–1108.

2. In the 2010 update from the Dutch MRISC Screening Study (Rijnsburger AI et al. *J Clin Oncol* 2010; 28: 5265–5273) the BRCA-1 gene-positive patients had a 32.3% rate of interval cancer, a definite outlier compared to all other studies. Still, it prompted many high-risk screening programs to stagger annual mammograms and annual MRI at 6-month intervals. In this same update, the BRCA-2 patients had a remarkably low 6.3% rate of interval cancers, while high risk patients had a 3.7% interval cancer rate, and modest risk patients 6.3%, all these numbers well below interval cancer rates with mammography alone.

3. Accessed 1/11/16: http://www.cancer.gov/types/breast/hp/breast-screening-pdq#link/_13_toc._

4. Zahl PH, Strand BH, Maehlen J. Incidence of breast cancer in Norway and Sweden during introduction of nationwide screening: prospective cohort study. *BMJ* 2004; 328:921–924.

5. In his book *Statistics Done Wrong* (San Francisco: No Starch Press; 2015), author Alex Reinhart describes a 2002 study where statistics students and their instructors overwhelmingly failed to interpret the correct definition of a p-value. Of the multiple choice options, none were true. Shockingly, the majority chose a wrong answer. The author provides many examples of wildly distorted conclusions drawn from p-values through failure to recognize the *base rate fallacy*. As an example, most early drug development trials fail, so when a trial does have "significant" results with a p-value under 0.05, the odds are that this, in fact, is a statistical fluke, rather than significant benefit.

6. For a fascinating look at the history of Bayes' Theorem from its origins to present day, read *The Theory That Would Not Die: How Bayes' Rule Cracked the Enigma Code, Hunted Down Russian Submarines, and Emerged Triumphant from Two Centuries of Controversy* by Sharon Bertsch McGrayne (New Haven: Yale University Press; 2011).

## Chapter 6

1. From: "Highlights from the History of Mammography" (Gold RH, Bassett LW, Widoff BE. *RadioGraphics* 1990; 10:1111–1131), without explanation as to the very high cancer yield in this study, approximately 3-fold what one would expect in screening a population of 2,000 women.

2. Philip Strax (1909–1999) is listed in his *New York Times* obituary as a "radiologist," though that same document points out he began his career as a "general practitioner with a small family practice in Manhattan." Without having done a radiology residency, it appears that the practice of Dr. Strax evolved into full-time mammographic screening, including the interpretation of the X-rays.

3. Feig SA, Shaber GS, Schwartz GF, et al. Thermography, mammography, and clinical examination in breast cancer screening: review of 16,000 studies. *Radiology* 1977; 122:123–127.

## Chapter 7

1. Miller AB, Baines CJ, To T, Wall C. Canadian National Breast Screening Study: 1. Breast cancer detection and death rates among women aged 40 to 49 years. *CMAJ* 1992; 15:1459–1476.

2. Yaffe MJ. Correction: Canada study. Letter to the editor. *J Natl Cancer Inst* 1993; 155:748–749.

3. Baines CJ, Miller AB, Kopans DB, et al. Canadian National Breast Screening Study: assessment of technical quality by external review. *AJR Am J Roentgenol* 1990; 155:743–747; discussion 748–749.

4. Much has been written about the overuse of military metaphors to describe cancer politics, both pertaining to activists and the medical profession. With that acknowledged, I'd gladly use another set of metaphors if I could think of one. Nothing else seems to capture the spirit of the times.

5. In 2005, Dr. Donald A. Berry and the CISNET collaborators, published an article in the *New England Journal of Medicine* (353:1784–1792) addressing the dual contributions of screening and systemic therapies as pertaining to the improved mortality in breast cancer over the past 25 years. The Cancer Intervention and Surveillance Modeling Network (CISNET) is an NCI-sponsored consortium designed to use biostatistics to guide recommendations for improving cancer interventions (for 5 cancer types) through mathematical modeling. In this case, the group used seven independent statistical models, and found that the proportion of reduced deaths from breast cancer attributed to screening ranged from 28% to 65%, with adjuvant systemic therapies responsible for the rest. Since the median in this range was 46%, it is fair to say that the benefits of screening and adjuvant systemic therapies contribute equally to the reduction in the death rates from breast cancer in the U.S.

6. Robert Egan, M.D., is usually referred to as the "father of mammography" due to his contributions while at MD Anderson. Some of these advances were facilitated through his background as a metallurgical engineer prior to medical school. After he was given the assignment to develop a practical and safe X-ray for the diagnosis of problems in the female breast, Dr. Egan endured the jokes of his colleagues that saddled him with monikers that one would incorrectly believe are limited to the boys' locker room in high school. Not only did he make vast improvements in the pre-existing technology, but he also found 53 "occult" cancers in asymptomatic women as discussed earlier, setting the stage for mass screening. Yet, he did not organize the large-scale prospective trials that followed. As for the "father of *screening* mammography," the other nod goes to Philip Strax, M.D., for his role as the engine behind the HIP study. For those disturbed by these "fathers" but no "mothers," consider the era, specifically the fact that few women entered the medical profession as physicians during this time period.

7. Tabár L, Vitak B, Chen TH, et al. Swedish two-county trial: impact of mammographic screening on breast cancer mortality during 3 decades. *Radiology* 2011; 260:658–663.

8. Larsson LG, Andersson I, Bjurstam N, et al. Updated overview of the Swedish Randomized Trials on Breast Cancer Screening with Mammography: age group 40–49 at randomization. *J Natl Cancer Inst Monogr* 1997;(22)57–61.

9. Tabár L, Fagerberg CJ, Gad A, et al. Reduction in mortality from breast cancer after mass screening with mammography. Randomised trial from the Breast Cancer Screening Working Group of the Swedish National Board of Health and Welfare. *The Lancet* 1985; 1(8433): 829–832.

10. Tabár L, Duffy SW, Burhenne LW. New Swedish breast cancer detection results for women aged 40–49. *Cancer* 1993; 72:1437–1448.

11. Fletcher SW, Black W, Harris R, Rimer BK, Shapiro S. Report of the International Workshop on Screening for Breast Cancer. *J Natl Cancer Inst* 1993; 85:1644–1656.

12. Baines CJ. The Canadian National Breast Screening Study: a perspective on criticisms. *Ann Intern Med* 1994; 120:326–334.

13. Tarone RE. The excess of patients with advanced breast cancer in young women screened with mammography in the Canadian National Breast Screening Study. *Cancer* 1995; 75:997–1003.

## Chapter 8

1. Hollingsworth AB. Chapter 1: Risk Assessement, in: *Breast Cancer: A New Era In Management*. Editors: Francescatti DS, Silverstein MJ. New York: Springer; 2014.

2. Tabár L, Vitak B, Chen TH, et al. Swedish two-county trial: impact of mammographic screening on breast cancer mortality during 3 decades. *Radiology* 2011; 260:658–663.

3. Dr. Stephen Feig is a pioneering breast radiologist and one of the founders of the Society of Breast Imaging. In 2009 and 2010, in one of many attempts nationwide to minimize the impact of the U.S. Preventive Services Task Force, the author of this book joined Dr. Feig and Dr. Gail Lebovic in authorship of an article on the cost-effectiveness of risks, screening, and prevention of breast cancer, published in the journal *Breast* (2010;19:260–267). At the time, lead author Gail Lebovic, M.D., was president of the American Society of Breast Disease, while Dr. Feig was president-elect of that same organization. Dr. Hollingsworth has never held political office.

4. Pace LE, Keating NL. A systematic assessment of benefits and risks to guide breast cancer screening decisions. *JAMA* 2014; 311:1327–1335.

## Chapter 9

1. Otis Webb Brawley and Paul Goldberg. *How We Do Harm: A Doctor Breaks Ranks About Being Sick in America* (New York: St. Martin's Griffin; 2012).

2. The most exhaustive coverage of the history of mammographic screening comes from the insightful book *The Breast Cancer Wars: Hope, Fear and the Pursuit of a Cure in Twentieth-Century America* by Dr. Barron H. Lerner, a public health expert and historian. Although credited here with insights about the BCDDP, Dr. Lerner's writings, both in his book and in a background paper he wrote for the Institute of Medicine, served as rich source material for this book throughout.

3. AFIP is the Armed Forces Institute of Pathology, once considered a premier site for consultative services when pathologists in the U.S. encountered rare and difficult cases. In fact, *radiology* residents across the country routinely rotated to the AFIP in order to learn how to correlate findings on X-ray to what the pathologist sees grossly and under the microscope. Nowhere is this correlation more important than in breast cancer. Sadly, Base Realignment and Closure forced the AFIP to be "disestablished" in September 2011. Dr. McDivitt's authorship of the "breast fascicle" is listed as: Tumors of the breast. By Robert W. McDivitt, M.D., New York: Fred W. Stewart, M.D., Ph.D., New York; and John W. Berg, M.D. Maryland. Pp. 156 with 120 illustrations. Washington, D.C.: Armed Forces Institute of Pathology; 1968.

4. Early Detection of Breast Cancer (p. 127, Chapter 5), in *Breast Diseases* (Editors: Harris JR, Hellman S, Henderson IC, Kinne DW) (Philadelphia: J. B. Lippincott; 1987).

## Chapter 10

1. Alan Sokal was a physics professor at New York University and University College London who was growing weary of postmodernists, some of them scientists, undermining the validity of the scientific process. His now-infamous article "Transgressing the Boundaries: Toward a Transformative Hermeneutics of Quantum Gravity" was published (without peer review) by the *Social Text* journal, a leading academic periodical of postmodern cultural studies. On the days of its publication in May 1996, he revealed in *Lingua Franca* that the article was a hoax.

2. Prior to his death in 2015, Dr. Dodd served as Emeritus Head, Division of Diagnostic Imaging; Emeritus Editor of *Breast Diseases: A Year Book® Quarterly*; and Moreton Chair Emeritus of Diagnostic Radiology at the University of Texas MD Anderson Cancer Center. In 1993, the author of this book would meet Dr. Dodd on the top floor of a Manhattan skyscraper, in the law offices of Penny & Edmonds, then considered one of the top intellectual property firms in the country, where most of the lawyers were also PhDs. The purpose of the meeting was most bizarre, in that two clinicians had been called to a strategy meeting with the firm, to relate how a proposed blood test for the detection of breast cancer would interface with breast imaging. Dr. Dodd was the authority on breast imaging, while the author was a clinician who had contacted the scientist at Tel Aviv University who was proposing the test. The author had earlier arranged for Dr. Chaya Moroz to travel from Israel to Oklahoma City where a strategy was proposed for implementing clinical trials for the blood test. In the end,

the placental ferritin blood test was a bust; however, the author, to this day, continues to collaborate with researchers working on this same agenda.

3. Bloche G, M.D., J.D. *The Hippocratic Myth: Why Doctors Have To Ration Care, Practice Politics, and Compromise Their Promise To Heal* (New York: Palgrave Macmillan; 2011).

4. Quoting the late Dick Lampton of Oklahoma City, a talented and witty armchair philosopher.

5. Feynman, RP. *The Meaning of It All: Thoughts of a Citizen-scientist* (New York: Helix Books; 1998).

## Chapter 11

1. Norman F. Boyd, M.D., was a researcher with the Ontario Cancer Institute, Princess Margaret Hospital in Toronto, when he wrote an editorial in the January 15, 1997, edition of the *Canadian Medical Association Journal*, raising his concern about the totality of randomization issues, rather than any single infraction. His article was in response to the review published in this same issue of the journal, which defended the randomization process in the CNBSS. Notably, the lead author of this CNBSS defense was Dr. John C. Bailar III who had been a leader in the anti–BCDDP movement. In Dr. Boyd's response to Dr. Bailar, he makes the interesting claim that he (Boyd) worked under the direction of the CNBSS head (Dr. Anthony Miller) from 1976 to 1978. Dr. Boyd points out that only some of the accusations have been addressed by Bailer and his co-author, Brian MacMahon. For instance, 78% of the alleged "name alterations" could be accounted for in some way, but the remaining 22% (101 names) could not, and the majority of alterations occurred in the mammography arm. In fact, 4 parameters of possible randomization flaws were studied, and all 4 had more of these events occurring in the mammography arm, 3 of which to the degree of statistical significance. Advanced breast cancer being "randomized" into the mammography arm was 1 of the 4 parameters (p-value = 0.003).

2. Gøtzsche PC, Olsen O. Is screening for breast cancer with mammography justifiable? *The Lancet* 2000; 355:129–134.

3. Olsen O, Gøtzsche PC. Cochrane review on screening for breast cancer with mammography. *The Lancet* 2001; 358:1340–1342.

4. Freedman DA, Petitti DB, Robins JM. On the efficacy of screening for breast cancer. *Int J Epidemiol* 2004; 33:43–55.

5. Fletcher SW, Elmore JG. Clinical practice: mammographic screening for breast cancer. *N Engl J Med* 2003; 348:1672–1680.

6. Dean PB. Gøtzsche's quixotic antiscreening campaign: nonscientific and contrary to Cochrane principles. *J Am Coll Radiol* 2004; 1:3–7.

## Chapter 12

1. Zackrisson S, Andersson I, Janzon L, Manjer J, Garne JP. Rate of over-diagnosis of breast cancer 15 years after end of Malmö mammographic screening trial: follow-up study. *BMJ* 2006; 332:689–692.

2. Welch HG, Schwartz LM, Woloshin S. Ramifications of screening for breast cancer: 1 in 4 cancers detected by mammography are pseudocancers. *BMJ* 2006; 332:727.

3. Feig SA. Overdiagnosis of invasive breast cancer and DCIS: why do estimates vary? *Breast Diseases: A Year Book® Quarterly* 2014; 25:196–201.

4. Puliti D, Zappa M, Miccinesi G, Falini P, Crocetti E, Pace E. An estimate of overdiagnosis 15 years after the start of mammographic screening in Florence. *Eur J Cancer* 2009; 45:3166–3171.

5. Bleyer A, Welch HG. Effect of three decades of screening mammography on breast-cancer incidence. *N Engl J Med* 2012; 367:1998–2005.

6. Smith RA. Counterpoint: overdiagnosis in breast cancer screening. *J Am Coll Radiol* 2014; 11:648–652.

## Chapter 13

1. Spontaneous regression of cancer has always been an intriguing possibility. Steven A. Rosenberg, M.D., PhD, is chief of the surgical branch of the National Cancer Institute and the pioneer of cancer immunotherapy. In interviews, he has stated that, early in his medical training, he witnessed the spontaneous regression of an advanced, incurable cancer. That single patient prompted him to spend his entire career developing the first cancer immunotherapies. In the past, a fair amount of effort was devoted to documenting these spontaneous regression events, but very few could be identified and validated. Estimates made in the 1950s placed the probability of regression at 1 out of every 80,000 to 100,000 patients with cancer. Still, in September 1956, two members of the Department of Surgery at the University of Illinois College of Medicine (Drs. Tilden C. Everson and Warren H. Cole) published their extraordinary effort (*Annals of Surgery*) to confirm or deny spontaneous cancer regression. More than 600 cases were reviewed dating back to the late 1800s when pathologic confirmation became the norm. However, only 47 patients were considered to have adequate documentation, including histologic confirmation, to accept as probable examples of spontaneous regression. Of the 47, only 4 were breast cancer patients. Two patients had complete regression of both local recurrences and metastases, one additional patient in this category had partial regression, and one patient had complete regression of a local recurrence that had occurred after mastectomy.

2. The explanation as to why DCIS appears on MRI is still debated, some citing animal models, while others claim "there is no angiogenesis with DCIS, so the explanation is unknown." However, the explanation may have come from a study done long before the introduction of breast MRI. In 1994, a team led by noted breast pathologist Stuart Schnitt, M.D. (Guidi AJ, Fischer L, Harris JR, Schnitt SJ. Microvessel density and distribution in DCIS of the breast. *J Natl Cancer Inst* 1994; 86:614–619) reported two distinct patterns of angiogenesis associated with DCIS. In one of these patterns, the angiogenesis closely hugs the outside of the duct, as if forming "insulation." This would translate to the "linear" pattern of enhancement on MRI for DCIS as described

by radiologists. Dr. Steven Harms took this one step further with very thin "cuts" through enhancing DCIS, revealing "tram tracks," or double, parallel lines as would be seen by cutting through the pipeline, with angiogenesis on the outside of the pipe. The second pattern of angiogenesis occurs as "filler" in between affected ducts grouped closely together. This would translate to the "clumped" pattern of enhancement seen on MRI with some DCIS, making it difficult to distinguish from invasive disease.

3. Sanders ME, Schuyler PA, Simpson JF, Page DL, Dupont WD. Continued observation of the natural history of low-grade ductal carcinoma in situ reaffirms proclivity for local recurrence even after more than 30 years of follow-up. *Modern Pathology* 2015; 28:662–669.

In this well-known series of patients from Nashville, 45 women with low-grade DCIS were followed for many years, with 36% of them developing invasive cancer near the site where they had previously undergone surgical biopsy (excision), but wherein the low-grade DCIS had originally gone undiagnosed (and untreated) beyond the biopsy. Of the 16 women who developed invasive cancer at the biopsy site, 11 occurred within 10 years of the biopsy, but 5 more occurred at 12, 23, 25, 29 and 42 years after the biopsy. Seven of these women, including one who developed invasive cancer 29 years after her DCIS biopsy, died of metastatic breast cancer. This should give pause when branding DCIS with benign-sounding names. Furthermore, it shows how remarkably long the natural history of DCIS can be, leading to many incorrect conclusions when only short-term follow-up is available. Furthermore, this was a study of low-grade DCIS. Many experts believe that high-grade DCIS has a stronger tendency to invade, and to do so more quickly than the low grade lesions.

4. In July 1962, an article was published in the *British Medical Journal* (by H.J.G. Bloom, W.W. Richardson, and E.J. Harries) entitled "Natural History of Untreated Breast Cancer," a review of the Middlesex Hospital in London where women with breast cancer were sent for mere custodial care from 1803 to 1933. Of 356 untreated cases overall, 250 women were studied in remarkable detail, with regard to their presenting stage, their longevity, and their cause of death (with autopsy confirmation in all 250). Many students of breast cancer draw from this database in trying to understand the natural history of the disease. 83% of patients presented with a palpable mass, but most were Stage III, given that ulceration was present in 68%. Even though the presentation of these patients was relatively late, the remarkable feature for our discussion here is that while mean survival was only 3 years, 5% survived more than 10 years, and one patient lasted 18 years, demonstrating the remarkably protracted course that breast cancer can take, making it very hard to proclaim "overdiagnosis" with certainty. Given that these patients were primarily Stage III, one can invoke even longer natural histories when the starting point is Stage I or Stage II. Without adequate follow-up and adjustment for lead time at the end of screening studies, overdiagnosis will be overestimated.

5. Elmore JG, Longton GM, Carney PA, et al. Diagnostic concordance among pathologists interpreting breast biopsy specimens. *JAMA* 2015; 313:1122–1132.

## Chapter 14

1. Humphrey LL, Helfand M, Chan BK, Woolf SH. Breast cancer screening: a summary of evidence for the U.S. Preventive Services Task Force. *Ann Int Med* 2002; 137:347–360.

2. Hendrick RE, Helvie MA. United States Preventive Services Task Force screening guidelines: science ignored. *AJR Am J Roentgenol* 2011; W112-W116.

In several publications, R. Edward Hendrick, PhD (Dept. of Radiology, University of Colorado) and Mark Helvie, M.D. (Dept. of Radiology, University of Michigan), used the CISNET data to come up with sharply different outcomes than the Task Force. One problem: they ended up mostly preaching to the choir in the *AJR American Journal of Roentgenology*, excellent for maintaining esprit de corps, but the world of primary care is still fairly naïve as to how much the data can be twisted and tortured. The first time one hears the "100,000 deaths" mantra coming from pro-screeners aimed at the Task Force, it can strike you as absurd. Yet, even back-of-the-envelope calculations indicate 2,000 more deaths every year if we exclude women in their 40s from screening and switch to biennial screening for others. Is this a drop in the bucket if one is dealing with 40,000 deaths a year anyway? Certainly, it depends on one's definition of a "drop." But consider that this 2,000 per year is, well, *per year*. Hendrick and Helvie calculated for the entire screening-life of patients, which is 44 years of screening. Now, the 100,000 doesn't seem such an alarmist number after all (99,829 to be exact). The saving grace here is compliance, the good-bad news being that many women are not very compliant with mammography. When Hendrick and Helvie assumed a 65% compliance rate, "only" 64,889 more deaths will occur in the current 30–39 age group if Task Force guidelines are followed.

3. The Health Insurance Plan study (HIP) and the Edinburgh trial also included clinical exam as part of the screening process. Critics have no problem singling out these two studies for their insufficiencies, often excluding them from analyses, while embracing the CNBSS in spite of its overt randomization flaws (starting with the fact that the Canadian trial identified lumps on exam *prior* to randomization). If one excludes all studies that included clinical exam (these two plus the CNBSS), one is left with the 4 Swedish studies (5 if Two-County study is divided) plus the U.K.'s AGE trial that have addressed "mammography alone" as a screening tool. This explains why one often hears about the "Swedish data," and that the benefit of mammography should be judged solely from the Swedish prospective trials and the Swedish Overview.

4. Siu AL: U.S. Preventive Services Task Force. Screening for breast cancer: U.S. Preventive Services Task Force recommendation statement. *Ann Intern Med* 2016; 164: 279–296.

## Chapter 15

1. Miller AB, Wall C, Baines CJ, Sun P, To T, Narod SA. Twenty five year follow-up for breast cancer incidence and mortality of the Canadian National Breast Screening Study: randomized screening trial. *BMJ* 2014; 348:g366.

2. Tarone RE. The excess of patients with advanced breast cancer in young women screening with mammography in the Canadian National Breast Screening Study. *Cancer* 1995; 5:997–1003.

3. Paraphrase taken from *Toy Story* (1995) when Woody watches in dismay as Buzz Lightyear demonstrates his aeronautical abilities to the rest of the toys. Woody tries to calm the enthusiasm with "That wasn't flying. That was falling with style."

4. Editorial by Dr. Paula Gordon, "It's Just Wrong," published in response to the 25-year update on the CNBSS, appearing on Dr. Tabár's web site for Mammography Education, Inc. She is also quoted in this chapter from the editorial "Shoddy Canadian Research Puts Women's Lives at Risk," published in the *Vancouver Sun* that had covered the CNBSS update.

5. Coldman A, Phillips N, Wilson C, et al. Pan-Canadian study of mammography screening and mortality from breast cancer. *J Natl Cancer Inst.* Oct. 1, 2014. Although not a prospective, randomized controlled trial, data were obtained on 2,796,472 screening participants representing areas with 85% of the Canadian population, and steps were taken to account for self-selection bias. Age at entry into screening did not greatly affect the magnitude of mortality reduction, ranging from 35% to 44%.

6. A confession: All of us in medicine read abstracts, and all of us, on occasion, read only the conclusion. The volume of medical literature is staggering, and one reads the abstract first to determine whether or not to pursue a more in-depth study. Often, a debater (me in this instance) will attempt to deride the opposition by stating, "This is not appreciated by those who only read abstracts," a smug condescension that is, simultaneously, self-incriminating. We all do it. The difference is when you are considered expert in an area, or if you plan on making public statements, you should read the entire article, including the domain of the devil—"Materials and Methods."

7. Smith RA. Counterpoint: overdiagnosis in breast cancer screening. *J Am Coll Radiol* 2014; 11:648–652.

8. *Ductal Carcinoma in Situ of the Breast* (Editor: Melvin J. Silverstein; Associate Editors: Abram Recht and Michael Lagios) (Philadelphia: Lippincott Williams & Wilkins, 2nd edition; 2002). The title of Chapter 2 sums up the very difficult challenges that follow the diagnosis of in situ disease: "Insanity of DCIS."

9. Zombies are variously defined, but are generally referred to as the "undead" or "reanimated corpses that hunger for human flesh." The 1968 movie *Night of the Living Dead* represents the American adoption of this horror craze that has been gaining momentum ever since. The author had a difficult time picking between *Night of the Living Dead* and *Invasion of the Body Snatchers* when it came time to draw a metaphor for the seemingly relentless social trend toward the anti-screening position.

## Chapter 16

1. Ioannidis JP. Contradicted and initially stronger effects in highly cited clinical research. *JAMA* 2005; 294:218–228.

2. Kalager M, Zelen M, Langmark F, et al. Effect of screening mammography on breast-cancer mortality in Norway. *N Engl J Med* 2010; 363:1203–1210.

3. van Schoor G, Moss SM, Otten JDM, et al. Increasingly strong reduction in breast cancer mortality due to screening. *Br J Cancer* 2011; 104:910–914.

4. Hellquist BN, Duffy SW, Abdsaleh S, et al. Effectiveness of population-based service screening with mammography for women ages 40 to 49 years: evaluation of the Swedish Mammography Screening in Young Women (SCRY) cohort. *Cancer* 2011; 117:714–722.

5. Puliti D, Miccinesi G, Collina N, et al. Effectiveness of service screening: a case-control study to assess breast cancer mortality reduction. *Br J Cancer* 2008; 99:423–427.

6. Allgood PC, Warwick J, Warren RM, et al. A case-control study of the impact of the East Anglian breast screening programme on breast cancer mortality. *Br J Cancer* 2008; 98:206–209.

7. Fielder HM, Warwick J, Brook D, et al. A case-control study to estimate the impact on breast cancer death of the breast screening programme in Wales. *J Med Screen* 2004; 11:194–198.

8. Coldman A, Phillips N, Wilson C, et al. Pan-Canadian study of mammography screening and mortality from breast cancer. *J Natl Cancer Inst*; Oct. 1, 2014.

9. Webb ML, Cady B, Michaelson JS, et al. A failure analysis of invasive breast cancer: most deaths from disease occur in women not regularly screened. *Cancer* 2014; 120:2839–2846.

10. Feig S. Editorial response to Ref #5: Effectiveness of service screening: a case-control study to assess breast cancer mortality reduction. *Breast Diseases: A Year Book® Quarterly* 2012; 22:377–378.

11. Smith RA. The value of modern mammography screening in the control of breast cancer: understanding the underpinnings of the current debate. *Cancer Epidemiol Biomarkers Prev* 2014; 23:1139–1146.

## Chapter 17

1. The irony here is that low volume centers, where expertise is less likely, have the leeway to do work-ups on the spot rather than schedule a call-back. Interestingly, however, there are published studies that indicate a higher cancer detection rate when radiologists turn out the lights, sip some coffee, and "get in the groove" by reading screening studies in bunches, without interruptions. I can't attest to the scientific solidity of those studies, but it takes little imagination to see how that might be true.

2. The 1000-square grid has become a popular way to represent mammography in a poor light. Probably "borrowed" from Dr. H. Gilbert Welch's presentation, some forms of this presentation will light up (or color-in) a grossly inflated number of squares up to 300, with the intent to render a saved life nearly meaningless, a solitary square that lights up as the punchline.

3. Sanders ME, Schuyler PA, Simpson JF, Page DL, Dupont WD. Continued observation of the natural history of low-grade ductal carcinoma in situ reaffirms proclivity for local recurrence even after more than 30 years of follow-up. *Modern Pathology* 2015; 28:662–669.

4. It would seem that the author is focused on a single

screening benefit—saving lives. And this would be true. A list of other benefits to mammographic screening is often proposed. For instance, women with screen-detected cancers are allegedly more likely to undergo conservation surgery, that is, lumpectomy and radiation therapy, rather than mastectomy. Studies, however, are mixed on this claim, with some showing no difference in the surgery performed. Certainly, the *option* of lumpectomy is more common for screen-detected cancers, but a trend today is toward bilateral preventive mastectomies even after early diagnosis. This has dulled the impact on breast conservation rates among screen-detected cancers. Another claim made by pro-screeners is that women with screen-detected cancers are less likely to require chemotherapy. While this was the case in the days when adjuvant therapy was restricted to larger tumors and those with positive lymph nodes, today's guidelines include chemotherapy and biotherapies for some tumors less than 1.0cm in size, so the effect of early detection by mammography is muted here as well. In the end, the author sticks to one claim for breast cancer screening—saved lives.

## Chapter 18

1. Oeffinger KC, Fontham ET, Etzioni R, et al. Breast cancer screening for women at average risk: 2015 guideline update from the American Cancer Society. *JAMA* 2015; 314:1599–1614.

2. Brawley O, Byers T, Chen A, et al. New American Cancer Society process for creating trustworthy cancer screening guidelines. *JAMA* 2011; 306:2495–2499.

3. Broeders M, Moss S, Nystrom L, et al. The impact of mammographic screening on breast cancer mortality in Europe: a review of observational studies. *J Med Screen* 2012; 19 Suppl 1:14–25.

4. Myers ER, Moorman P, Gierisch JM, et al. Benefits and harms of breast cancer screening: a systematic review. *JAMA* 2015; 314:1615–1634.

5. Gøtzsche PC, Jørgensen KJ. Screening for breast cancer with mammography. *Cochrane Database Syst Rev* 2013; Jun 4;6:CD001877.

6. Gøtzsche PC. Time to stop mammography screening? *CMAJ* 2011; 183:1957–1958.

7. Webb ML, Cady B, Michaelson JS, et al. A failure analysis of invasive breast cancer: most deaths from disease occur in women not regularly screened. *Cancer* 2014; 120:2839–2846.

In this study of 7,301 patients diagnosed with breast cancer between 1990 and 1999, medical records were reviewed in detail to learn the screening habits of the 609 women from this group who had died specifically of breast cancer. 71% of the deaths occurred in unscreened women, while only 29% of the women had been screened. A disproportionate number of deaths occurred in women under 50 (50%), implicating more aggressive tumors and a greater need to screen. In the 40–49 age group, 70% of the deaths were in unscreened women, comparable to the overall 71%, but with a larger proportion of younger women. In comparison, in the over 70 group, only 47% of the deaths occurred in unscreened women.

8. Hollingsworth AB, Singletary SE, Morrow M,

et al. Current comprehensive assessment and management of women at increased risk for breast cancer. *Am J Surg* 2004; 187:349–362.

## Chapter 19

1. Dupont WD, Page DL. Risk factors for breast cancer in women with proliferative breast disease. *N Engl J Med* 1985; 312:146–151.

2. Hartmann LC, Degnim AC, Santen RJ, Dupont WD, Ghosh K. Atypical hyperplasia of the breast—risk assessment and management options. *N Engl J Med* 2015; 372:78–89.

3. Fisher B, Costantino JP, Wickerham DL, et al. Tamoxifen for prevention of breast cancer: report of the National Surgical Adjuvant Breast and Bowel Project P-1 Study. *Journal of the National Cancer Institute* 1998; 90:1371–1388.

4. Lambird PA, Shelley WM. The spatial distribution of lobular in situ mammary carcinoma: implications for size and site of biopsy. *JAMA* 1969; 210:689–693.

5. Bodian CA, Perzin KH, Lattes R. Lobular neoplasia: long term risk of breast cancer and relation to other factors. *Cancer* 1996; 78:1024–1034.

6. Hollingsworth AB. Risk assessment. In DS Francescatti, MJ Silverstein (Eds.), *Breast Cancer: A New Era in Management* (pp. 3–30) (New York: Springer Science+Business Media; 2014).

7. Saslow D, Boetes C, Burke W, et al for the American Cancer Society Breast Cancer Advisory Group. American Cancer Society guidelines for breast screening with MRI as an adjunct to mammography. *CA Cancer J Clin* 2007; 57:75–79.

8. King TA, Pilewskie M, Muhsen S, et al. Lobular carcinoma in situ: a 29-year longitudinal experience evaluating clinicopathologic features and breast cancer risk. *J Clin Oncol* 2015; 33:3945–3952.

9. Page DL, Kidd TE, Dupont WD, Simpson JF, Rogers LW. Lobular neoplasia of the breast: higher risk for subsequent invasive cancer predicted by more extensive disease. *Hum Pathol* 1991; 22:1232–1239.

10. Fadare O, Dadmanesh F, Alvarado-Cabrero I, et al. Lobular intraepithelial neoplasia (LCIS) with comedo-type necrosis: a clinicopathologic study of 18 cases. *Am J Surg Pathol* 2006; 30:1445–1453.

11. Hollingsworth AB, Stough RG. Multicentric and contralateral invasive tumors identified with pre-op MRI in patients newly diagnosed with ductal carcinoma in situ of the breast. *Breast J* 2012; 18:420–427. As of this writing in 2016, nearly 15 years after the clinical introduction of breast MRI, this was the only published study using MRI to identify the risk of invasive cancer "elsewhere," unrelated to the site of newly diagnosed DCIS.

12. Dawood S, Broglio K, Gonzalez-Angulo AM, et al. Development of new cancers in patients with DCIS: the MD Anderson experience. *Ann Surg Oncol* 2008; 15:244–249.

13. Narod SA, Iqbal J, Giannakeas V, Sopik V, Sun P. Breast cancer mortality after a diagnosis of ductal carcinoma in situ. *JAMA Oncol* 2015; 1:888–896.

14. Silverstein MJ, ed. *Ductal Carcinoma in Situ of the Breast*, 1st ed. (Philadelphia: Lippincott Williams & Wilkins; 1997).

15. Silverstein MJ, Lagios MD. Treatment selection for patients with ductal carcinoma in situ (DCIS) of the breast using the University of Southern California/Van Nuys (USC/VNPI) Prognostic Index. *Breast J* 2015; 21:127–132.

16. Lagios MD, Westdahl PR, Margolin FR, Rose MR. Duct carcinoma in situ. Relationship of noninvasive disease to the frequency of occult invasion, multicentricity, lymph node metastases, and short-term treatment failures. *Cancer* 1982: 50:1309–1314.

17. Fisher B, Dignam J, Wolmark N, et al. Tamoxifen in treatment of intraductal breast cancer: National Surgical Adjuvant Breast and Bowel Project B-24 randomised controlled trial. *The Lancet* 1999; 353:1993–2000.

18. Rosai J. Borderline epithelial lesions of the breast. *Am J Surg Pathol* 1991; 15:209–221.

19. Schnitt SJ, Connolly JL, Tavassoli FA, et al. Interobserver reproducibility in the diagnosis of ductal proliferative breast lesions using standardized criteria. *Am J Surg Pathol* 1992; 16:1133–1143.

20. Page DL, Anderson TJ. *Diagnostic Histopathology of the Breast* (New York: Churchill Livingstone; 1987).

21. Masood S. A call for change in the diagnosis and treatment of patients with ductal carcinoma in situ: an opportunity to minimize overdiagnosis and overtreatment. *Breast J* 2015: 21:575–578.

## Chapter 20

1. In 2000, the author published the first lay book on breast cancer risk assessment, intended as a local fund-raiser. (In fact, it was a "tie" for first. Patricia T. Kelly, PhD, published a similar book the same month— *Assess Your True Risk of Breast Cancer* [New York: Holt; 2000]). *The Truth About Breast Cancer Risk Assessment* (Aurora, CO: National Writers Press; 2000) was discovered by a visiting physician who gave a copy to Victor Vogel, M.D., arguably the nation's leading authority on breast cancer risk assessment and pharmacologic interventions. From there, the author was asked to serve as editor of a national risk assessment working group that published its guidelines in 2004 (Hollingsworth AB, Singletary SE, Morrow M, et al.... Vogel VG. Current comprehensive assessment and management of women at increased risk for breast cancer. *Am J Surg* 2004; 187: 349–362.)

2. The author hopes to update that original book on risk assessment and genetics, in which he will demonstrate the frailties of using lifetime risks as a guide to interventions.

3. Hollingsworth AB, Stough RG. An alternative approach to selecting patients for high-risk screening with breast MRI. *Breast J* 2014; 20: 192–197.

4. Webb ML, Cady B, Michaelson JS, et al. A failure analysis of invasive breast cancer: most deaths from disease occur in women not regularly screened. *Cancer* 2014; 120:2839–2846.

5. Price ER, Keedy AW, Gidwaney R, Sickles EA, Joe BN. The potential impact of risk-based screening mammography in women 40–49 years old. *AJR Am J Roentgenol* 2015; 205:1360–1364.

6. Mavaddat N, Pharoah PDP, Michailidou K, et al (200-PLUS authors). Prediction of breast cancer risk

based on profiling with common genetic variants. *J Natl Cancer Inst.* 2015; 107(5).

## Chapter 21

1. Although the concept of randomization and control groups dates back hundreds of years, the first published RCT in medicine was a study using streptomycin in the treatment of tuberculosis in 1948. Austin Bradford Hill, one of the investigators in that study, was given credit for the design, thereby becoming the originator of the modern RCT.

2. Today, patients with positive margins have the option of returning to the operating room to remove more tissue, and in most cases, this is successful and thus, mastectomy is not required. However, when the idea of lumpectomy was new, criteria for performing successful surgery were much more conservative. In the breast conservation trials where "standardization" was important, you couldn't allow some surgeons to re-excise tissue for wider margins while others were doing mastectomy after a positive margin.

3. Moss SM, Cuckle H, Evans A, et al. Effect of mammographic screening from age 40 years on breast cancer mortality at 10 years' follow-up: a randomized trial. *The Lancet* 2006; 368:2053–2060.

4. Moss SM, Wale C, Smith R, et al. Effect of mammographic screening from age 40 years on breast cancer mortality in the UK Age Trial at 17 years' follow-up: a randomized controlled trial. *Lancet Oncology* 2015; 16:1123–1132.

## Chapter 22

1. Pisano ED, Gatsonis C, Hendrick E, et al. Diagnostic performance of digital versus film screen mammography for breast-cancer screening. *N Engl J Med* 2005; 353:1773–1783. Although this reference was the initial announcement of results, the sub-group analysis was published later as Pisano ED, Hendrick RE, Yaffe MJ, et al. in *Radiology* 2008; 246:376–383. By the time this trial was broken up into 10 sub-groups, each group having both types of mammography, the number of cancers in any group was relatively small even though the trial began with 49,528 women.

2. Humphrey LL, Helfand M, Chan BK, Woolf SH. Breast cancer screening: a summary of the evidence for the U.S. Preventive Services Task Force. *Ann Int Med* 2002; 137:347–360.

3. Shen Y, Zelen M. Screening sensitivity and sojourn time from breast cancer early detection clinical trials: mammograms and physical examinations. *J Clin Oncol* 2001; 3490–3499.

4. Sensitivity for all screening rounds in the #3 reference above was reported as sub-groups in the Swedish Two-County and the Stockholm trial, rather than a single number. Swedish Two-County Sensitivity for all rounds was 53% for women in their 40s, 75% for women in their 50s, 69% for women in their 60s, and 92% for women in their 70s. In the Stockholm Trail, Sensitivity was 64% for women in their 40s and 89% for women in their 50s.

5. Hollingsworth AB, Taylor LDH, Rhodes DC. Establishing a histologic basis for false-negative mammograms. *Am J Surg* 1993; 166:643–647.

6. Ursin G, Hovanessian-Larsen L, Parisky YR, Pike MC, Wu AH. Greatly increased occurrence of breast cancers in areas of mammographically dense tissue. *Breast Cancer Res* 2005; 7:605–608. In 28 patients with a solitary focus of DCIS, only one patient was found to have calcium in a black zone. In 21 patients, the DCIS was clearly in a white zone, while 6 patients were indeterminate. The problem here is the chicken-egg scenario, as DCIS can elicit a inflammatory and fibrotic reaction that creates white patches on X-ray. Still, it is remarkable that more work along this line has not made it to the clinical literature (though basic scientists are pursuing the biologies of breast cancers that arise in fatty vs. dense tissue).

## Chapter 23

1. Wolfe JN. Breast patterns as an index of risk for developing breast cancer. *AJR* 1976; 126:1130–1139. Dr. John Wolfe (1923–1993) was a professor of radiology at Wayne State University School of Medicine in Detroit when he published his landmark paper. His N1 pattern today would be called "predominantly fatty" (estimated lifetime risk for breast cancer—2%), with the P-1 pattern being less than 25% prominent ducts, P-2 being greater than 25% prominent ducts, and DY (*dysplastic*) for dense fibro-glandular tissue. Acknowledgment for the "boy who cried Wolf" pun goes to Karla Kerlikowske, M.D., who wrote a *New England Journal of Medicine* editorial in 2007 titled "The Mammogram That Cried Wolfe." I should have known a pun so obvious would not be original on my part, but in truth, I found Dr. Kerlikowske's editorial in my files after I had written this chapter. So it probably was not an original thought on my part, but instead, extracted from a subliminal repository.

2. While all pioneering authors on breast ultrasound screening deserve mention, space limits us to the first authors on papers that led to the Society of Breast Imaging recommendations: Paula Gordon, Thomas M. Kolb, W. Buchberger, Stuart S. Kaplan, Isabelle Leconte, Pavel Crystal, V. Corsetti, W. Berg (see Ref. #5), and Kevin Kelly. Dr. Thomas Stavros played a key role in the development of breast ultrasound, as well as many others.

3. Hollingsworth AB, Stough RG. Breast MRI screening for high-risk patients. *Semin Breast Dis* 2008; 11:67–75. In this article, we gave our initial experience with MRI screening, using a point system that selected patients for auxiliary imaging equally weighted for risk and density. The scoring system also delineated the MRI interval, that is, MRI performed annually, every 2 years, or every 3 years. While this approach was intended for MRI, the principles are the same for ultrasound. Our preliminary findings were unsettling in that our MRI-discovered cancers were almost entirely in patients who would later prove to *not* qualify for MRI based on American Cancer Society guidelines introduced in 2007.

4. Cummings SR, Tice JA, Bauer S, et al. Prevention of breast cancer in postmenopausal women: approaches to estimating and reducing risk. *J Natl Cancer Inst* 2009; 101:384–398.

5. Berg WA, Zhang Z, Lehrer D, et al. for the ACRIN 6666 Investigators. Detection of breast cancer with addition of annual screening ultrasound or a single screening MRI to mammography in women with elevated cancer risk. *JAMA* 2012; 307:1394–1404.

6. Dr. Berg joined with JoAnn Pushkin and Cindy Henke-Sarmento to form their activist group called DENSE (website: DenseBreast-info.org).

## Chapter 24

1. A confession—In all its years of popularity, I never watched a single Oprah show in its entirety, or even more than 15 minutes while channel flipping. It was a complete fluke that I happened to see this segment on my way to work one morning, ruining my entire day.

2. As with ultrasound trials, I offer the lead authors in the publications from the 7 international trials—Warner (Canada), Kriege (the Netherlands), Kuhl (Germany), Leach (United Kingdom), Sardanelli (Italy), Riedl (Austria), and Lehman (United States).

3. Hillman BJ, Harms SE, Stevens G, et al. Diagnostic performance of a dedicated 1.5-T breast MR Imaging system. *Radiology* 2012; 265:51–58.

4. Sardanelli F, Podo F. Breast MR imaging in women at high-risk of breast cancer: is something changing in early breast cancer detection? *Eur Radiol* 2007; 17:873–887.

5. These counter-intuitive results came from a subset analysis in the Canadian MRI trial where all patients were at comparable risk since they were all BRCA-positive. With this variable held steady, the Sensitivity of mammography was evaluated in the over 50 vs. under 50 group and published in the *Proc Am Soc Clin Oncol* 2004: 23:841 (abstract), while the low density Sensitivity of 33% was published in *Cancer Epidemiol Biomarkers Prev* 2008; 17:706–711.

6. Hollingsworth AB, Stough RG. An alternative approach to selecting patients for high-risk screening with breast MRI. *The Breast Journal* 2014; 20:192–197.

7. Ikeda DM, Birdwell RL, O'Shaughnessy KF, et al. Analysis of 172 subtle findings on prior normal mammograms in women with breast cancer detected at follow-up screening. *Radiology* 2003; 226:494–503. In this study, 286 women out of 493 (58%) had something going on at the cancer site one year earlier. The 172 in the title refers to those changes that were "too subtle" to fault the radiologist, but the other 114 could be construed as mammographic misses through interpretation.

8. Schrading S, Strobel K, Kuhl C. University Hospital RWTH Aachen, Aachen, Germany. MRI screening of women at average risk of breast cancer. General Session, 36th Annual San Antonio Breast Cancer Symposium, 2013.

9. Shen Y, Zelen M. Screening sensitivity and sojourn time from breast cancer early detection clinical trials: mammograms and physical examinations. *J Clin Oncol* 2001; 3490–3499.

## Chapter 25

1. Mandelblatt JS, Cronin KA, Bailey S, et al. Effects of mammography screening under different screening schedules: model estimates of potential benefits and harms. *Ann Intern Med* 2009; 151:738–747.

2. Hendrick RE, Helvie MA. United States Preventive Services Task Force screening mammography recommendations: science ignored. *AJR* 2011; 196:W112–W116.

3. Dr. Harms' name on the speakers docket was so common that many of us non-radiologists believed that RODEO® MRI (Rotating Delivery of Excitation Off-Resonance) was the only method of breast MRI in existence. Breast MRI was delayed by 20 years compared to the rest of the body. Many problems had stalled the development of breast MRI, most notably the "biopsy problem," or how to perform a biopsy so that the needle doesn't interfere with the image being generated on the MRI.

4. Moroz C, Shamai G, Kupfer B, Urca I. Ferritin-bearing lymphocytes and T-cell levels in peripheral blood of patients with breast cancer. *Cancer Immunology and Immunotherapy* 1977; 3:101–105.

5. Matritech, CeMines, Fred Hutchinson Cancer Center, A&G Pharmaceuticals, Power3 Medical Technologies, DiaGenic (Norway), OncImmune (U.K.), University of Ferrara (Italy), and Provista Diagnostics (Scottsdale/New York). Provista Diagnostics, Inc. is the biotechnology company that has converted a multiple marker approach into a blood test (Videssa®) that predicts when further clinical action is appropriate in the diagnostic setting. Financial disclosure: the author serves as a consultant to Provista Diagnostics.

6. The sites for the Provista blood test study were The Cleveland Clinic, Mayo Clinic Rochester, Mayo Clinic Scottsdale, St. Joseph's (Phoenix, AZ), Sinai Grace (Detroit, MI), Scripps (San Diego, CA), Henry Ford (Detroit, MI), Sutter (Sacramento, CA), Rhode Island Hospital (Providence, RI), Avera Cancer Institute (Sioux Falls, SD), Banner—University Medical Center (Phoenix, AZ), Sansum Clinic (Santa Barbara, CA), Lahey Clinic (Peabody, MA), Summit Medical Group Breast Center (Berkeley Heights, NJ) and Mercy Breast Center (Oklahoma City, OK).

7. Reese DE, Silver M, Henderson MC et al. Age-related variations: A retrospective analysis of 851 prospectively collected patient samples to determine the benefit of combining combinatorial protein biomarker assay for risk assessment in women with dense breast. J Clin Oncol 2015; 33:Suppl 27 (abstract)

8. Hollingsworth AB, Reese DE. Potential use of biomarkers to augment clinical decisions for the early detection of breast cancer. *Oncology and Hematology Review* 2014; 10:103–109.

9. Gladwell M. *Outliers* (Boston: Little, Brown; 2008).

10. Zheng B, Tan M, Ramalingam P, Gur D. Association between computed tissue density asymmetry in bilateral mammograms and near-term breast cancer risk. *The Breast Journal* 2014; 20:249–257.

11. National Cancer Institute Grant #1R01CA197150-01. Hollingsworth A, Liu H, Zheng B. Increasing Cancer Detection Yield Using Breast MRI Screening Modality. Awarded July 2015.

## Chapter 26

1. Let me apologize for glossing over MBI, or "molecular breast imaging," in this book which, if it weren't

for the total body radiation exposure, would very likely have already replaced breast MRI. Sensitivity is about the same as MRI (90+%), while Specificity seems to be better (fewer false-positives). "Molecular breast imaging" is a nuclear medicine scan that involves the injection of a radionuclide that "lights up" cancer, similar to the gadolinium "enhancement" on MRI (the latter, however, without radiation exposure). The radiation exposure for a single "molecular imaging" study is harmless, but my hesitancy has been to use this technology for yearly screening studies over a lifetime. Pre-op staging, or evaluating a diagnostic problem, is where this technology will probably find its home. While development of PEM (PET mammography) and MBI have occurred in tandem, it's the latter that is gaining momentum. The Mayo Clinic has been heavily focused on MBI and is responsible for a good portion of the development. In the early days of both MRI and MBI, I was presenting my "90% Sensitivity talk" (it had a novelty aspect to it, sort of like juggling chainsaws for entertainment) at a meeting of radiologists, where a PhD who was developing MBI at the Mayo Clinic was on the program as well. She came up after my talk and said, "I wanted to stand up and clap. No one will talk about the true sensitivity of mammography." Of course, her MBI was based on the identical premise that I had proposed—the Sensitivity of mammography is not nearly as high as we've thought, now that we have other imaging methods for direct comparisons.

2. Certainly, oncologists could use a blood test to guide breast cancer management, unrelated to screening. A blood test could be used for prognosis and to predict response to therapies (as opposed to the older markers that were used to check for recurrences, but without guiding treatment). The detection of circulating tumor cells (CTCs) is commercially available, and cell-free DNA in blood samples is being studied as well. Then, when you move into microRNAs and a host of other candidate biomarkers, there might be some that are applicable both for screening as well as monitoring treatment and detecting recurrences. Obviously, this is a hotbed of rapid developments, but if you are inclined to follow the research here, it is important to distinguish the exact strengths and weaknesses of proposed biomarkers, as we probably won't see an all-purpose blood test. The host reaction changes as cancer gains a foothold, and the biomarkers for early detection could easily prove to be different than those that guide therapy, which could be different still than those that detect recurrences.

# Bibliography

Agency for Healthcare Quality and Research. http://www.ahrq.gov/cpi/about/index.html. Accessed July 16, 2015.

Allgood PC, Warwick J, Warren RM, et al. A case-control study of the impact of the East Anglian breast screening programme on breast cancer mortality. Br J Cancer 2008; 98:206–209.

American Cancer Society. Cancer Facts & Figures 2015. Atlanta: American Cancer Society; 2015.

Are You Dense, Inc. http://www.areyoudense.org/. Accessed October 12, 2015.

Author of Canadian breast cancer study retracts warnings. JNCI, 1992; 84:832–833.

Baines CJ. The Canadian National Breast Screening Study: a perspective on criticisms. Ann Intern Med 1994; 120:326–334.

Baines CJ, Miller AB, Kopans DB, et al. Canadian National Breast Screening Study: assessment of technical quality by external review. AJR Am J Roentgenol 1990; 155:743–747.

Berg WA, Zhang Z, Lehrer D, et al. for the ACRIN 6666 Investigators. Detection of breast cancer with addition of annual screening ultrasound or a single screening MRI to mammography in women with elevated cancer risk. JAMA 2012; 307:1394–1404.

Berry DA. Breast cancer screening: controversy of impact. The Breast 2013; 22:S73-S76.

Berry DA, Cronin KA, Plevritis SK, et al. Cancer Intervention and Surveillance Modeling Network (CISNET) Collaborators: effect of screening and adjuvant therapy on mortality from breast cancer. N Engl J Med 2005; 353:1784–1792.

Bevers, Therese B. Flaws in CNBSS are vast, impact on screening recommendations is nil. The ASCO Post 2014; 5.

Bigenwald RZ, Warner E, Gunasekara A, et al. Is mammography adequate for screening women with inherited BRCA mutations and low breast density? Cancer Epidemiol Biomarkers Prev 2008; 17:706–711.

Bland, Kirby I., Copeland, Edward M. The Breast: Comprehensive Management of Benign and Malignant Diseases. Philadelphia: W.B. Saunders; 1998.

Bleyer A, Welch HG. Effect of three decades of screening mammography on breast-cancer incidence. N Engl J Med 2012; 367:1998–2005.

Bloche, Gregg. The Hippocratic Myth: Why Doctors Have to Ration Care, Practice Politics, and Compromise Their Promise to Heal. New York: Palgrave Macmillan; 2011.

Bloom HJ, Richardson WW, Harries EJ. Natural history of untreated breast cancer (1805–1933). Comparison of untreated and treated cases according to histological grade of malignancy. Br Med J 1962; 2:213–221.

Bodian CA, Perzin KH, Lattes R. Lobular neoplasia: long term risk of breast cancer and relation to other factors. Cancer 1996; 78:1024–1034.

Boyd NF. The review of randomization in the Canadian National Breast Screening Study. Is the debate over? Can Med Assoc J 1997; 156:207–209.

Boyd NF, Guo H, Martin LJ, et al. Mammographic density and the risk and detection of breast cancer. N Engl J Med 2007; 356:227–236.

Brawley, O. Guest commentary: the benefits and harms of cancer screening. NCI Cancer Bulletin 2012; 9/.

Brawley O, Byers T, Chen A, et al. New American Cancer Society process for creating trustworthy cancer screening guidelines. JAMA 2011; 306:2495-2499.

Brawley, O, Goldberg, Paul. How We Do Harm: A Doctor Breaks Ranks About Being Sick in America. New York: St. Martin's Griffin; 2012.

Breast Cancer Screening for Health Professionals (PDQ®), National Cancer Institute. http://www.cancer.gov/types/breast/hp/breast-screening-pdq#link/_13_toc. Accessed January 11, 2016.

Broeders M, Moss S, Nystrom L, et al. The impact of mammographic screening on breast cancer mortality in Europe: a review of observational studies. J Med Screen 2012; 19 Suppl 1:14–25.

Brower, Vicki. Breast density gains acceptance as breast cancer risk factor. Journal of the National Cancer Institute News 2010; 102:374–375.

Burstein, H. Editorial: expert opinion vs guideline based care: the St. Gallen Case study. The Breast 2013; 22: S1-S2.

Cassidy J, Rayment T. Breast scans boost risk of cancer death. The Sunday Times, London, June 2, 1991.

Charles B. Huggins - Biographical. Nobelprize.org. Nobel Media AB 2014. http://www.nobelprize.org/nobel_prizes/medicine/laureates/1966/huggins-bio.html. Accessed April 13, 2015.

Coldman A, Phillips N, Wilson C, et al. Pan-Canadian study of mammography screening and mortality from breast cancer. *J Natl Cancer Inst* 2014; 106. doi: 10. 1093/jnci/dju261.

Cummings SR, Tice JA, Bauer S, et al. Prevention of breast cancer in postmenopausal women: approaches to estimating and reducing risk. *J Natl Cancer Inst* 2009; 101:384–398.

Davis, AM. Lung cancer screening. JAMA clinical guidelines synopsis. *JAMA* 2014; 312:1248–1248.

Dawood S, Broglio K, Gonzalez-Angulo AM, et al. Development of new cancers in patients with DCIS: the M.D. Anderson experience. *Ann Surg Oncol* 2008; 15:244–249.

Dean PB. Gøtzsche's quixotic antiscreening campaign: nonscientific and contrary to Cochrane principles. *J Am Coll Radiol* 2004; 1:3–7.

DenseBreast-info, Inc. http://densebreast-info.org/. Accessed November 16, 2015.

Department of Health and Human Services. http://www.hhs.gov/. Accessed June 2, 2015.

Dodd GD. Editorial response to Kopans DB, Feig SA. The Canadian National Breast Screening Study: a critical review (*AJR Am J Roentgenol* 1993; 161:755–760), published in *Breast Diseases: A Year Book® Quarterly* 1994; 5:46–47.

Dupont WD, Page DL. Risk factors for breast cancer in women with proliferative breast disease. *N Engl J Med* 1985; 312:146–151.

Eapen ZJ, Lauer, MS, Temple RJ. The imperative of overcoming barriers to the conduct of large, simple trials. *JAMA* 2014; 311:1397–1398.

Elmore JG, Longton GM, Carney PA, et al. Diagnostic concordance among pathologists interpreting breast biopsy specimens. *JAMA* 2015; 313:1122–1132.

Fadare O, Dadmanesh F, Alvarado-Cabrero I, et al. Lobular intraepithelial neoplasia (LCIS) with comedotype necrosis: a clinicopathologic study of 18 cases. *Am J Surg Pathol* 2006; 30:1445–1453.

Feig SA. Editorial response: Effectiveness of service screening: a case-control study to assess breast cancer mortality reduction. *Breast Diseases: A Year Book® Quarterly* 2012; 22:377–378.

Feig SA. Overdiagnosis of invasive breast cancer and DCIS: why do estimates vary? *Breast Diseases: A Year Book® Quarterly* 2014; 25:196–201.

Feig SA. U.S. Preventive Services Task Force screening recommendations: a step backwards to less effective screening. *Breast Diseases: A Year Book® Quarterly* 2010; 21:105–108.

Feig SA, Shaber GS, Schwartz GF, et al. Thermography, mammography, and clinical examination in breast cancer screening: review of 16,000 studies. *Radiology* 1977; 122:123–127.

Feynman, Richard P. *The Meaning of It All: Thoughts of a Citizen-scientist*. New York: Helix Books; 1998.

Fielder HM, Warwick J, Brook D, et al. A case-control study to estimate the impact on breast cancer death of the breast screening programme in Wales. *J Med Screen* 2004; 11:194–198.

Firestein, Stuart. What science wants to know: an impenetrable mountain of facts can obscure the deeper questions. *Scientific American* 2012; April: 10.

Fisher B, Costantino JP, Wickerham DL, et al. Tamoxifen for prevention of breast cancer: report of the National Surgical Adjuvant Breast and Bowel Project P-1 Study.

*Journal of the National Cancer Institute* 1998; 90:1371–1388.

Fisher B, Dignam J, Wolmark N, et al. Tamoxifen in treatment of intraductal breast cancer: National Surgical Adjuvant Breast and Bowel Project B-24 randomised controlled trial. *The Lancet* 1999; 353:1993–2000.

Fletcher SW, Black W, Harris R, Rimer BK, Shapiro S. Report of the International Workshop on Screening for Breast Cancer. *J Natl Cancer Inst* 1993; 85:1644–1656.

Fletcher SW, Elmore JG. Clinical practice: mammographic screening for breast cancer. *N Engl J Med* 2003; 348:1672–1680.

Freedman DA, Petitti DB, Robins JM. On the efficacy of screening for breast cancer. *Int J Epidemiol* 2004; 33:43–55.

Haas GP, Delongchamps N, Brawley OW, Wang CY, de La Roza, G. The worldwide epidemiology of prostate cancer: perspectives from autopsy studies. *Can J Urol* 2008; 15: 3866–3871.

Gladwell M. *Outliers: The Story of Success.* Boston: Little, Brown; 2008.

Gold RH, Bassett LW, Widoff BE. Radiologic history exhibit: highlights from the history of mammography. *RadioGraphics* 1990; 10:1111–1131.

Goldberger JJ, Buxton AE. Personalized medicine vs guideline-based medicine. *JAMA* 2013; 309:2559–2560.

Goldman, SL. *Science Wars: What Scientists Know and How They Know It.* Chantilly, VA: The Great Courses; 2006. Audio.

Gordon, Paula. Canadian National Breast Screening Study—Flaws. *BCMJ* 2014; 56:126–127.

Gordon, P. Editorial: it's just wrong. Mammography Education, Inc. http://www.mammographyed.com/Resources/15266/FileRepository/ItsJustWrong_DrPaulaGordon.pdf. Accessed November 12, 2015.

Gordon, P. Opinion: shoddy Canadian research is putting women's lives at risk. Regular mammography screenings detect cancer, despite what flawed study reported. Special to the *Vancouver Sun*, February 13, 2014.

Gøtzsche PC. Time to stop mammography screening? *CMAJ* 2011; 183:1957–1958.

Gøtzsche PC, Jørgensen KJ. Screening for breast cancer with mammography. *Cochrane Database Syst Rev* 2013; Jun 4;6:CD001877.

Gøtzsche PC, Olsen O. Is screening for breast cancer with mammography justifiable? *The Lancet* 2000; 355:129–134.

Guidi AJ, Fischer L, Harris JR, Schnitt SJ. Microvessel density and distribution in DCIS of the breast. *J Natl Cancer Inst* 1994; 86:614–619.

Güth U, Huang DJ, Huber M, et al. Tumor size and detection in breast cancer: self-examination and clinical breast exam are at their limit. *Cancer Detect Prev* 2008; 32:224–228.

Harms SE. Introduction to the International Working Groups on Breast MRI. *Breast J* 2004; 10 Suppl 2: S1–2.

Harms SE, Radensky P, Sunshine J, et al. MRI efficacy and effectiveness research: who needs it and who pays for it? *J Magn Reson Imaging* 1996; 6:4–6.

Hartmann LC, Degnim AC, Santen RJ, Dupont WD,

Ghosh K. Atypical hyperplasia of the breast—risk assessment and management options. *N Engl J Med* 2015; 372:78–89.

Hellman S. Karnofsky Memorial Lecture. Natural history of small breast cancers. *J Clin Oncol* 1994; 12: 2229–2234.

Hellquist BN, Duffy SW, Abdsaleh S, et al. Effectiveness of population-based service screening with mammography for women ages 40 to 49 years: evaluation of the Swedish Mammography Screening in Young Women (SCRY) cohort. *Cancer* 2011; 117:714–722.

Henderson MC, Silver M, Yeh S, et al. Use of serum biomarkers to differentiate benign breast lesions from invasive breast cancer in women with a BI-RADS 3 or 4. *J Clin Oncol* 2014; 32 (Suppl) (September 10), 20 (abstract).

Hendrick RE, Helvie MA. United States Preventive Services Task Force screening guidelines: science ignored. *AJR Am J Roentgenol* 2011; W112-W116.

Hillman BJ, Harms SE, Stevens G, et al. Diagnostic performance of a dedicated 1.5-T breast MR Imaging system. *Radiology* 2012; 265:51–58.

Hitti, Miranda. Breast self-exams: no survival benefit. *WebMD Health News*. http://www.webmd.com/breast-cancer/news/20080715/breast-self-exam-no-survival-benefit. Accessed August 25, 2008.

Hollingsworth AB. Chapter 1: Risk Assessement, in: *Breast Cancer: A New Era In Management*. Editors: Francescatti DS, Silverstein MJ. New York: Springer; 2014.

Hollingsworth AB, Reese DE. Potential use of biomarkers to augment clinical decisions for the early detection of breast cancer. *Oncology and Hematology Review* 2014; 10:103–109.

Hollingsworth AB, Singletary SE, Morrow M, et al. Current comprehensive assessment and management of women at increased risk for breast cancer. *Am J Surg* 2004; 187:349–362.

Hollingsworth AB, Stough RG. An alternative approach to selecting patients for high-risk screening with breast MRI. *Breast J* 2014; 20: 192–197.

Hollingsworth AB, Stough RG. Breast MRI screening for high-risk patients. *Semin Breast Dis* 2008; 11:67–75.

Hollingsworth AB, Stough RG. Multicentric and contralateral invasive tumors identified with pre-op MRI in patients newly diagnosed with ductal carcinoma in situ of the breast. *Breast J* 2012; 18:420–427.

Hollingsworth AB, Taylor LDH, Rhodes DC. Establishing a histologic basis for false-negative mammograms. *Am J Surg* 1993; 166:643–647.

Horn SD, Gassaway J, Pentz L, James R. Practice-based evidence for clinical practice improvement: an alternative study design for evidence-based medicine. *Stud Health Technol Inform* 2010; 151:446–460.

Humphrey LL, Helfand M, Chan BK, Woolf SH. Breast cancer screening: a summary of evidence for the U.S. Preventive Services Task Force. *Ann Int Med* 2002; 137:347–360.

Ikeda DM, Birdwell RL, O'Shaughnessy KF, et al. Analysis of 172 subtle findings on prior normal mammograms in women with breast cancer detected at follow-up screening. *Radiology* 2003; 226:494–503.

Ioannidis JP. Contradicted and initially stronger effects in highly cited clinical research. *JAMA* 2005; 294: 218–228.

Jatoi I, Miller AB. Breast cancer screening in elderly women: primum non nocere. *JAMA* 2015; 150:1107–1108.

Kalager M, Zelen M, Langmark F, et al. Effect of screening mammography on breast-cancer mortality in Norway. *N Engl J Med* 2010; 363:1203–1210.

Kent DM, Shah ND. Risk models and patient-centered evidence. Should physicians expect one right answer? *JAMA* 2012; 307:1585–1586.

King TA, Pilewskie M, Muhsen S, et al. Lobular carcinoma in situ: a 29-year longitudinal experience evaluating clinicopathologic features and breast cancer risk. *J Clin Oncol* 2015; 33:3945–3952.

Kinsinger L, Harris R, Karnitschnig J. Interest in decision-making about breast cancer screening in younger women. *J Gen Intern Med* 1998; 13(Suppl):98. Abstract.

Kolata G. Vast study casts doubts on value of mammograms. *New York Times*, February 11, 2014.

Kopans DB. Mammography still saves lives. Medscape Ob/Gyn 2014 (online). http://www.medscape.com/viewarticle/820705_print. Accessed February 25, 2014.

Kopans, DB. Review of papers in current oncology on the CNBSS women ages 40–49. Society of Breast Imaging (online). http://www.sbi-online.org/Portals/0/downloads/DOCUMENTS/pdfs/Kopans%20Critique%20(2)%20(2).pdf. Accessed August 16, 2015.

Kopans DB. The 2009 U.S. Preventive Services Task Force Guidelines ignore important scientific evidence and should be revised or withdrawn. *Radiology* 2010; 256:15–20.

Kopans DB, Feig SA. The Canadian National Breast Screening Study: a critical review. *AJR Am J Roentgenol* 1993; 161:755–760.

Kuhl CK. The "coming of age" of nonmammographic screening for breast cancer. *JAMA* 2008; 299:2203–2205.

Lagios MD, Westdahl PR, Margolin FR, Rose MR. Duct carcinoma in situ: relationship of noninvasive disease to the frequency of occult invasion, multicentricity, lymph node metastases, and short-term treatment failures. *Cancer* 1982: 50:1309–1314.

Lambird PA, Shelley WM. The spatial distribution of lobular in situ mammary carcinoma. Implications for size and site of biopsy. *JAMA* 1969; 210:689–693.

Larsson LG, Andersson I, Bjurstam N, et al. Updated overview of the Swedish Randomized Trials on Breast Cancer Screening with Mammography: age group 40–49 at randomization. *J Natl Cancer Inst Monogr* 1997; 22:57–61.

Lerner, Barron H. *To See Today with the Eyes of Tomorrow: A history of screening mammography*. Background paper for the Institute of Medicine report: "Mammography and Beyond: Developing Technologies for the Early Detection of Breast Cancer," March 2001. Published in *Can Bull Med Hist* 2003; 20:299–321.

Lerner, Barron H. *The Breast Cancer Wars: Hope, Fear and the Pursuit of a Cure of Twentieth-Century America*. Oxford: Oxford University Press; 2001.

Linton, Otha. *Moments in Radiology History: Part 15—Mammography's Roots*, May 9, 2014. http://www.aunt

minnie.com/index.aspx?sec=ser&sub=def&pag=dis&ItemID=107358. Accessed March 3, 2015.

Lowenfels, AB. Nobel-honored Surgeons. Medscape General Surgery (online), 2009. http://www.medscape.com/viewarticle/704979_2. Accessed May 19, 2015.

Mandelblatt JS, Cronin KA, Bailey S, et al. Effects of mammography screening under different screening schedules: model estimates of potential benefits and harms. *Ann Intern Med* 2009; 151:738–747.

Masood S. A call for change in the diagnosis and treatment of patients with ductal carcinoma in situ: an opportunity to minimize overdiagnosis and overtreatment. *Breast J* 2015: 21:575–578.

Mavaddat N, Pharoah PDP, Michailidou K, et al. Prediction of breast cancer risk based on profiling with common genetic variants. *J Natl Cancer Inst* 2015; 107(5).

McDivitt, RW, Stewart FW, Berg, JW. *Tumors of the Breast*. Washington, D.C.: Armed Forces Institute of Pathology; 1968.

McGrayne, SB. *The Theory That Would Not Die: How Bayes' Rule Cracked the Enigma Code, Hunted Down Russian Submarines, and Emerged Triumphant from Two Centuries of Controversy*. New Haven: Yale University Press; 2011.

Merkow R, Ko CY. Evidence-based medicine in surgery: the importance of both experimental and observational study designs. *JAMA* 2011; 306:436–437.

Miller, A. Early detection of breast cancer, chapter 5. *Breast Diseases*. Harris JR, Hellman S, Henderson IC, Kinne D. Philadelphia: J.B. Lippincott; 1987.

Miller AB, Baines CJ, To T, Wall C. Canadian National Breast Screening Study: 1. Breast cancer detection and death rates among women aged 40 to 49 years. *CMAJ* 1992; 15:1459–1476.

Miller AB, Wall C, Baines CJ, Sun P, To T, Narod SA. Twenty five year follow-up for breast cancer incidence and mortality of the Canadian National Breast Screening Study: randomized screening trial. *BMJ* 2014; 348:g366.

Misconduct in science: an array of errors. *Economist*. Sept. 10, 2011.

Moroz C, Shamai G, Kupfer B, Urca I. Ferritin-bearing lymphocytes and T-cell levels in peripheral blood of patients with breast cancer. *Cancer Immunology and Immunotherapy* 1977; 3:101–105.

Moss SM, Cuckle H, Evans A, et al. Effect of mammographic screening from age 40 years on breast cancer mortality at 10 years' follow-up: a randomized trial. *The Lancet* 2006: 368:2053–2060.

Moss SM, Wale C, Smith R, et al. Effect of mammographic screening from age 40 years on breast cancer mortality in the UK Age Trial at 17 years' follow-up: a randomized controlled trial. *Lancet Oncology* 2015; 16:1123–1132.

Mukherjee, Siddhartha. *The Emperor of All Maladies: A Biography of Cancer*. New York: Scribner; 2010.

Myers ER, Moorman P, Gierisch JM, et al. Benefits and harms of breast cancer screening: a systematic review. *JAMA* 2015; 314:1615–1634.

Narod SA, Iqbal J, Giannakeas V, Sopik V, Sun P. Breast cancer mortality after a diagnosis of ductal carcinoma in situ. *JAMA Oncol* 2015; 1:888–896.

National Guideline Clearinghouse, Agency for Healthcare Research and Quality. https://www.guideline.gov/. Accessed August 2, 2015.

O'Conner, S. What if I decide to just do Nothing? *TIME*, October 12, 2015.

Oeffinger KC, Fontham ET, Etzioni R, et al. Breast cancer screening for women at average risk: 2015 guideline update from the American Cancer Society. *JAMA* 2015; 314:1599–1614.

Olsen O, Gøtzsche PC. Cochrane review on screening for breast cancer with mammography. *The Lancet* 2001; 358:1340–1342.

Pace LE, Keating NL. A systematic assessment of benefits and risks to guide breast cancer screening decisions. *JAMA* 2014; 311:1327–1335.

Page DL, Anderson TJ. *Diagnostic Histopathology of the Breast*. New York: Churchill Livingstone; 1987.

Page DL, Kidd TE, Dupont WD, Simpson JF, Rogers LW. Lobular neoplasia of the breast: higher risk for subsequent invasive cancer predicted by more extensive disease. *Hum Pathol* 1991; 22:1232–1239.

Park, A. Screening Cancer: a new study reveals mammograms may not be doing much good. *TIME*, page 18, February 24, 2014.

Park A, Picket K. The mammogram melee: why the furor over the new screening guidelines could be a sign of things to come. *TIME*, December 7, 2009.

Pisano ED, Gatsonis C, Hendrick E, et al. Diagnostic performance of digital versus film screen mammography for breast-cancer screening. *N Engl J Med* 2005; 353:1773–1783.

Pisano ED, Hendrick RE, Yaffe MJ, et al. DMIST Investigators Group. Diagnostic accuracy of digital versus film mammography: exploratory analysis of selected population subgroups in DMIST. *Radiology* 2008; 246:376–383.

Price ER, Keedy AW, Gidwaney R, Sickles EA, Joe BN. The potential impact of risk-based screening mammography in women 40–49 years old. *AJR Am J Roentgenol* 2015; 205:1360–1364.

Puliti D, Miccinesi G, Collina N, et al. Effectiveness of service screening: a case-control study to assess breast cancer mortality reduction. *Br J Cancer* 2008; 99: 423–427.

Puliti D, Zappa M, Miccinesi G, Falini P, Crocetti E, Pace E. An estimate of overdiagnosis 15 years after the start of mammographic screening in Florence. *Eur J Cancer* 2009; 45:3166–3171.

Ransohoff DF, Pignone M, Sox H. How to decide whether a clinical practice guideline is trustworthy. *JAMA* 2013; 309:139–140.

Reese DE, Silver M, Henderson MC, et al. Age-related variations: a retrospective analysis of 851 prospectively collected patient samples to determine the benefit of combining combinatorial protein biomarker assay for risk assessment in women with dense breasts. *J Clin Oncol* 2015; 33: Suppl 27 (abstract).

Reinhart, Alex. *Statistics Done Wrong*. San Francisco: No Starch Press; 2015.

Rosai J. Borderline epithelial lesions of the breast. *Am J Surg Pathol* 1991; 15:209–221.

Rosenbaum L. Invisible risks, emotional choices—mammography and medical decision making. *N Engl J Med* 2014; 371:1549–1552.

Saey, TH. Come again, research results? Scientists tackle the irreproducibility problem. *Science News*, December 26, 2015.

Sanders ME, Schuyler PA, Simpson JF, Page DL, Dupont WD. Continued observation of the natural history of low-grade ductal carcinoma in situ reaffirms proclivity for local recurrence even after more than 30 years of follow-up. *Modern Pathology* 2015; 28:662–669.

Sardanelli F, Podo F. Breast MR imaging in women at high-risk of breast cancer. Is something changing in early breast cancer detection? *Eur Radiol* 2007; 17: 873–887.

Saslow D, Boetes C, Burke W, et al for the American Cancer Society Breast Cancer Advisory Group. American Cancer Society guidelines for breast screening with MRI as an adjunct to mammography. *CA Cancer J Clin* 2007; 57:75–79.

Schnitt SJ, Connolly JL, Tavassoli FA, et al. Interobserver reproducibility in the diagnosis of ductal proliferative breast lesions using standardized criteria. *Am J Surg Pathol* 1992; 16:1133–1143.

Schrading S, Strobel K, Kuhl C. University Hospital RWTH Aachen, Aachen, Germany. MRI screening of women at average risk of breast cancer. General Session, 36th Annual San Antonio Breast Cancer Symposium, 2013.

Shapiro S, Venet W, Strax P, et al. Selection, follow-up, and analysis in the Health Insurance Plan Study: a randomized trial with breast cancer screening. *Natl Cancer Inst Monogr* 1985; 67:65–74.

Shaw DM. Beyond conflicts of interest: disclosing medical biases. *JAMA* 2014; 312:697–698.

Shen Y, Zelen M. Screening sensitivity and sojourn time from breast cancer early detection clinical trials: mammograms and physical examinations. *J Clin Oncol* 2001; 3490–3499.

Silverstein MJ, ed. *Ductal Carcinoma in Situ of the Breast*, 1st edition. Baltimore: Williams and Wilkins; 1997.

Silverstein, MJ, ed. Recht A, Lagios M, associate eds. *Ductal Carcinoma in Situ of the Breast*. Philadelphia: Lippincott Williams & Wilkins, 2nd edition; 2002.

Silverstein MJ, Lagios MD. Treatment selection for patients with ductal carcinoma in situ (DCIS) of the breast using the University of Southern California/Van Nuys (USC/VNPI) Prognostic Index. *Breast J* 2015; 21:127–132.

Simpson, David. Francis Bacon (1561–1626). Internet Encyclopedia of Philosophy: A Peer-Reviewed Academic Resource. http://www.iep.utm.edu/bacon/. Accessed July 2015.

Siu AL: U.S. Preventive Services Task Force. Screening for breast cancer: U.S. Preventive Services Task Force recommendation statement. *Ann Intern Med* 2016; 164:279–296.

Skloot R. Taboo organ: How a Pitt alum refused to let mammography be ignored. *PittMed: University of Pittsburgh School of Medicine Magazine* 2001; 3.

Smith R, Rennie D. Evidence-based medicine—an oral history. *JAMA* 2014; 311:365–367.

Smith RA. Counterpoint: overdiagnosis in breast cancer screening. *J Am Coll Radiol* 2014; 11:648–652.

Smith RA. The value of modern mammography screening in the control of breast cancer: understanding the underpinnings of the current debate. *Cancer Epidemiol Biomarkers Prev* 2014; 23:1139–1146.

Sniderman, AD, Furberg CD. Why guideline-making requires reform. *JAMA* 2009; 301:429–431.

Squiers LB, Holden DJ, Dolina SE, et al. The public's response to the U.S. Preventive Services Task Force's 2009 recommendations on mammography screening. *Am J Prev Med* 2011; 40:497–504.

Sullivan P, Goldmann D. The promise of comparative effectiveness research. *JAMA* 2011; 305:400–401.

Tabár L. Mammography Education, Inc. http://www.mammographyed.com. Accessed September 2, 2015.

Tabár L, Duffy SW, Burhenne LW. New Swedish breast cancer detection results for women aged 40–49. *Cancer* 1993; 72:1437–1448.

Tabár L, Fagerberg CJ, Gad A, et al. Reduction in mortality from breast cancer after mass screening with mammography. Randomised trial from the Breast Cancer Screening Working Group of the Swedish National Board of Health and Welfare. *Lancet* 1985; 1(8433):829–832.

Tabár L, Vitak B, Chen TH, et al. Swedish two-county trial: impact of mammographic screening on breast cancer mortality during 3 decades. *Radiology* 2011; 260:658–663.

Tarone RE. The excess of patients with advanced breast cancer in young women screened with mammography in the Canadian National Breast Screening Study. *Cancer* 1995; 75:997–1003.

*This Month in Physics History: November 8, 1895—Roentgen's Discovery of X-rays*. APS Physics (online)—American Physical Society. http://www.aps.org/publications/apsnews/200111/history.cfm. Accessed February 5, 2016.

Thompson IM, Goodman PJ, Tangen CM, et al. The influence of finasteride on the development of prostate cancer. *N Engl J Med* 2003; 349:215–224.

Topol EJ. Topol: time to end routine mammography. Mammography is a recipe for net harm. *Medscape Pathology and Lab Medicine*. May 6, 2015. http://www.medscape.com/viewarticle/844153?nlid=81024_1021&src=wnl_edit_medp_pa. Accessed May 12, 2015.

United States Preventive Services Task Force. http://www.uspreventiveservicestaskforce.org/. Accessed January 30, 2016.

Ursin G, Hovanessian-Larsen L, Parisky YR, Pike MC, Wu AH. Greatly increased occurrence of breast cancers in areas of mammographically dense tissue. *Breast Cancer Res* 2005; 7:605–608.

van Schoor G, Moss SM, Otten JDM, et al. Increasingly strong reduction in breast cancer mortality due to screening. *Br J Cancer* 2011; 104:910–914.

Webb ML, Cady B, Michaelson JS, et al. A failure analysis of invasive breast cancer: most deaths from disease occur in women not regularly screened. *Cancer* 2014; 120:2839–2846.

Welch HG, Black WC. Using autopsy series to estimate the disease "reservoir" for ductal carcinoma in situ of the breast: how much more breast cancer can we find? *Ann Intern Med* 1997; 127: 1023–1028.

Welch HG, Schwartz LM, Woloshin S. Ramifications of screening for breast cancer: 1 in 4 cancers detected by mammography are pseudocancers. *BMJ* 2006; 332:727.

Williams, R. Thomas L. Dao (obituary). *The Lancet* 2009; 374:1060.

Wingo PA, Tong T, Bolden S. Cancer Statistics, 1995. *CA Cancer J Clin* 1995; 45:8–30.

Wolfe JN. Breast patterns as an index of risk for developing breast cancer. *AJR* 1976; 126:1130–1139.

Woolf S, Campos-Outcalt D. Severing the link between coverage policy and the US Preventive Services Task Force. *JAMA* 2013; 309:1899–1900.

Yaffe MJ. Correction: Canada study. Letter to the editor. *J Natl Cancer Inst* 1993; 155:748–749.

Zackrisson S, Andersson I, Janzon L, Manjer J, Garne JP. Rate of over-diagnosis of breast cancer 15 years after end of Malmö mammographic screening trial: follow-up study. *BMJ* 2006; 332:689–692.

Zahl PH, Strand BH, Maehlen J. Incidence of breast cancer in Norway and Sweden during introduction of nationwide screening: prospective cohort study. *BMJ* 2004; 328:921–924.

Zheng B, Tan M, Ramalingam P, Gur D. Association between computed tissue density asymmetry in bilateral mammograms and near-term breast cancer risk. *The Breast Journal* 2014; 20:249–257.

# Index